Contributions to Psychology and Medicine

# Contributions to Psychology and Medicine

The Psychology of Childhood Illness
*Christine Eiser*

Psychological Aspects of Early Breast Cancer
*Colette Ray/Michael Baum*

Medical Thinking: The Psychology of Medical Judgment and Decision Making
*Steven Schwartz/Timothy Griffin*

Women With Cancer: Psychological Perspectives
*Barbara L. Anderson, Editor*

The Somatizing Child: Diagnosis and Treatment of Conversion and Somatization Disorders
*Elsa G. Shapiro/Alvin A. Rosenfeld with Norman Cohen and Dorothy Levine*

Individual Differences, Stress, and Health Psychology
*Michel Pierre Janisse, Editor*

The Psychology of the Dentist Patient Relationship
*Stephen Bochner*

Prospects of Heart Surgery: Psychological Adjustments to Coronary Bypass Grafting
*Alan Radley*

Assessing Chronic Pain: A Multidisciplinary Clinic Handbook
*Paul M. Camic/Frederick D. Brown, Editors*

Paul M. Camic   Frederick D. Brown

Editors

# Assessing Chronic Pain

## A Multidisciplinary Clinic Handbook

With 46 Illustrations

Springer-Verlag
New York Berlin Heidelberg
London Paris Tokyo

Paul M. Camic, Ph.D.
Clinical Assistant Professor of Psychiatry
Division of Clinical Psychology
and
Clinical Director of Pain Treatment Service
Department of Neurosurgery
Northwestern University Medical School
448 East Ontario Street, Suite 510
Chicago, IL 60611, U.S.A.

Frederick D. Brown, M.D.
Associate Professor of Surgery
Department of Surgery, Section of Neurosurgery
University of Chicago Medical Center
Chicago, IL 60637, U.S.A.

*Advisor*
J. Richard Eiser
Department of Psychology
Washington Singer Laboratories
University of Exeter
Exeter EX4 4QG, England

Library of Congress Cataloging-in-Publication Data
Assessing chronic pain : a multidisciplinary clinic handbook / Paul M. Camic, Frederick D. Brown, editors
p. cm. — (Contributions to psychology and medicine)
1. Intractable pain—Handbooks, manuals, etc. 2. Intractable pain—Diagnosis—Handbooks, manuals, etc. I. Camic, Paul Marc, 1955- . II. Brown, Frederick D. (Frederick David), 1947- III. Series.
[DNLM: 1. Chronic Disease. 2. Pain—therapy. WL 704 A846]
RB127.A85 1988
616'.0472—dc 19
DNLM/DLC
for Library of Congress 88-36752

Printed on acid-free paper



Typeset by Publishers Service, Bozeman, Montana.

9 8 7 6 5 4 3 2 1

ISBN-13:978-1-4613-8870-8 e-ISBN-13:978-1-4613-8868-5
DOI: 10.1007/978-1-4613-8868-5

# Preface

Assessment and treatment of acute and chronic pain has become an area of specialization within anesthesiology, clinical psychology, dentistry, neurology, neurosurgery, and physical therapy. This has occurred in part, due to major advancements in both assessment and treatment procedures over the past decade that have further developed the art and science of clinical pain management. Initially, these advancements were reported solely within their respective disciplines. It was the rare exception that a psychologist knew about anesthesiological treatments or a neurosurgeon about cognitive and behavioral aspects of chronic pain. As each discipline developed their respective subspecialty in chronic pain, the limitations of each discipline became apparent.

The founding of the International Association for the Study of Pain in May 1974 brought together the scientists and clinicians of the various disciplines working in the area of pain management on an international level. Since its inception, this association has been a leading proponent of integrating advances in the treatment of acute and chronic pain between disciplines. As a health care problem, pain affects the physical and psychological well-being of our patients. Due in part to the integration of the mind and body in the experience of pain, no single discipline has been able to provide us with all the answers in managing pain.

This book provides the reader with an up-to-date perspective about integrative treatment approaches from a multidisciplinary assessment and approach. It was edited by a psychologist and a neurosurgeon with contributions from others in these fields in addition to anesthesiology, dentistry, psychiatry, and social work. It is a volume written by practicing clinicians who have collectively worked with thousands of patients in hospital clinics at The University of Chicago, Universität Göttingen, Case Western Reserve University, and the University of Illinois/Illinois Masonic Medical Center.

A volume such as this can serve many purposes without losing sight of its primary goal, which is to advance further an understanding and appreciation of the work of a multidisciplinary pain clinic. Although the term "multidisciplinary pain clinic" has become a fashionable concept to disseminate as we enter the last decade of this century, it is also a treatment perspective that has begun to bear fruit. Simply listing various disciplines on a clinic's letterhead or brochure does not assure the patient or insurance company or regulatory agency that integrative assessment and treatment is, in fact, taking place. The organization and development of a clinic's philosophy of assessment and treatment, together with a coherent rationale for such assessment and treatment, does set that clinic apart from the dreaded and now infamous "pain doctor" who was content to prescribe narcotics and schedule questionable surgeries.

This handbook provides a clear, concise, step-by-step approach to the evaluation of a patient within a multispecialty clinic practice. It provides the physician with the basis of clinical decision making utilizing available treatments from medicine, surgery, and psychology. It provides the psychologist with an in-depth understanding of the assessment procedures and treatment options of the other members of the pain clinic treatment team. This handbook further provides the insurance company claims executive with a look at the appropriate assessment and treatment tools considered to be relevant components of pain management. Finally, this volume provides the hospital administrator with a detailed overview of clinical operations that are sound and ethical.

Many of us have worked side by side in the clinics for several years before the idea for this volume was conceived. While we are excited by the work we have accomplished and by the many successes we have experienced, there remains much to be done to help further the patient manage his or her pain. The recent decision to admit psychologists to institutes of psychoanalytic training in the United States will help advance research in psychodynamic treatment of pain as well as a host of other psychophysiological problems. This will hopefully allow psychoanalytic research on patients presenting with physical complaints to equal the outstanding contributions of behavioral researchers. As medical science advances and imaging techniques take us into new areas of the human body, we may uncover yet-unknown physical mechanisms that contribute to the continuation of pain. As these advances in research translate into clinical practice, refinements in chronic pain assessment will be needed.

In a final note, we thank the many secretaries who worked diligently in typing the manuscript; Jean E. Rhodes, Ph.D., for her invaluable comments; and Glenn M. Deacon (PMC) and Mary Jo Brown (FDB) for their personal support and encouragement.

Paul M. Camic
Frederick D. Brown

# Contents

# Contributors

MICHAEL T. BAUTZ, Dipl. Psych.
Clinical Psychologist, Department of Anesthesiology, Georg-August Universität Göttingen, D-3400 Göttingen, Federal Republic of Germany

RUTH M. BENCA, M.D., Ph.D.
Assistant Professor of Psychiatry and Neurology, Departments of Psychiatry, Neurology and The College, University of Chicago Medical Center, Chicago, Illinois 60637, USA

MARGIT I.D. BRENIG, Dipl. Psych.
Clinical Psychologist, Department of Psychiatry, Georg-August Universität Göttingen, D-3400 Göttingen, Federal Republic of Germany

FREDERICK D. BROWN, M.D.
Associate Professor of Surgery, Section of Neurosurgery, and Director, Pain Evaluation and Treatment Service, University of Chicago Medical Center, Chicago, Illinois 60637, USA

PAUL M. CAMIC, Ph.D.
Clinical Assistant Professor of Psychiatry, Division of Clinical Psychology, and Clinical Director of Pain Treatment Service, Department of Neurosurgery, Northwestern University Medical School, Chicago, Illinois 60611, USA; Adjunct Assistant Professor of Psychology, Department of Psychiatry, University of Illinois, College of Medicine, Chicago, Illinois 60612, USA (Formerly at the University of Chicago Medical School, Pain Service)

Terri L. Dallas, M.D.
Assistant Professor of Anesthesiology, Department of Anesthesia and Critical Care, University of Chicago Medical Center, Chicago, Illinois 60637, USA

Dirk B. Eggebrecht, Dipl. Psych.
Clinical Psychologist, Department of Anesthesiology, Georg-August Universität Göttingen, D-3400 Göttingen, Federal Republic of Germany

Robert K. Erickson, M.D.
Assistant Professor of Surgery, Section of Neurosurgery, University of Chicago Medical Center, Chicago, Illinois 60637, USA

LaDeane Fattore, D.D.S., M.S.
Geriatric Resident, West Side Veterans Administration Medical Center Dental Service, University of Illinois, Chicago, Illinois 60612, USA

Richard G. Fessler, M.D., Ph.D.
Chief Resident, Section of Neurological Surgery, University of Chicago Medical Center, Chicago, Illinois 60637, USA

Richard S. Finn, M.D.
Fellow in Clinical Pain, Department of Anesthesia and Critical Care, University of Chicago Medical Center, Chicago, Illinois 60637, USA

Carmen Franz, Dipl. Psych.
Chief Clinical Psychologist, Department of Anesthesiology, Georg-August Universität Göttingen, D-3400 Göttingen, Federal Republic of Germany

Michael Pfingsten, Dipl. Psych.
Clinical Psychologist, Department of Anesthesiology, Georg-August Universität Göttingen, D-3400 Göttingen, Federal Republic of Germany

Kathleen Blindt Segraves, Ph.D.
Assistant Professor of Psychiatry, Director of Behavioral Medicine, Cleveland Metropolitan General Hospital, Case Western Reserve University, Cleveland, Ohio 44106, USA

Robert A. Strauss, D.D.S.
Assistant Professor of Dental Surgery, Department of Oral and Maxillofacial Surgery, Medical College of Virginia, Richmond, Virginia 23298, USA

# 1

# Introduction to Multidisciplinary Pain Assessment

*Paul M. Camic*

Chronic pain as a clinical and research problem is well documented in the literature of medicine, surgery, and clinical psychology. The treatment of chronic pain has often been a frustrating and evasive experience for physicians and psychologists alike. Issues concerning measurement and intensity of pain, appropriate pharmacological intervention, physical disability determination, psychogenic versus organic etiology, and effectiveness of invasive procedures confront every clinician working with the chronic pain patient. Partly because of the allusiveness of treatment success and partly because so many disciplines have an interest in treating chronic pain patients, questions have arisen regarding appropriate assessment criteria. In addition to assessment indecision within a discipline, the problem of effective multidisciplinary assessment procedures is also present.

The multidisciplinary approach to assessment and treatment of chronic pain has been heralded at regional, national, and international meetings of various professional pain associations as an alternative to the solo discipline approach to treatment. Simply put, no single discipline, be it anesthesia, dentistry, neurology, neurosurgery, physical therapy, psychiatry, or psychology, has, on their own, been highly effective in treating the problems of chronic, nonmalignant, pain. The interaction of multidisciplinary treatments, occurring either sequentially or concurrently, has however, yielded success at helping patients manage the problem of pain. Whether success is judged by reductions in medication, fewer days hospitalized, return to work, progressive fiscal compensation packages, or increased activity levels, fewer "pain behaviors" have been the result. While each discipline has well-developed textbooks on pain treatment, an integrated multidisciplinary handbook on assessment procedures does not exist.

We have written a handbook, rather than a textbook. Each chapter offers a current, state-of-the-art evaluation of each specialties' assessment process and how that specialty interacts with other specialties to produce a truly multidisciplinary evaluation. Without presenting a "cookbook" or a formula assessment package, our aim is to suggest strategies for thinking about the patient in pain and to systematically evaluate medical, psychological, and surgical treatments from the perspective of a clinical treatment team.

Treatment teams, like sports teams, need leadership and an organizational structure. Whether developing a new pain clinic or reorganizing an existing one, the formulation and design of the pain treatment team are important. Effective collaboration between disciplines should not be left to chance. Defining the goals of the pain clinic and operationalizing the clinic's structure permits multidisciplinary clinical work to be carried out more effectively and in a more secure fiscal environment. Dr. Kathleen Segraves elaborates on clinical team development in Chapter 12, our "bringing-it-all-together" chapter.

After a clear and concise review of the physiology, anatomy, and pharmacology of pain perceptions by Dr. Richard Fessler in Chapter 2, we have decided to begin at the beginning in Chapter 3, with a detailed description of the physical examination of the patient presenting with pain as a primary symptom. Dr. Robert Erickson's chapter goes beyond the details of a physical examination, however, by laying the groundwork for the foundation of the many possible steps in clinical decision making. His examination of the patient offers, in addition to a diagnosis, information about functional impairment and a first look at pain-related behaviors. This is where hypothesis generation begins and the most likely place for the patient to enter the pain clinic.

If the patient has had pain for a six month or longer period, an assessment by the clinical psychologist is the next step in the clinical decision process. The psychological assessment should not be considered a litmus test to answer the question of organic versus psychogenic etiology; it cannot accomplish this. The psychiatric examination of the patient, which is different from the psychological assessment, and presented by Dr. Ruth Benca in Chapter 8, also cannot clearly establish a psychogenic etiology; this can only be determined by the work of a physical exam and appropriate diagnostic medical tests. A psychiatric examination by a psychiatrist or clinical psychologist can determine if a psychiatric disorder is present concurrently with the symptom of pain. This examination evaluates specifically for the various psychiatric problems associated with pain. This need not be a general psychiatric examination complete with mental status exam and thorough childhood and adult history. Unless there is clinical indication that this is necessary, as with suicidal ideation, cognitive distortion, or psychotic symptoms, a focused psychiatric examination is appropriate. It is important that we not lose sight of the purpose of the patient's visit: The patient is being seen for the symptom of chronic pain. A long and detailed psychiatric examination may uncover psychopathology, but unless the pathology is connected with the pain symptom we are not assisting the multidisciplinary assessment.

The goal of the psychological assessment, as outlined by Dr. Paul Camic in Chapter 4, is to determine how effectively the patient is coping with chronic pain, what psychological and environmental factors may be exacerbating the pain, and to decide if a psychiatric examination or psychometric testing is necessary. As previously stated, the psychological assessment is a routine part of the multidisciplinary assessment for all chronic pain patients with pain present at least six months or longer.

Psychometric testing should be seen as distinct from the psychological assessment and requested only as indicated. Dr. Dirk Eggebrecht and associates offer a thorough review of what psychological testing can and cannot offer in Chapter 5. Although it is gradually becoming accepted that the MMPI should not be used to diagnose a pain-prone personality (because one does not exist!), it remains a useful test to evaluate psychological functioning of more complicated patients where somatization disorder may be contributing to the patient's description of pain or when there is a question of a psychotic disorder.

Evaluation of functional status begins during the physical examination and continues during the third part of the routine portion of the multidisciplinary assessment with the physical therapist. The physical therapist, upon recommendation by a physician, further determines current functional status of the patient in relation to job-related requirements of movement as well as movement requirements at home, for transportation, etc. This is discussed in Chapter 9 on conservative medical management by Dr. Robert Erickson.

This completes the routine evaluation of patients who enter the pain clinic: a physical examination and review of previous diagnostic tests, a psychological assessment, psychometric testing and psychiatric examination when indicated, and an evaluation by a physical therapist. The patient is then discussed at a clinical case conference. It is at this point, during the discussion of the patient by these three team members, that further evaluative work is requested or treatment initiated.

If necessary, further requests for evaluation are made to other members of the chronic pain treatment team. In Chapter 6 Drs. Terri Dallas and Richard Finn outline the role the anesthesiologist can play. In Chapter 7, Dr. Richard Fessler describes pharmacologic diagnostic and treatment options. Dr. Frederick Brown, in Chapter 10, discusses evaluating the patient for neurosurgical treatment and in Chapter 11 Drs. LaDeane Fattore and Robert Strauss exhaustively assess dental pain syndromes.

Finally, the treatment setting where a pain clinic is organized is an important consideration. Many current pain treatment programs are inpatient based. Outpatient programs, however, have taken a firm footing in both North America and Europe. While many of the assessment strategies discussed in the following chapter are applicable for an inpatient treatment setting, the focus of this volume is on outpatient assessment procedures. The shift from inpatient to outpatient assessment and treatment is based on two important factors. The more expensive inpatient programs have not shown end-of-treatment results to be superior to the far less costly outpatient clinics. Insurance companies and workman's compensation agencies have taken note and have become reluctant to pay for inpatient treatment other than for certain anesthesia or surgical procedures. Lack of superior treatment results and high cost of care are requiring many inpatient pain treatment programs to either cease operations or adapt to an outpatient model. This volume is oriented toward the outpatient treatment model and is based on the authors' experience in developing and working within that model.

# 2

# Physiology, Anatomy, and Pharmacology of Pain Perception

*Richard G. Fessler*

Our current understanding of pain perception is a synthesis of neurophysiology, neuropharmacology, and neuroanatomy. Neurophysiologic concepts developed in the late 19th century and refined over the last 20 years have provided a strong conceptual framework through which rigorous scientific methodology has been applied to analyze how our central nervous system receives and analyzes information regarding pain. Moreover, neuropharmacologic and neuroanatomic data gathered over the last several decades has extended our knowledge of somatosensory information processing to relatively sophisticated levels regarding neurochemical events within specific neuroanatomic structures. The goal of this chapter is to review these three fields as they relate to nociceptive (i.e., pain) information processing, and to integrate them into a framework that will enable a logical approach to the analysis and treatment of pain. This will be achieved by reviewing the major neurophysiologic theories of pain perception and examining how current neurophysiologic and neuroanatomic data support or detract from these theories. We will then review the neuroanatomy relevant to pain perception, and, where appropriate, discuss the neurochemistry that appears relevant to nociception. In doing this, what emerges is a circuit involved in the perception and modulation of pain that can be briefly described and easily comprehended.

## Theories of Pain Perception

In 1894, von Frey wrote the most complete formulation of what has since come to be known as the "specificity" theory of pain perception.[1] In this hypothesis, which explained the sensory-discriminative aspects of pain quality, location, intensity, etc.), it was proposed that free nerve endings located within the skin responded only to specific modalities of sensation and conveyed this information to the brain along pathways exclusively activated by such stimuli. Although modern analysis has contributed some evidence in support of this hypothesis, in general our knowledge of anatomy and physiology does not support this theory.

Two types of nociceptors have been found widely in mammalian skin. High-threshold mechanoreceptive units (HTMs) are nociceptors that respond only to strong pressure, applied to discrete points spread over an area of skin up to 1 $cm^2$, and have axons of 1 to 5 $\mu$ in diameter (Table 2.1).[2] Responses are slowly adapting and have little or no dynamic firing during stimulus onset. HTM units in normal skin do not respond to chemical irritants and only rarely respond to heat stimulation, and therefore could be considered "modality specific."[3] Polymodel nociceptive units (PMNs), on the other hand, are high threshold units that respond to mechanical pressure, noxious heating, and chemical irritants applied over smaller areas of skin (2 $mm^2$), and have axons less than 1 $\mu$ in diameter.[4]

In addition to these two common nociceptive units, several studies have demonstrated the existence of another nociceptor that produces pain in response to heat stimuli, but also responds to other stimuli (e.g., mechanical force).[5] Similar to the mechanical force nociceptor (A-$delta_1$), the axons of these A-$delta_2$ units are lightly myelinated, 1 to 5 $\mu$ in diameter, and conduct impulses in the 2.5 to 36 m/s range. These are believed to be responsible for "first-pain" sensations of early stinging, sharp, well-localized pain (compared to the diffuse, burning "second-pain" sensations of C-fiber origin). Since it has been reported that activation of these units alone can produce pain, it has been suggested that these represent the first direct evidence in support of the specificity theory.[6] Lynn,[7] however, reports that most of these nociceptors do respond to other stimuli at higher thresholds, and therefore are "PMNs" and not truly "modality specific." Similar arguments have been made for the HTM receptor discussed above.

Beyond the difficulty in demonstrating an anatomical substrate for the specificity theory, there are several other serious problems with this theory. First, "nonmodality specific" units, which respond in both the A-delta and C-fiber diameter range, are easily identified. Second, whereas pain evoked by repeated heat stimulation at 3-second intervals increases the magnitude of perceived "second pain," it has been clearly shown that this stimulation *decreases* the activity in PMN afferents.[8] This has been interpreted as evidence that "central summation" (see below) must be responsible for the perceived increase in pain. Third, single neurons in the dorsal horn are known to receive convergent input from modalities. Finally, the specificity theory cannot explain several characteristics of clinical pain syndromes. For example:

**Table 2.1.** Peripheral Nerves Involved in Conducting Painful Stimuli

| Group | Diameter | Conduction Velocity | Effective Stimuli | Threshold | Myelination |
|---|---|---|---|---|---|
| A-beta | 2–22 μ | 40 –80 m/s | hair movement, light pressure | low | ⊕ |
| A-delta$_1$ | 1–5 μ | 2.5–36 m/s | mechanical force | high | ⊕ |
| A-delta$_2$ | 1–5 μ | 2.5–36 m/s | thermal mechanical force nociceptor | high | ⊕ |
| C | ≤1 μ | .5–1.7 m/s | polymodal | high | ⊖ |

1. It cannot explain the delayed pain of post-herpetic neuralgia produced by innocuous stimulation.
2. It cannot explain referred pain triggered by innocuous stimulation of normal skin.
3. It cannot explain the paroxysms of pain produced by mild stimulation of trigger zones in trigeminal neuralgia.
4. It cannot explain the failure of specific surgical lesions of known "pain pathways" to alleviate pain.
5. It cannot explain causalgic pain.
6. It cannot explain phantom pain.

Dissatisfaction with the specificity theory led to several proposals that are generally referred to as "pattern" theories. Goldscheider[9] first proposed that stimulus intensity and central summation, rather than sensory discrimination, were the critical determinants of pain perception. Nafe[10] and Weddell[11] extended the pattern aspect of this theory to propose that all fiber endings were alike, and that pain resulted from spatiotemporal patterns of excessive stimulation of nonspecific receptors. As discussed above, pain fibers (and receptors) demonstrate significant (but not absolute) specialization; thus in failing to account for physiological specialization this theory is not an acceptable model of pain perception. Moreover, this pattern theory also could not explain the pain of the clinical syndromes listed above.

Livingston[12] stressed the "central summation" aspect of Goldscheider's theory in proposing that intense stimulation sets up "reverberating circuits" in spinal internuncial neurons that can then be triggered by normally nonpainful stimuli. This generates abnormal neural activity that is interpreted as pain. Related to this concept is the theory that a specialized input-controlling mechanism exists as an interaction between rapidly conducting (myelinated) and slowly conducting (unmyelinated) fiber tracts. In pathologic conditions the slowly conducting system establishes dominance over the rapidly conducting system, resulting in burning dysesthesia and hyperalgesia.[13]

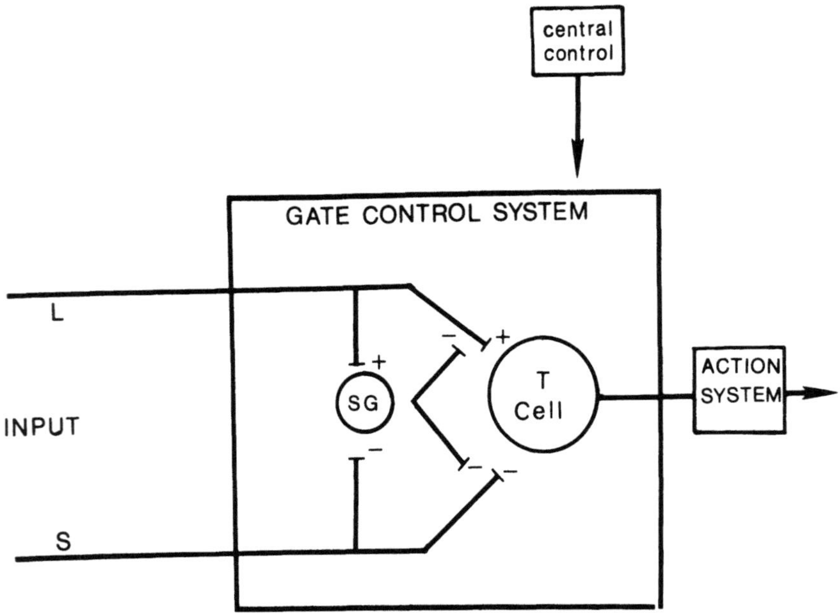


**Figure 2.1.** Schematic representation of "Gate Control Theory of Melzack and Wall. See text for discussion.

These theories provided explanations for several of the known clinical pain syndromes. Hyperalgesia following peripheral nerve trauma or post-herpetic neuralgia, for example, results from a relatively greater loss of large to small fibers. Moreover, failure of surgical lesions to completely relieve pain is explained on the basis of diffuse connections within ascending multisynaptic pathways. The strength of the theory, therefore, is its considerable interaction between nociceptive and non-nociceptive pathways. Its major limitation is its failure to recognize the importance of receptor specialization in response to noxious stimuli.

In 1965, Melzack and Wall proposed a theory that recognized and combined the strengths of both the specificity and pattern theories (convergence, summation, and inhibition).[14] In their "gate control" theory, afferent impulses were transmitted to the substantia gelatinosa layer of the spinal cord where modulation of their input occurred prior to central transmission. The "gate" referred to the net effect of two parallel systems of incoming peripheral fibers, and a system of descending control, on a theoretical transmission (T)-cell. Large fibers (A-beta), activated by low threshold, non-noxious stimuli, tended to inhibit transmission, while small fibers (A-delta, C), activated by intense, noxious stimuli, tended to facilitate transmission. When the output of the T-cells exceeded a critical level (central summation), neural systems were activated that initiated the complex behaviors of escape and avoidance of the stimuli (Fig. 2.1). Since its inception, the gate-control theory has undergone considerable revision as our knowledge of neuroanatomy and neurophysiology have disproved various details of the theory.[15] The strength of this theory has remained its conceptual framework which provides a mechanism for understanding the multidimensionality of the experience of pain.

## Neuroanatomy and Neuropharmacologic Anatomy of Pain Transmission

### Peripheral Nerve Fibers Dorsal Root and Spinal Cord

In general, receptors and afferent fibers can be evaluated according to several criteria: (1) Size and conduction velocity (A vs. C fibers), (2) modalities to which the receptors respond, (3) threshold for response initiation, and (4) characteristics of the response (e.g., rate of adaptation).

Information regarding the sensation of pain is received by "nociceptors" located in peripheral body tissues. Nociceptors are high threshold receptors, usually identified as free nerve endings, with relatively small receptor fields. Their afferent fibers are small A-delta and C fibers, and are variably polymodal in that they can frequently be activated by mechanical as well as nociceptive information (see Table 2.1). Several lines of evidence support the concept that painful stimuli are transmitted by C fibers: (1) the threshold for C-fiber activation and human pain thresholds to heat are similar (43° C);[16,17] (2) selective C-fiber block (local anesthetic) vs. A-fiber block (ischemia) indicates that C-fiber function is sufficient for thermal pain perception;[18] (3) stimulus interaction effects observed in psychophysical data are also demonstrable in C-fiber electrophysiologic recordings;[16] (4) the latency to pain sensation from skin stimulation is sufficiently long to be mediated by C fibers;[19] (5) intraneural C-fiber stimulation in humans causes pain;[20] and (6) a linear relationship exists between C-fiber recordings and human ratings of pain over the temperature of 39° to 55° C.[21]

A fibers also conduct painful stimuli. Fibers that have been identified in the A-delta range have been divided into two groups, HTM-I (high-threshold mechanoceptors-I) and HTM-II units.[22] Table 2.2 lists the characteristics of these units. HTM-I units have long response latencies from stimulus initiation, slow rates of adaptation, high thermal and mechanical thresholds, but rapid rates of conduction.[23,24] Based on the observation that HTM-I units respond vigorously beginning several seconds after the onset of a painful stimulus (whereas C fibers respond only during the first few seconds after stimulus onset) and maintain a prolonged output, it has been suggested that these units have an important role in signalling sustained pain.[25] On the other hand, the low threshold and short latency of

**Table 2.2.** Comparison of the Characteristics of HTM-I and HTM-II Units

| Characteristic | HTM-I | HTM-II |
|---|---|---|
| Location | glabrous skin of hand hairy skin of hand and forearm | hairy skin of hand and forearm |
| Response latency | >500 m/sec | <200 m/sec |
| Date of adaptation | slow | rapid |
| Heat threshold | 49°C (A-delta, of Table 2.1) | 43°C (A-delta) |
| Mechanical threshold | 1.3 gm | 0.4 gm |

HTM-II units has resulted in the suggestion that they may subserve "first-pain" responses.[24]

Electrical stimulation of A fibers results in the perception of a sharp, pricking pain. Stimulation of C fibers, on the other hand, evokes a prolonged dull or burning pain.

Upon entering the spinal cord, the central processes of these afferent fibers are segregated in a precise laminar fashion (Fig. 2.2). Small myelinated and unmyelinated fibers, which are activated by noxious stimuli, constitute the lateral border of the dorsal root. These fibers enter the Tract of Lissauer and travel for one or two segments before terminating in layer I (marginal zone) and layer II of Rexed (substantia gelatinosa).[27] Within layer II polymodal nociceptors project to its outer region whereas C fibers generally appear to terminate in its inner region.[26,28,29] Several lines of evidence have suggested that Substance P (SP), an 11-amino acid peptide, is the neurotransmitter released from these small myelinated and unmyelinated afferents. First, immunohistochemical and radioimmunoassay experiments have demonstrated that SP is distributed primarily in layers I and II.[30,31] Second, it is contained in vesicles within synaptosomal fractions.[32] Third, it is releasable in vitro by local depolarization and its release is inhibited by morphine.[33] Fourth, iontophoretic application of SP produces a prolonged depolarization of functionally identified dorsal horn nociceptive neurons.[34] Finally, intrathecal injection of SP produces behavioral signs of irritation[35] and depletion of SP produces prolonged elevation of nociceptive threshold.[36]

In contrast to the above afferents, low threshold myelinated fibers that innervate hair follicles and mechanoreceptive afferents terminate primarily in laminae III and IV.[37] High threshold, myelinated, mechanoreceptors terminate in lamina I and have collaterals that extend to lamina II.[26]

Axons of cell bodies that arise in lamina I, transmit information to the ipsilateral, and, via the anterior white commissure, the contralateral ascending spinothalamic tract. They do this either directly, or through small inhibitory interneurons located in lamina II and III. These interneurons also send axons back to lamina I. Cells in lamina V also con-

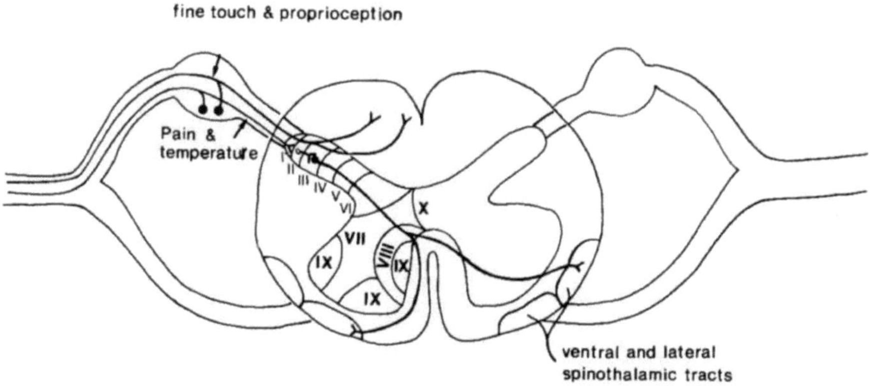


**Figure 2.2.** Laminar segregation of afferent sensory information in spinal cord. See text for discussion.

tribute axons to ipsilateral and contralateral spinothalamic tracts. Cells that arise in lamina I and lamina II utilize enkephalin[38] and gamma-amino-butyric acid (GABA)[39] as inhibitory neurotransmitters that synapse upon thalamic projection neurons.

## Ascending Spinal Pathways and Thalamocortical Projections

Four pathways convey the majority of afferent sensory information from the spinal cord to the thalamus (Fig. 2.3). First, the tract of Lissauer (or dorsolateral fasciculus) contains primary afferent fibers from the dorsal root as well as axons from layers II and III. HRP studies reveal that few individual fibers project for more than two or three segmental levels within this tract, however, as an identifiable structure lamina I extends throughout the length of the spinal cord.

The dorsal columns (fasciculus cuneatus and gracilus) are composed of heavily myelinated fibers derived from the medial aspect of the dorsal horn. As these fibers enter the posterior columns and begin their ipsilateral ascent, the lower lumbar and sacral fibers are pushed progressively more medially as more fibers enter at successively higher levels. Therefore, these fiber tracts are roughly somatotopically organized. They conduct information about fine-touch, pressure, vibration, two-point discrimination and kinesthesia (positions of body-parts in space). As the fibers in these tracts reach the medulla they synapse somatotopically within the nucleus gracilus and cuneatus. Axons of the cells arising within these nuclei sweep ventromedially as "internal arcuate fibers," cross midline, and form the medial lemniscus. This tract ascends through the medulla, pons, and midbrain to terminate somatotopically in the ventro-postero-lateral nucleus of the thalamus (VPL). Relay neurons then arise

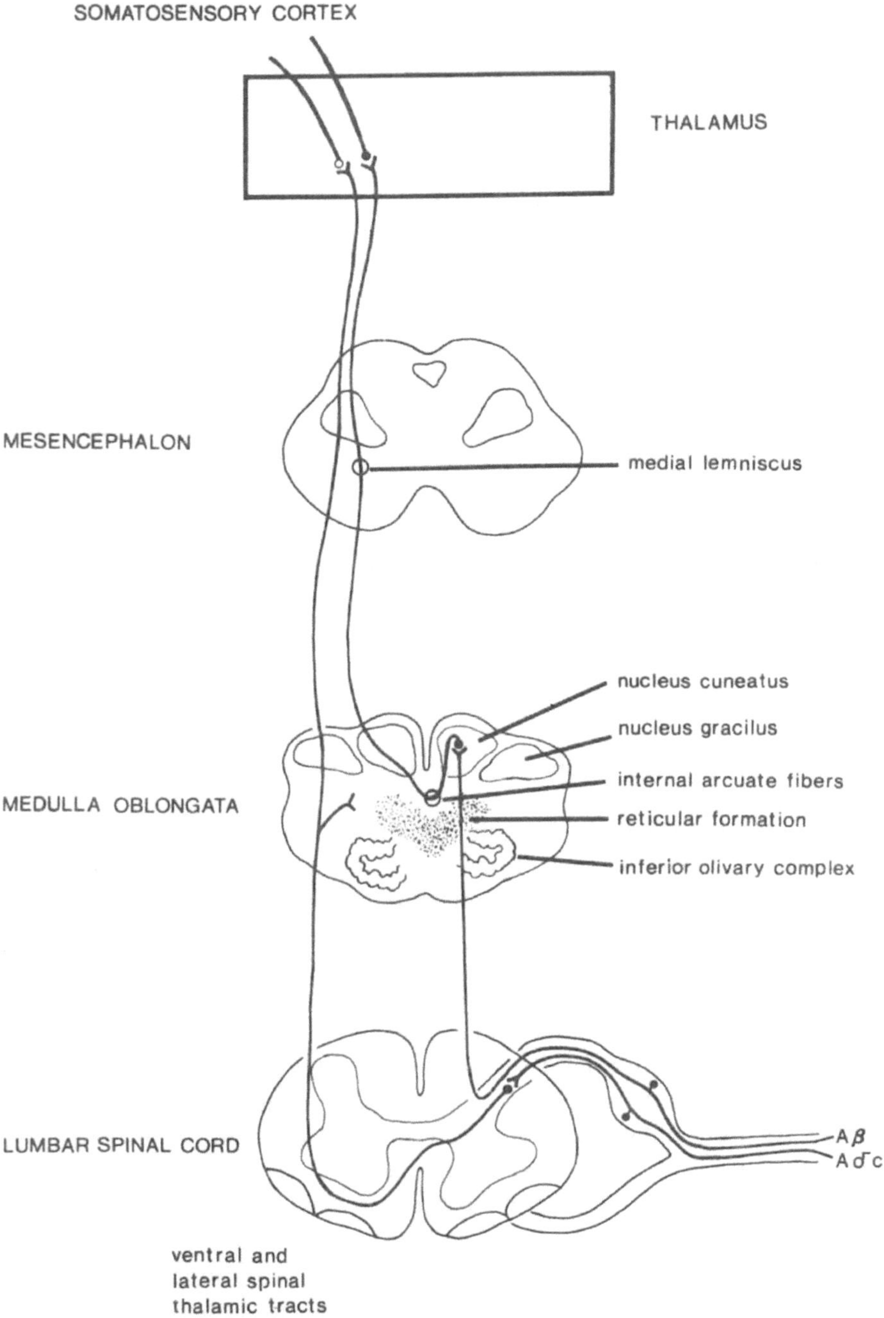


**Figure 2.3.** Ascending sensory pathways from dorsal root to somatosensory cortex. See text for discussion.

from this nucleus, traverse the posterior limb of the internal capsule, and terminate in the appropriate sensory areas of the cortex.

The anterior spinothalamic tract arises from cell bodies in layers I, IV, and V of Rexed,[40] decussate through the anterior white commissure over several spinal segments, and ascend contralaterally in the anterior funiculus. In the medulla the tract is located dorsolateral to the inferior olivary nucleus, along with the lateral spinothalamic tract. At this level a large number of fibers project to and terminate in the reticular formation and lateral reticular nucleus (a cerebellar relay nucleus). In the upper pons and midbrain the tract becomes closely associated with the medial lemniscus. Finally, in the mesencephalon the tract divides into medial and lateral components. The lateral components terminate in the posterior thalamic nucleus and caudal aspects of the VPL. Several fibers cross midline and terminate in the same nuclei on the other side. The medial component projects to the periaquaductal gray and bilaterally to the paralaminar nuclei of the thalamus. Axons reaching the VPL terminate somatotopically on cells which then project to the post-central gyrus of the cortex. Fibers of the anterior spinothalamic tract transmit information regarding light touch. However, since deep touch (pressure) information is carried in the dorsal columns, loss of the anterior spinothalamic tracts are of minimal clinical significance. It is believed that anterior spinothalamic fibers reaching the VPL are concerned with discriminatory functions, while those reaching the periaqueductal gray and posterior thalamic nucleus are concerned with nociception.[41]

Fibers of the lateral spinothalamic tract also arise from cells located in laminae I, III, and V.[40] The fibers decussate medial to those of the anterior spinothalamic tract in the anterior white commissure, form a more compact bundle within the segment of entry, and ascend in the lateral funiculus. In their ascent these fibers assume an anteromedial/posterolateral arrangement with the most lateral and posterior fibers representing the lowest portion of the body, and the anterior-medial fibers representing the upper extremities and neck. Sensory modalities are also segregated in this tract, thermal sensation is located posteriorly, whereas pain is located predominantly anteriorly. As it ascends through the medulla, pons, and midbrain, the lateral spinothalamic tract follows the same path as the anterior spinothalamic tract, and terminate somatotopically in the ipsilateral VPL and bilaterally in several intralaminar nuclei and the posterior thalamic nucleus. The cells terminating in the posterior thalamic nucleus, but not the VPL, are known to respond to noxious stimuli.[42] Clinically, unilateral section of this tract produces complete loss of pain and thermal sensation on the opposite side of the body, extending to one level below the injury. The anesthesia includes superficial and deep muscular, but not visceral, pain. Anogenital pain is not markedly reduced by unilateral lesions.

In addition to these major pathways, several other systems transmit nociceptive information. The spinoreticular system, alluded to while discussing the anterior spinothalamic tract, arises from posterior horn cells, ascends ipsilaterally, and terminates upon cells of the nucleus reticularis gigantocellularis and lateral reticular nucleus. It has been suggested that these fibers may be involved in motivation and affective responses to pain.[43] Although the cells of origin of the spinotectal tract are unknown, they are presumed to arise from the dorsal horn. The tract ascends contralaterally in the anterolateral part of the spinal cord in close association with the spinothalamic tract. At midbrain levels the tract projects medially to terminate somatotopically in the caudal superior colliculus. Evidence indicating that this tract transmits nociceptive information includes elicitation of evoked potentials in this region by noxious stimuli as well as behavioral responses consistent with severe pain when this area is electrically stimulated.[44]

## Trigeminal System

Conceptually, the organization of the trigeminal somesthetic system (for the face, sinuses, nasal mucous membranes, and dura) is very similar to that discussed above. All cell bodies of afferent peripheral nerves are located in the trigeminal ganglion. These afferent fibers terminate in the principal sensory trigeminal nucleus, the spinal trigeminal nucleus (upward continuation of the substantia gelatinosa), and the mesencephalic trigeminal nucleus. Neurons found within these nuclei receive input from large, myelinated fibers signalling touch, pressure, and joint position (and, therefore, are analogous to the dorsal columns) in a somatotopically organized fashion. The face is represented in an inverted manner with the jaw (mandibular nerve) represented dorsally, and the forehead (ophthalmic nerve) ventrally. Second-order neurons arising from these nuclei decussate in the pons and ascend as the ventral trigeminal lemniscus in close association with the medial lemniscus. These fibers then terminate somatotopically within the ventral posteromedial nucleus and intralaminar nuclei of the thalamus. A smaller group of fibers ascends ipsilaterally in the dorsal pontine tegmentum as the dorsal trigeminal lemniscus to a similar somatotopic termination.

Afferent fibers conveying nociceptive information enter the brainstem in the trigeminal (V), facial (VII), and vagus (X) cranial nerves. The fibers descend in the spinal trigeminal tract and terminate in the caudal spinal trigeminal nucleus. The second-order neurons cross the median raphe and become associated with the medial lemniscus as discussed above.

## Descending Pain Control Systems

Over the last two decades our understanding of the anatomy and pharmacology of descending pain modulatory systems has advanced significantly.

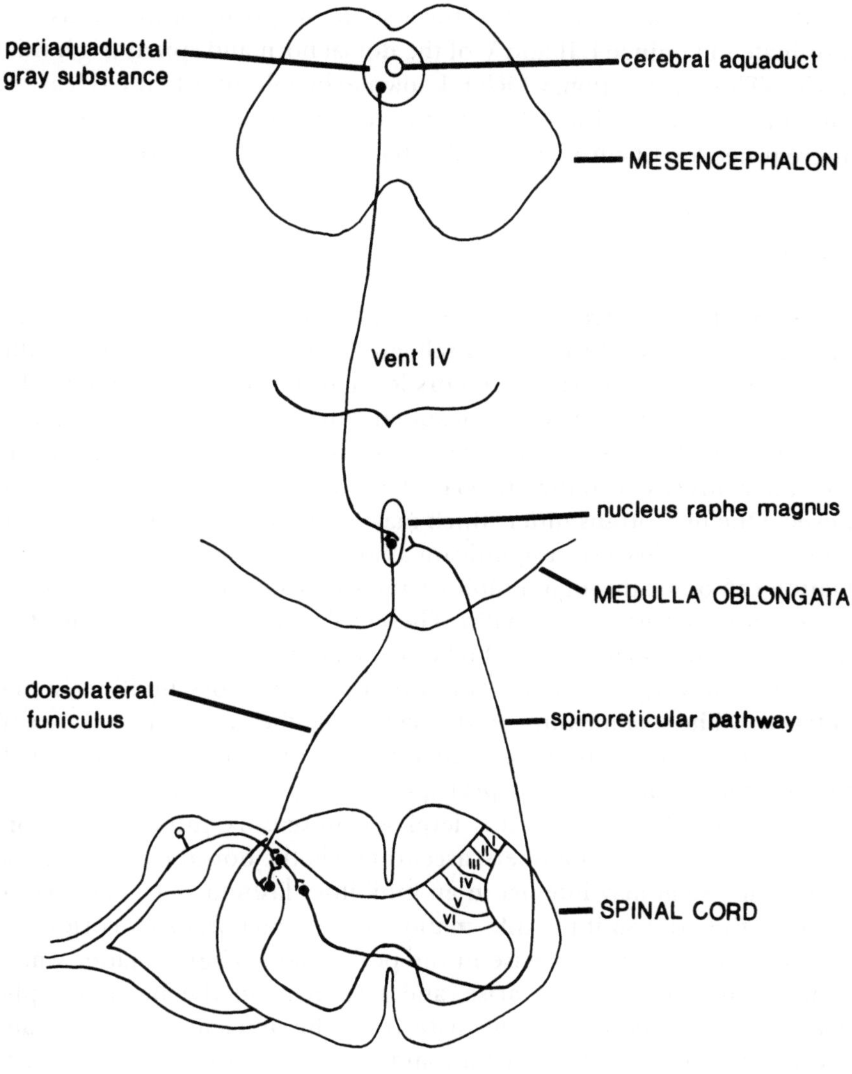


**Figure 2.4.** Descending influences on pain sensation afferent to spinal cord. See text for discussion.

We now appreciate that enkehalin containing neurons in the periaquaductal (PAG) region of the midbrain (Fig. 2.4) are activated by a variety of stimuli, including pain, opiate micro-injection, and electrical stimulation.[45] The periaquaductal gray has a large efferent pathway to the nucleus raphe magnus (NRM) that is activated by PAG activity, and this in turn excites neurons of the NRM. Excitation of NRM reduces behavioral responses to pain and increases the concentration of serotonin (5-HT) in spinal superperfusates.[46] Both these effects are reversed by 5-HT antagonist administration.[47] These results indicate that the pain modulatory effects of PAG stimulation are transmitted to the spinal cord via the

NRM. This pathway is known to traverse the dorsolateral funiculus and terminate in laminae I, II and V of the dorsal horn and spinal trigeminal nucleus.This termination, which is known to be inhibitor to the release of substance P, can be either directly an incoming primary somatosensory afferent neuron or through an enkephalin containing interneuron.

## Summary

Our current knowledge of the anatomy, physiology, and chemistry of pain perception suggests the following scheme. Information regarding painful stimuli is received by pain receptors located throughout the body. This information is transmitted to the spinal cord via thinly myelinated and nonmyelinated fibers that enter via the dorsal root. These axons terminate either directly or indirectly via interneurons, in layers I, II, and V of Rexed. One neurotransmitter which may be released by these neurons is Substance P. At this level a significant amount of modulation of the information can occur through inhibitory interneurons some of which utilize the neurotransmitter enkaphalin. These cells may also be influenced by descending information from higher centers.

Axons carrying nociceptive information then cross midline in the anterior white commissure and ascend via the anterior and lateral spinothalamic tracts to the brainstem where connections are made with the reticular formation, and periaquaductal gray and ventral-posterior nuclei of the thalamus. At this level somatosensory information from large, myelinated A delta fibers, ascending via the dorsal column-medial lemniscal system may interact in an inhibitory fashion. Thalamocortical neurons then transmit the information to the somatosensory cortex.

Descending influences arise in the periaquaductal gray matter where β-endorphinergic neurons arise, and terminate in the nucleus raphe magnus. Serotonergic neurons arise from this nucleus, travel caudally within the dorsolateral funiculus, and terminate directly, or indirectly via enkephalin interneurons, on incoming somatosensory fibers in laminae I, II, and V.

### References

1. Boring, E.G. (1942). *Sensation and Perception in the History of Experimental Psychology.* New York: Appleton-Century.
2. Burgess, P.R., & Perl, E.R. (1967). Myelinated afferent fibers responding specifically to noxious stimulation of the skin. *Journal of Physiology* 190:541–562.
3. Fitzgerald, M., & Lynn, B. (1977). The sensitization of high threshold mechanoreceptors with myelinated axons by repeated heating. *Journal of Physiology* 265: 549–563.
4. Bessou, P., & Perl, E. (1969). Response of cutaneous sensory units with unmyelinated fibers to noxious stimuli. *Journal of Neurophysiology* 32:1025–1043.

5. Beck, P.W., Handwerker, H.O., & Zimmermann, M. (1974). Nervous outflow from the cat's footpad during noxious radiant heat stimulation. *Brain Research* 67:373–386.
6. Dubner, R. (1978). Neurophysiology of pain. *Dental Clinics of North America* 22:11–30.
7. Lynn, B. (1984). The detection of injury and tissue damage. In: *Textbook of Pain.* (Eds.) P.D. Wall and R. Melzack. Edinburgh: Churchill Livingstone, pp. 19–33.
8. Price, D.D., & Dubner, R. (1977). Neurons that subserve the sensory-discriminative aspects of pain. *Pain* 3:307.
9. Goldscheider, A. (1894). *Ueber den Schmerz in physiologischer und klinischer Hinsicht.* Berlin: Hirschwold.
10. Nafe, J.P. (1934). In: *Handbook of General Experimental Psychology* (Ed.) C. Murchison. Worcester, Mass.: Clark University Press.
11. Weddell, G. (1955). Somesthesis and chemical senses. *Annual Review of Psychology* 6:119–136.
12. Livingston, W.K. (1943). *Pain Mechanisms.* New York: Macmillan.
13. Bishop, G.H. (1959). The relation between nerve fiber size and sensory modality: Phylogenetic implications of the afferent innervation of cortex. *Journal of Nervous & Mental Disease* 128:89–114.
14. Melzack, R., & Wall, P.D. (1965). Pain mechanisms: A new theory. *Science* 150: 971–979.
15. Nathan, P.W. (1976). The gate-control theory of pain. A critical review. *Brain* 99:123.
16. LaMotte, R.H., & Campbell, J.N. (1978). Comparison of responses of warm and nociceptive C-fiber afferents in monkey with human judgments of thermal pain. *Journal of Neurophysiology* 41:509–528.
17. Van Hees, J., & Gybels, J. (1981). C nociceptor activity in human nerve during painful and non-painful skin stimulation. *Journal of Neurology, Neurosurgery and Psychiatry* 44:600–607.
18. Sinclair, D.C., & Hinshaw, J.R. (1950). A comparison of the sensory dissociation produced by procaine and by limb compression. *Brain* 73:480–498.
19. Campbell, J.N., & LaMotte, R.H. (1983). Latency to detection of first pain. *Brain Research* 226:203–208.
20. Torebjork, H.E., & Ochoa, J. (1980). Specific sensations evoked by activity in single identified sensory units in man. *Acta Physiologica Scandinavica* 110: 445–447.
21. Torebjork, H.E., LaMotte, R.H., & Robinson, C.J. (1984). Peripheral neural correlates of magnitude of cutaneous pain and hyperalgesia. Simultaneous recordings in humans of sensory judgments of pain and evoked responses in nociceptors with C-fibers. *Journal of Neurophysiology* 51:325–339.
22. Dubner, R., & Bennett, G.J. (1983). Spinal and trigeminal mechanisms of nociception. *Annual Review of Neuroscience* 6:381–418.
23. Campbell, J.N., Meyer, R.A., & LaMotte, R.H. (1979). Sensitization of myelinated nociceptive afferents that innervate monkey hand. *Journal of Neurophysiology* 42:1669–1679.
24. Dubner, R., Price, D.D., Beitel, R.E., & Hu, J.W. (1977). Peripheral neural correlates of behavior in monkey and human related to sensory-discriminative aspects of pain. In: *Pain In The Trigeminal Region.* (Eds.) D.J. Anderson and B. Matthews. Amsterdam: Elsevier, pp. 57–66.

25. Meyer, R.A., Campbell, J.N., & Raja, S.N. (1985). Peripheral neural mechanisms of cutaneous hyperalgesia. In: *Advances in Pain Research and Therapy.* Vol. 9. (Eds.) H.L. Fields, R. Dubner, and F. Cervero. New York: Raven Press, pp. 53–71.
26. Light, A.R., Trevino, D.L., & Perl, E.R. (1979). Morphological features of functionally defined neurons in the marginal zone and substantia gelatinosa of the spinal dorsal horn. *Journal of Comparative Neurology* 186:151–172.
27. Rethelyi, M. (1977). Preterminal and terminal axon arborizations in the substantia gelatinosa of cat's spinal cord. *Journal of Comparative Neurology* 172:511–528.
28. Ralston, J.H., III (1979). Distribution of dorsal root axons in laminae I, II, and III of the macaque spinal cord. *Journal of Comparative Neurology* 184: 643–684.
29. Rebiero DaSilva, A., & Coimbra, A. (1982). Two types of synaptic glomeruli and their distribution in laminae I–III of the rat spinal cord. *Journal of Comparative Neurology* 209:176–189.
30. Barber, R.P., Vaughn, J.E., Slemmon, J.R., Salvatena, P.M., Roberts, E., & Leeman, S.E. (1979). The origin, distribution, and synaptic relationship of substance P axons in rat spinal cord. *Journal of Comparative Neurology* 184:331–352.
31. Hokfelt, T., Kellerth, J-O., Nilsson, G., & Pernow, B. (1975). Experimental immunohistochemical studies on the localization and distribution of substance P in cat primary sensory neurons. *Brain Research.* 100:235–252.
32. Duffy, M.J., Mulhall, D., & Powell, D. (1975). Subcellular distribution of substance P in bovine hypothalamus and substantia nigra. *Journal of Neurochemistry* 25:305–307.
33. Jessell, T.M., & Iversen, L.L. (1977). Opiate analgesics inhibit substance P release from rat trigeminal nucleus. *Nature* 268:549–551.
34. Henry, J.L. (1976). Effects of substance P on functionally identified units in cat spinal cord. *Brain Research* 114:439–451.
35. Hylden, J.L.K., & Wilcox, G.L. (1981). Intrathecal substance P elicits a caudally directed biting and scratching behavior in mice. *Brain Research* 217:212–215.
36. Yaksh, T.L., Farb, D., Leeman, S., & Jessell, T. (1979). Intrathecal capsaicin depletes substance P and produces prolonged thermal analgesia. *Science* 206: 481–483.
37. Brown, A.G. (1982). The dorsal horn of the spinal cord. *Quarterly Journal of Experimental Physiology* 67:193–212.
38. Ruda, M.A. (1982). Opiates and pain pathways: Demonstration of enkephalin synapses on dorsal horn projection neurons. *Science* 215:1523–1525.
39. Barber, R.P., Vaughn, J.E., & Roberts, E. (1982). The cytoarchitecture of gabaergic neurons in rat spinal cord. *Brain Research* 238:305–308.
40. Trevino, D.L., & Carstens, E. (1975). Confirmation of the location of spinothalamic neurons in the cat and monkey by retrograde transport of horseradish peroxidase. *Brain Research* 98:177–182.
41. Kerr, F.W.L. (1975). The ventral spinothalamic tract and other ascending systems of the ventral funiculus of the spinal cord. *Journal of Comparative Neurology* 159:335–356.
42. Perl, E.R., & Whitlock, D.G. (1961). Somatic stimuli exciting spinothalamic projections in thalamic neurons in the cat and monkey. *Experimental Neurology* 3:256–296.

43. Dash, M.S., & Deshpande, S.S. (1976). Human skin nociceptors and their chemical response. In: *Advances in Pain Research and Therapy, Vol. 1* (Eds.) J.J. Bonica and D. Albe-Fessard. New York: Raven Press, pp. 47–51.
44. Spiegel, E.A., Kletzkin, M., & Szekely, E.G. (1954). Pain reactions upon stimulation of the tectum mesencephali. *Journal of Neuropathology and Experimental Neurology* 13:212–220.
45. Yaksh, T.L., Yeung, J.C., & Rudy, T.A. (1976). Systematic examination in the rat of brain sites sensitive to the direct application of morphine: Observation of differential effect within the periaquaductal gray. *Brain Research* 114:83–103.
46. Yaksh, T.L., Hammond, D.L., & Tyce, G.M. (1981). Functional aspects of bulbospinal monoaminergic projections in modulating processing of somatosensory information. *Federation Proceedings* 40:2786–2794.
47. Yaksh, T.L. (1978). Opiate receptors for behavioral analgesia resemble those related to the depression of spinal nociceptive neurons. *Science* 199:1231–1223.

# 3

# The Physical Examination of the Patient in Pain

*Robert K. Erickson*

The diagnostic explanation of many chronic pain states proves elusive, despite continuing advances in neurophysiologic measurement and radiologic imaging. All too often, patients undergo overly brief physical examinations, after which expensive tests or specialized evaluations are obtained in series. A thorough history and physical examination can provide essential diagnostic information that cannot be obtained in any other way; the examination becomes the proper groundwork for a properly orchestrated clinical decision-making process. In addition to pure diagnosis, the examination of the patient offers a valuable estimate of functional impairment, and a preliminary description of pain-related behavior. The present chapter will highlight those aspects of the history, physical, and neurological examination that are particularly pertinent to the chronic pain complaint; we will then discuss the role of ancillary diagnostic testing.

## General Considerations

Before proceeding to an outline of the examination of the patient with intractable pain, it is important to briefly review the general categories of pain, which most often are characterized by the location, distribution, and quality of the sensation. This categorization will be employed throughout the following discussion. It should be noted that these categories overlap somewhat; a particular constellation of symptoms may be described by several of the terms defined below.

## Nociceptive (Somatic) vs. Deafferentation Pain

It is generally accepted that chronic pain in humans is sustained by central neural pathways that differ significantly from those pathways that signal and provide awareness of acute noxious stimuli.[26] It is intriguing that almost any form of nerve injury that alters somatic sensation, whether it be in the peripheral or central nervous system, has a 1 to 5% chance of leading to chronic pain.[27] This pain, which is secondary to neural trauma and often termed deafferentation pain, is not associated in any consistent fashion with lesions of specific tracts or with lesions at specific levels in the nervous system. Indeed, there is no known lesion in the peripheral or central nervous system that uniformly leads to persistent pain in all patients. It is felt that deafferentation pain is a consequence of reverberating neuronal circuits set up by hyperactive pools of neurons which in fact may be quite remote from the original lesion.[16,27] Deafferentation pain is characterized by a wide variety of sensory phenomena and stimulation effects.

Nociceptive pain, on the other hand, is sensation referable to ongoing tissue damage detected by thermal receptors and mechanoreceptors leading to A-gamma and C-fiber axons. Nociceptive or somatic pain generally responds well to narcotic medication, while pain due to chronic nerve injury and presumed deafferentation typically does not. The terms patients use to describe their pain again are often more unusual and variable in cases of deafferentation than in cases of nociception (e.g., "burning," "crawling," "cold," "gnawing"). Both deafferentation and nociceptive pains may be increased by stress and improved by relaxation.

## Projected (Transmitted) Pain

Pain transmitted along the course of a nerve that is either segmental or peripheral in distribution is termed projected pain. Common examples of this type of pain are trigeminal neuralgia, brachial plexus neuralgia, herpes zoster, and meralgia paresthetica.

## Referred Pain

It is a well-known clinical fact that irritation of deep somatic or visceral structures may provoke sensation of pain in distant regions innervated by the same neural segment. This pain may or may not be accompanied by hyperesthesia, deep tenderness, muscle spasm, or autonomic disturbances. Common examples of referred pain include angina referred to the left arm or jaw, acute pancreatitis or perforated duodenal ulcer referred to the spine, and cervical spine disease with referral of sensation to the retro-orbital area. Referred pain may be particularly confusing in those instances in which tenderness and hyperesthesia are largely absent in the area of disease.

### Reflex Pain (Causalgic Pain)

Reflex pain is marked by striking hyperalgesia, hyperesthesia as well as vasomotor, sudomotor, and trophic changes. Major syndromes in this category are causalgia and the other reflex sympathetic dystrophies. Typically these sensations do not conform to any segmental or peripheral nerve distribution, often involving an entire extremity. The extremity may be so exquisitely sensitive that it is held immobile, eventually undergoing atrophy and osteoporosis.

### Nonorganic Pain (Psychologic Factors Affecting Pain Sensation)

Painful sensations in central, segmental, or peripheral distributions may be related to anxiety states, depression, conversion syndromes, and somatization disorders. These complaints may or may not be associated with somatic or autonomic changes. Inasmuch as these pain complaints mimic deafferentation or nociceptive pain, they may greatly obscure the subsequent diagnostic process. Long-term chronic pain states may also alter character structure, and affect normal coping and adaptation strategies.

## The History

The history is the cornerstone of the initial evaluation of the patient with persistent pain and all subsequent evaluations. In most cases the diagnosis will depend to a lesser degree on the physical examination and laboratory evaluations. The successful history will gather detailed information regarding the chronology, intensity, and incapacitation of the pain while establishing rapport with the patient in the initial stages of the interview. The physician should intervene as little as possible, allowing patients to relate their entire stories from the beginning with whatever details they deem relevant. During a patient's spontaneous narrative, the examiner has the opportunity to evaluate attitude, affect, and pain-associated behavior.

After the patient has been allowed sufficient time to recount his or her story, it is often necessary to focus the patient's account by leading questions that are presented in a conversational manner. The examiner must emerge from the interview with details and specific information regarding the onset, course, and present status of the pain. The exact location and the distribution of the pain, the presence of referred symptoms, the quality of the sensation, and the temporal characteristics of the pain must be determined exactly. It is important to note whether or not the patient is in pain at the time of the interview, and to have the patient compare the intensity of the pain to other more familiar sensations. Of course, if any interventions have been made previously, their effectiveness should be assessed by the patient; any relieving or exacerbating actions should be noted. A complete history of medication use must be included in the record.

The diagnosis of several chronic pain states is arrived at solely on the basis of a typical history. Examples of such conditions are trigeminal neuralgia, classical migraine, and post-herpetic neuralgia. However, a great number of cases referred to the pain clinic do not fall into discrete diagnostic categories. This is the difficult situation faced when beginning the evaluation of a patient with chronic low back pain who is in the throes of delayed compensation or litigation, or whose pain has persisted despite multiple interventions. These patients may have undergone unsuccessful surgery and may be suffering from some degree of denervation. At this point in the illness, psychologic factors are almost always intertwined with the problem. Although the examiner may not emerge from the interview with the precise diagnosis, he or she should begin to form an opinion as to whether the problem is predominantly organic or functional.

If the pain complaint has an organic basis, one must decide whether it represents continuous irritation (nociception) or a lesion within the nervous system (deafferentation). The most common event preceding the onset of deafferentation pain is trauma to the nervous system. The history is usually consistent with the pathology; pain due to metabolic or neoplastic disease is slowly progressive, and pain due to most vascular lesions or traumatic injuries arises suddenly. There is no uniform manner in which patients suffering from deafferentation describe their discomfort. In general, however, the terms used to describe the pain differ from those used to describe the more familiar sensations of nociception. The most common description in cases of deafferentation usually include words such as burning, gnawing, numb, or crawling. The patient often remarks that this pain is different than any felt previously. One salient feature of many of these pains is their frequent exacerbation by otherwise innocuous touch or temperature stimulation. Deafferentation pain may or may not respond to transcutaneous electrical nerve stimulation; indeed, this treatment often causes distinct discomfort. Both nociceptive and deafferentation pains are usually made worse by stress and improved by relaxation. In fact, any pain complaint that is not influenced whatsoever by stress or relaxation might raise the question of underlying malingering, depression, or other psychologic factors that may influence the painful condition. Diagnostic nerve blocks may result in temporary abolition of the pain whether or not the pain is caused by nociception or injury to the nervous stem.[14,27] Nerve blocks do not reliably predict the outcome of lesion-generating or stimulating procedures and may not help distinguish deafferentation pain from nociceptive pain. An exception to this rule is reflex pain (causalgia) in which a favorable result of sympathetic blockade usually portends a good result following definitive sympathectomy. Deafferentation pain is coincident with sensory loss in 79% of this group of patients; some of these patients describe their discomfort as a painful numbness.[27] Of interest is the fact that 61% of patients with deafferentation pain report delayed onset of their pain, with the discomfort starting months or years after the causative event.[27]

Faced with an atypical history, the examiner frequently entertains the possibility that the primary illness may be a result of nonorganic disease. Organic and nonorganic disease may exist simultaneously; either kind of disease may precipitate, color, or exacerbate the other. An especially difficult situation is one in which organic symptoms are exaggerated or extended by nonorganic disease. If the examiner has strong evidence that the illness is nonorganic, he or she must then decide the extent to which psychological factors exacerbate the problem, including the possibility of malingering and abnormal illness behavior.

Malingering exists in several forms, all of which may be seen in the pain clinic. *Malingering (misrepresentation)* is deliberate simulation of disease or disability. It may include false allegation that symptoms exist, or a conscious imitation of known disease symptoms. *Exaggeration (overreporting)* is the magnification or intensification of symptoms that do already exist. This exaggeration may be conscious or unconscious. *False imputation* refers to the ascribing of symptoms to a cause that bears no relationship to the symptoms, and may only be coincident. In fact, the symptom may have preceded the incident in question.[5]

Malingering should be distinguished from those conditions that include depression, hysteria, conversion reaction, psychophysiologic, or somatization disorders. Either abnormal illness behaviors or simulated symptoms may follow injuries or industrial accidents, but malingering is most apt to follow incidents in which symptoms are related in any way to compensation. The status of ongoing litigation or delayed compensation must be ascertained. In general, psychophysiologic disorders are associated with psychological, behavioral, or emotional factors that exacerbate pain complaints. In the patient with abnormal illness behaviors, there may be a past history of psychosomatic symptoms starting at an early age that might include anxiety attacks, tachycardia, anorexia nervosa, vomiting, constipation or diarrhea, or palpitations. A past history that includes patterns of behavior including repetitive minor trauma, poor employment records, or prior litigation raises the possibility of both malingering and abnormal illness behavior. This sort of information should be obtained not only from the patient but also from relatives and friends if at all possible. Their comments regarding the patient's reactions to prior illness and employment or familial stresses may prove invaluable.

## The Physical Examination

The general appearance of the patient, including the affect, posture, and nutritional status, is recorded. Anxiety, pallor, apathy, or tears are important concomitants of pain and should be noted. These general aspects should be looked for immediately upon making initial contact or, if possible, observed covertly. The nails, hair, and skin should be examined for dryness, hair loss, or trophic changes, particularly if there is a question of reflex sympathetic dystrophy or causalgia.

Attention is next directed to the painful region itself. The area in question should be inspected, palpated, and percussed. Inspection may disclose cyanosis or flushing, hyperhydrosis, pigmentary changes, atrophy, or asymmetry. Palpation should be carried out not only in the painful area but also on the opposite side to provide a standard of comparison. The presence of palpation tenderness should be verified by repeated palpations that approach the region from a different direction each time. The appropriateness of the affective response upon painful palpation should be judged. In general, organically based pain is attended by changes in pulse rate, blood pressure, breathing pattern, pupillary diameter, and autonomic function. Any groaning or reflex muscle spasm should be noted. Palpation may provoke theatrical gestures or facial expressions that seem out of proportion to the severity of the symptoms described in the interview. The patient should be asked whether palpation of the painful area provokes radiation of a discomfort to a remote area. An exaggerated response to superficial palpation of the painful area may reflect anxiety, malingering, hyperesthesia, or hyperpathia.

The hyperpathic response to stimulation has been described in detail by Foerster,[9] and more recently by Noordenbos.[18] Those patients with hyperpathic pain may note that the pain occurs spontaneously in some cases, while at other times the pain seems triggered by cutaneous stimulation. These patients generally have evidence of trophic changes or sensory loss implying a partial nerve lesion. Otherwise innocuous stimuli cause pain in this situation; a distinctive characteristic of the hyperpathic response is the often prolonged refractory period, that is, the time interval between onset of the stimulus and onset of the painful response (Fig. 3.1). If the stimulation in question does not continue long enough, the overshooting or hyperesthetic response may be missed. Such an area may be mistakenly described as anesthetic or analgesic, and wrongly characterized as analgesia dolorosa (Fig. 3.2). It has also been noted that the patient often has difficulty in localizing the stimulus precisely. An absence of delay in the hyperesthetic response to stimulus is characteristic of a heterotopic area of referred pain. Of course, in cases of pure pain referral, there should be no local evidence of sensory loss.

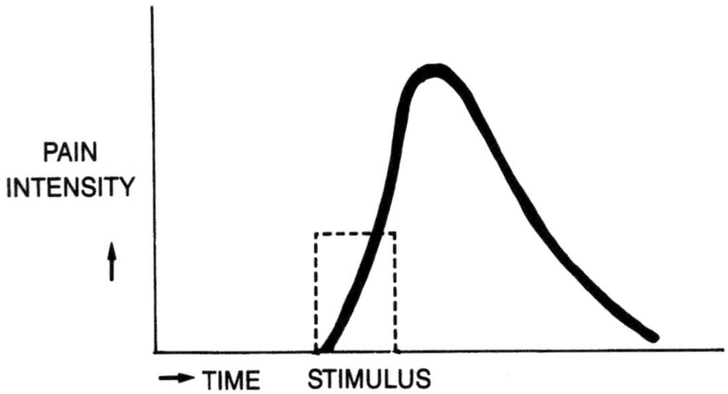


**Figure 3.1.** Graphic representation of stimulus duration versus pain intensity (after Noordenbos). The pain threshold is indicated by the top of the dotted rectangle. As the stimulus is continued, the pain threshold is exceeded, and the patient reports painful sensation.

The evaluation of an area rendered painful by palpation or percussion may be aided by the local injection of procaine or saline. In the saline-procaine test,[25] saline is first injected into the tender area around the nerve through a skin wheal made with local anesthetic. In ten to fifteen minutes, the area is palpated again and the patient observed for signs of discomfort. Nonorganic disorders may be dramatically relieved with saline injection alone. If the pain is persistent, procaine is infiltrated locally. Relief of pain with this supplementary injection in a patient with a negative response to saline infiltration points to a somatic basis for the complaint. When neither injection is effective, some degree of malingering or abnormal illness behavior may be present. In interpreting the result of such a test, it should be remembered that patients with functional disease sometimes react normally to injection of these substances, and that saline alone has been reported to be effective in breaking up cycles of somatic pain thought secondary to trigger points. Additionally, injection of any substance may act as a placebo. The intradermal procaine wheal test[25] consists of injecting dilute local anesthetic intradermally in the entire hyperalgesic area. If the discomfort is secondary to cutaneous hypersensitivity that is solely a referred manifestation of disease located at some distance, palpation of the area after infiltration evokes no pain. On some body surfaces, the outer margin of hypersensitive skin may be pulled aside so that a normal portion is brought over the sore spot and palpation then carried out to determine any deep tenderness. The persistent presence of deep soreness to palpation gives information as to whether the underlying structure is also tender. Ethyl chloride spray is an acceptable alternative to intradermal injection.

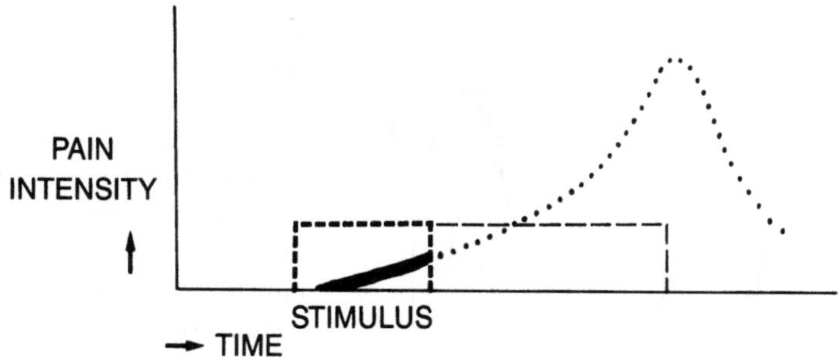


**Figure 3.2.** Graphic representation of stimulus duration versus pain intensity (after Noordenbos). In this instance, the stimulus is not of sufficient duration to exceed the pain threshold. This event may mimic complete anesthesia of the painful area.

The combination of systematic palpation and local injection in many cases indicates a myofascial pain syndrome. Indeed, the majority of patients referred to most pain clinics eventually are diagnosed as suffering from a form of myofascial pain.[8,10,24,28] This diagnosis is based primarily on history and physical examination. Most experts in myofascial pain syndromes feel that the pain is secondary to the presence of trigger points in specific muscles.[22,23,29] The somewhat controversial hypothesis is that pain due to active myofascial trigger points often begins suddenly in an acute episode of stress overload of the muscle. Alternatively, the pain may develop gradually because of chronic or repetitive muscle strain. In the absence of repetitive trauma, these active trigger points revert to a latent state, only to be exacerbated by future incidents. The pain caused by a trigger point is typically referred to a remote point. Typically, the patterns of these referred pains do not correspond to nerve distributions, but rather correspond quite well to the topography of the muscle involved. This concept of trigger points and resultant myofascial pain dates to 1938 in which Kellgren reported that pain is referred to various remote locations after intramuscular injection of hypertonic saline.[13] The hallmark of the syndrome is relief of the referred pain upon injection of the trigger point with local anesthetic. Travell and Rinzler[28] summarized the specific pain patterns referred from trigger points in the most commonly involved muscles (Fig. 3.3a and 3.3b). On examination, there may be palpable hardening of a taut band of muscle fibers at the point of tenderness. An additional local twitch response of this taut band of muscle fibers may occur on brisk palpation or needle penetration.

During the general physical examination, one should specifically determine the effect on the pain of extended range of motion, coughing, sneezing, straining, and the Valsalva maneuver. The patient should be asked to

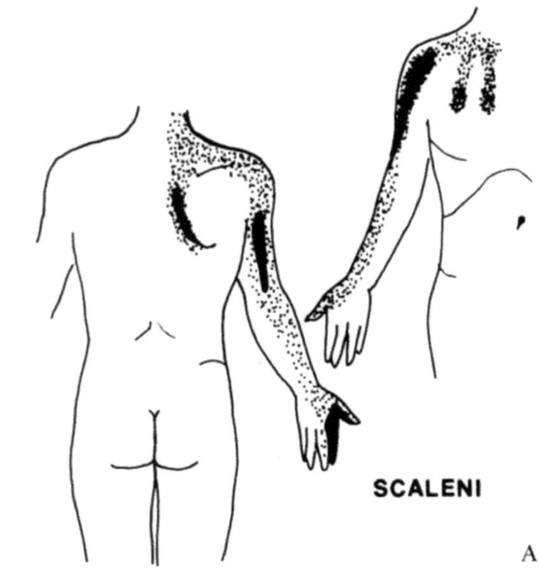


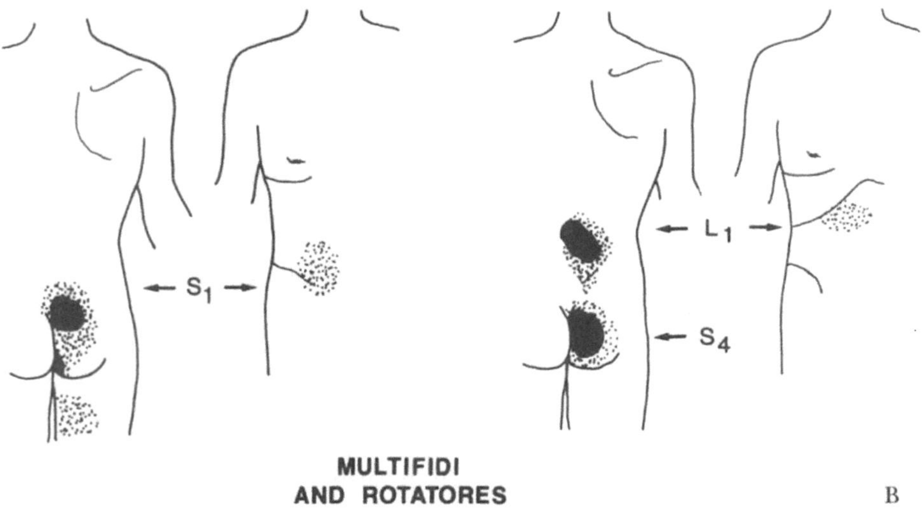


**Figure 3.3A,B.** Examples of referred pain patterns associated with trigger points in the multifidi, rotatores, and scaleni (after Travell and Simons). Muscular inflammation may closely resemble radicular or peripheral nerve compression syndromes.

assume the prone, seated, and upright positions and also to demonstrate what manner of activity is hampered by the pain, rather than depending on a verbal report by the patient. The presence of overdramatization in this circumstance may be quite significant.

## Neurological Examination

No attempt will be made here to exhaustively review the neurological examination in detail. However, a careful sensory examination centered about the painful complaint is mandatory. The examinations of the motor system, deep tendon and superficial reflexes, cranial nerves, and cerebellar function will be contributory inasmuch as they help localize a nervous system lesion.

In cases of chronic pain secondary to arthritis, fascitis, or other myofascial syndromes, the diagnosis may be evident following the history and general physical examination. However, in most cases, it is necessary either to rule out the presence of a nervous system lesion, or if one is suspected, to localize that lesion.

## "Upper Motor Neuron" vs. "Lower Motor Neuron"

In consideration of a possible nervous system lesion contributing to a painful syndrome, it is helpful to distinguish the concept of the "upper motor neuron" lesion from that of the "lower motor neuron" lesion. The concept of the upper motor neuron is more a physiological one than an anatomical entity. It was originally defined anatomically as the pyramidal or corticospinal tract that arises from the Betz cells and the precentral gyrus of each frontal lobe. The signs described to injury to this tract are called pyramidal signs, although many aspects of the syndrome seem extrapyramidal in nature. Damage to the system anywhere along its course from the cerebral cortex to the internal capsule and brain stem to the termination of its axons along the lateral white columns of the spinal cord results in weakness that tends to affect discrete movements of the distal limb segments. Associated with the weakness are spasticity or the clasp-knife phenomenon, hyperactive deep tendon reflexes, loss of the cutaneous abdominal and cremasteric reflexes on the paretic side, Babinski's toe sign, and relative lack of atrophy of the involved muscles. The lower motor neuron system refers to the aggregate of motor neurons in the body that include the motor nuclei of the cranial nerves and those motor cells that reside in the anterior gray horn of the spinal cord. Each neuron of this system is the final common pathway that influences motor function. A lesion anywhere from the motor neurons in the anterior horn to their endpoint at the motor end plates produces a weakness characterized by paralysis of individual muscles or group of muscles, a persistent loss of muscle tone, loss of deep tendon reflexes, early muscular atrophy, variable amounts of muscle fasciculations, and the absence of a Babinski sign or other pathological reflexes. Thus, the concept of the "lower motor neuron" lesion includes radiculopathy, plexopathy, and peripheral neuropathy.

## Spinal Canal Syndromes

Because many pain problems seem to involve the spine, it is necessary to possess a working knowledge of the cross-sectional and longitudinal anatomy of the spinal cord, the spinal roots and nerves within the canal, and meninges. It should be remembered that the spinal cord extends from the foramen magnum of the skull to the interspace between the first and

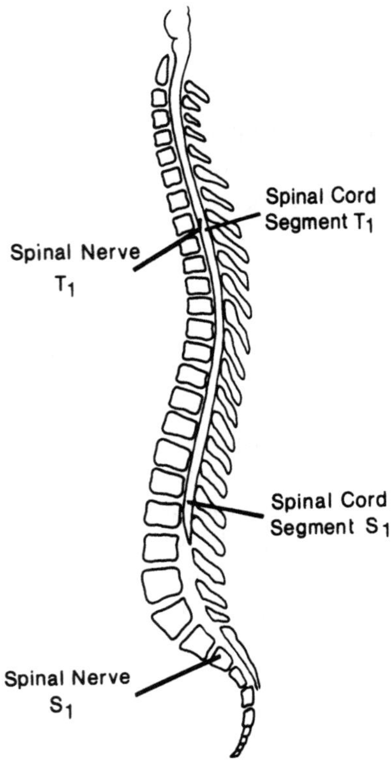


**Figure 3.4.** Diagramatic representation of the spinal canal and spinal cord. Whereas the spinal cord segment T1 is closely associated with the exit of the spinal nerve T1 from the spinal canal, relative lengthening of the spinal canal results in a significant disparity in location between the spinal cord segment and the spinal nerve exit of S1.

second lumbar vertebra. In the absence of congenital anomalies, lesions of the spinal canal caudal to the first lumbar vertebra will produce only signs referable to the spinal roots that constitute the cauda equina. Because of the discrepancy between the length of the spinal cord and that of the spinal canal, the segments of the spinal cord do not always coincide in the horizontal plane with their corresponding vertebrae (Fig. 3.4). Therefore, in describing the location of the lesion in the spinal canal, particularly one located in the thoracic or lumbar area, one must specifically designate whether one is referring to the spinal cord segment or the vertebral level of the lesion.

Each segment of spinal cord is represented topographically by an area of skin called the dermatome from which it receives sensory innervation. Although the dermatome maps commonly in use generally agree regarding major dermatomal distributions, it must be emphasized that there may be small variations between individuals. Because of overlap of nerve supply between adjacent dermatomes, no demonstrable sensory deficit is usually found unless two or more adjacent posterior roots or spinal nerves are interrupted.

Two related terms should be defined to avoid confusion. The myotome refers to those muscles innervated by a single spinal segment. While the majority of skeletal muscles receive their motor innervation from multiple spinal segments, in each group one segment predominates. For example, the C5 myotome consists primarily of the periscapular muscles, deltoid, pronator teres, and brachioradialis. The sclerotome comprises all of the tissue of embryonic mesodermal origin, including muscle, fascia, and connective tissue innervated by the spinal segment. Thus, pain originating in root compression or from soft tissue injuries is often wrongly described as being referred within the affected dermatome. It is well known that the referred pain is felt not only in the skin but in the deeper tissues within the affected sclerotome.[30] Despite the inaccuracy in terminology, the term dermatome is most commonly used when speaking of segmental reference of pain.

Within the spinal cord, the structural components of greatest and diagnostic usefulness are:

1. The descending motor tracts in the lateral white columns (lateral cord of the spinal tract).
2. The ascending fibers in the posterior white columns, which convey position and vibratory sensation (fasciculus gracilis and fasciculus cuneatus).
3. The ascending tracts in the anterior part of each lateral white column which convey cutaneous pain and temperature sensation (spinothalamic tracts).
4. The autonomic descending fibers in each lateral white column and autonomic cell groups of the intermediate gray column in the thoracic segments that give rise to preganglionic sympathetic fibers.
5. Cervical and lumbar enlargements of the spinal cord that correspond to segments innervating the upper and lower extremities.

A detailed discussion of long-tract lesions is beyond the scope of this chapter. The reader is referred to textbooks of neuroanatomy and the neurologic examination by DeJong[5] and Brodal.[2] Briefly, interruption of the lateral cortical spinal tract produces the syndrome of "upper motor neuron" paralysis below the level of the lesion. It should be remembered that both the lateral cortical spinal tract and the posterior columns cross approximately at the level of the foramen magnum. The lateral spinothalamic tract arises as a crossed tract as it originates within the spinal cord. Therefore, a unilateral lesion involving the spinothalamic tract on one side within the spinal canal or above the foramen magnum will produce a deficit of pain and temperature sensation contralaterally below the level of the lesion. It should also be remembered that the long tracts of the spinal cord are laminated in such a way that in the spinothalamic tracts and corticospinal tracts the sacral fibers are located most laterally while the cervical fibers are located most medially. For this reason, a progressive extramedullary lesion may lead to the findings of a sensory level on the trunk that are not reliable in indicating the exact level of the lesion, although one would know that the lesion probably lies in the spinal canal above that level. In contrast, an intramedullary spinal cord lesion may exert pressure upon only the most medial fibers of these tracts, which produces loss of pain and temperature sensation limited to a few segments, with a relative sparing of the sensations both above and below. This finding is referred to as a suspended sensory level or segmental sensory loss, and is indicative of lesion within the parenchyma of the spinal cord such as an intramedullary tumor or syrinx.

The intermediate gray column that gives rise to the paravertebral sympathetic chain is located in the T1 through L2 spinal cord segments. These preganglionic neurons are subject to control by the higher centers that include the cortex, hypothalamus, and brain stem reticular formation. Therefore, lesions at the cervical and upper thoracic levels of the canal are likely to alter vasomotor activity and sweating. Horner's syndrome (ptosis, miosis, and anhydrosis) may occur on the same side of the lesion at or above the T1 segment. The presence of Horner's syndrome may also indicate a lesion of the sympathetic fibers as they ascend cranially with the carotid artery.

The cauda equina syndrome results from lesions within the spinal canal located below the level of the first lumbar vertebra. Again, these lesions will not produce findings referable to the spinal cord tracts, as the spinal cord terminates at L1-2. The findings, therefore, will be limited to those of involvement of the lumbar and sacral spinal nerve roots making up the cauda equina. Any motor loss will be of the lower motor neuron type. Sensory loss will be limited to the lower extremities and the sacral saddle area. In severe cases, impairment of bladder control may be associated with the painful complaint.

The examiner should be familiar with the classical manifestations of partial spinal cord transection in the cross-sectional plane, although these syndromes are seen uncommonly in patients with chronic pain. These syndromes include complete transection of the spinal cord (transverse myelitis), the Brown-Sequard syndrome (transverse hemisection of the spinal cord), the anterior spinal artery syndrome (anterior cord syndrome), and the central cord syndrome. A working knowledge of these classical syndromes will help organize the sensory examination, particularly those in which bizarre sensory patterns emerge.

## Peripheral Nerve Lesions

The peripheral nerves are generally mixed nerves that include axons conveying motor, sensory, and autonomic impulses. As a particular nerve courses peripherally, its axons branch into more specialized components. Thus, the more proximally a nerve is affected, the more likely one is to find disturbance of all three functions in its territory. The peripheral nerve territories differ markedly from the dermatomal pattern. Because there is considerable overlap between adjacent peripheral nerve territories, the sensory deficit seen on examination in cases of a single peripheral nerve lesion is usually less extensive than that shown on a somatic map. The peripheral nerve problem may fall into several patterns of distribution such as plexus syndromes, mononeuropathy, polyneuropathy, or mononeuropathy multiplex. In mononeuropathy, an isolated peripheral nerve is injured. In polyneuropathy, multiple adjacent peripheral nerves are involved simultaneously in a pattern that is often quite symmetric. Mononeuropathy multiplex refers to a relatively rare condition in which two or more individual peripheral nerves are paralyzed simultaneously.

Mononeuropathies and plexopathies may be due to compressive, toxic, metabolic, or inflammatory problems. Polyneuropathy and mononeuropathy multiplex, on the other hand, are invariably due to medical disease. In the case of bilaterally symmetric lesions, polyneuropathies may simulate compressive problems. In general, the motor and sensory manifestations of polyneuropathy generally begin in the distal parts of the involved extremities. The proximal musculature becomes involved only late in the course of such disease. Truncal sensory levels do not occur. Most painful polyneuropathies are associated with selected small fiber loss. The most common example of this condition is diabetic neuropathy. Similar changes are seen in amyloid neuropathy, Fabry's disease, and hereditary sensory neuropathy. Examples of painful polyneuropathies in which both small and large fibers are lost are alcoholic neuropathy and the neuropathy associated with multiple myeloma. Painful polyneuropathies may also be associated with selective loss of large fibers, as in isoniazid neuropathy and pellagra. The pains of herpes zoster, diabetic mononeuropathy and amyotrophy, ischemic neuropathy, idiopathic brachial plexus neuropathy, and carcinomatous causalgia are best categorized as mononeuropathies. Again, the hallmark of these peripheral nerve problems is the distribution of the complaint that conforms to the known peripheral nerve topography. For further information regarding the manifestations of plexopathy and neuropathy, the reader is referred to the monograph entitled *Peripheral Nerve Injuries* by Haymaker and Woodhall.[12]

## The Sensory Examination

Even the sensory portion of the neurologic examination cannot directly assess pain, since there is no necessary physical concomitant of chronic pain. However, in many patients the neurological findings will give evidence of a nervous system lesion that is causative. The neurological examination in the chronic pain patient should generally begin with the sensory examination, as it is likely to be a tedious and somewhat uncomfortable procedure. Since the results of the examination depend entirely upon the verbal report of the patient, the patient must be alert, reasonably intelligent, and informed at each step. The sensory examination will be most difficult if the patient is suffering greatly at the time. The patient should be instructed to respond quickly each time he or she perceives a sensation and counseled that cooperation is necessary for a satisfactory result. The examiner must consciously avoid leading questions that may cause the suggestible patient to report sensations consistent with a preconceived notion of the examiner. Often hypochondriacal or overly cooperative patients may make too much of small differences and report sensory changes that are not present. Some areas of the body such as the neck, supraclavicular fossa, and inner forearm are more sensitive than others and the apparent sensory changes over these areas may lead to a false interpretation. There is a tendency to report the last in series of identical stimuli as the strongest stimulus. On occasion, a patient may be able to identify a sharp stimulus with a pin in an area where pain and temperature sensibility is absent. This phenomenon is called sensory dissociation, and is a typical finding in syringomyelia.

Any notable changes on the sensory examination should be mapped on a sensory chart that will become part of the medical record. In referring to an area of sensory alteration, it is important to use standardized terminology when indicating the impairment of sensory modalities. Analgesia, hypalgesia, and hyperalgesia should denote loss of pain sensation, diminished pain sensation, or increased pain sensation, respectively. The terms anesthesia, hypesthesia, and hyperesthesia should be used in the description of touch. Paresthesia refers to abnormal sensation that may include cold, prickling, tingling, or itching in the absence of specific stimulation, whereas the term dysesthesia is generally reserved for atypical sensations such as crawling, burning, or tingling. If delayed in onset following a stimulus, these may be properly described as hyperpathia. The term thigmanesthesia specifically denotes loss of light touch, while loss of sensation or movement of the skin hairs is known as trichoanesthesia. Topoanesthesia and graphanesthesia refer to loss of tactile localization. Graphanesthesia specifically denotes the inability to recognize letters or numbers written on the skin by the examiner. These latter two functions, along with two-point discrimination, are examples of cerebral sensory functions.

Superficial pain sensation may be evaluated by several physical methods, the simplest of which is to use a sharp pin with which the skin is systematically pricked beginning with the least sensitive area. For very accurate measurement of the amount of pressure exerted to elicit pinprick pain, one may use either the Von Frey hairs or other algesimeters. In general, however, it is possible to use the simple pin method reliably. One convenient method is simply to place the pinpoint at the level of the examiner's fingertip so that the examiner is able to feel the pressure as the pinprick is applied. It is also helpful to draw the point of the pin across the skin in a superficial scratching manner, again beginning in the area of least sensitivity.

Deep pain sensibility is tested by the application of pressure to muscles or tendons. Pressure may be conveniently applied with the finger or dull objects such as the rounded end of a pen. An alternative method is to slightly overextend the joints of the digits; the absence of pain with such a maneuver also signifies impairment of deep pain sensation.

Temperature sensibility is best tested by the use of test tubes containing cold and hot water. The two tubes should be visibly identical. The water should not either be so cold or so warm that it evokes discomfort.

Tactile sensibility is rapidly tested by using a wisp of cotton, applicator tip, or small brush. Any pressure should be avoided to isolate tactile sensibility. The patient should easily identify the direction of a light stroke on the skin.

Position and vibratory sense should be tested in concert. Testing for position sense is most sensitive when done at the fingertips or toes. Care must be taken not to cue the direction of movement by the application of pressure in the direction of movement. Vibration sense, termed pallesthesia, is tested by using a tuning fork at 128 vibrations per second. If a question of vibration sensibility emerges, this can be conveniently quantified by striking the tuning fork maximally and timing the duration of the sense vibration from joint to joint and from side to side. When losses of position and vibration sense co-exist, disease of the posterior columns of peripheral nerves is indicated. When a loss of position sense is isolated, parietal lobe dysfunction must be expected. Relatively isolated loss of vibratory sensation is typical in the peripheral sensory neuropathies, such as diabetic neuropathy.

It should be stressed that sensory findings may vary significantly between examinations. This variation is not necessarily a result of poor examination technique, nor is it necessarily a result of nonorganic pathology. Damage to any part of the peripheral nervous system is followed by sprouting of the damaged nerve, or gradual recovery of a neuropractic injury. The sprouting axons may become quite sensitive to mechanical stimulation, manifest as Tinel's sign, in which percussion over the nerve may produce paresthesias. Excitation may occur as a result of an electrical cross talk between bare axons that are in close apposition.[21] Localized areas of demyelination secondary to nerve compression may give rise to spontaneous action potentials that might travel proximally or distally. Normally produced action potentials may provoke sustained after-discharges.[20] There exists the possibility of abnormal communication between sympathetic afferent fibers and nociceptive primary afferents; this is supported by the experimental observation that stimulation of the sympathetic chain that supplies efferents to a traumatic neuroma can result in afferent discharge coming out of the neuroma.[6] This sympathetic innervation of neuromas may account for cases in which sympathetic block gives dramatic relief.[15] In addition to the formation of abnormal connections, a zone of denervation may change from week to week, based

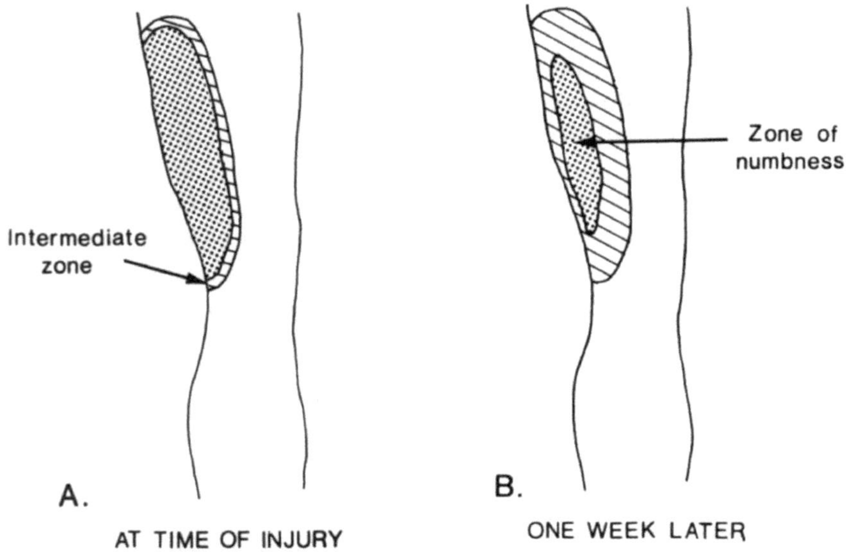


**Figure 3.5.** Diagram of sensory examination following a peripheral nerve injury (after Finneson). The area of complete anesthesia to pinprick or light touch may change quite rapidly during the days immediately following the injury. The intermediate zone is the area in which partial sensation is retained.

on the plasticity of central mechanisms (Fig. 3.5).[7] The sensory mapping done at the time of initial evaluation is of paramount importance.

## Examination of the Motor System

A degree of weakness is often intertwined with the chronic pain complaint. An examination of strength, tone, coordination, and volume may serve to localize a neurological lesion, or may indicate a fibromyalgic basis for the complaint. Detailed discussion of individual muscle testing will not be undertaken here; briefly, it should be recalled that most skeletal muscles receive multisegmental innervation. Therefore, involvement of a single root or segment is likely to be reflected by partial paralysis in several individual muscles. It is important to note whether a weakness is spastic or flaccid in nature. Spastic paralysis reflects a lesion of the upper-motor neuron variety, and is associated with increased deep tendon reflexes, diminished superficial reflexes, and the presence of pathological reflexes. There is a relative absence of atrophy. In flaccid paralysis, signs of lower-motor neuron dysfunction are evident. There is a decrease or complete loss of deep tendon reflexes, and often striking atrophy. The presence of visible fasciculations is quite significant. In addition to giving information about the particular reflex involved, examination of the reflexes as noted above may signal the presence of pyramidal tract disease vs. the presence of radiculopathy or neuropathy (lower motor neuron). In lesions of the pyramidal tract, the superficial reflexes are diminished or absent. Major examples of the superficial reflexes are those provoked by the stimulation of the cornea, pharynx, abdomen, and inner thigh (cremasteric). The appearance of pathological reflexes in the examination, however, signals pyramidal tract lesions. The most important of these reflexes is the Babinski response, whereupon plantar stimulation leads to abnormal extension of the great toe and fanning of the remainder of the toes. A similar response may be obtained by the other maneuvers about the foot and lower leg: the Oppenheim maneuver (stroking downward on the medial side of the tibia), Gordon maneuver (compression of the calf muscle), Chaddock maneuver (stroking around the external malleolus), and the Schaefer maneuver (pinching the Achilles tendon). In cases of pyramidal tract disease, ankle clonus may be elicited by briskly dorsiflexing the foot. If this maneuver is followed by a clonic repetition of the normal ankle jerk, it is taken as a sign of spasticity. In contrast to the superficial and pathological reflexes, the increase, absence, or asymmetry of a deep tendon reflex is in itself not sufficient to indicate the character or presence of organic disease unless it is correlated with other findings. In provoking deep reflex responses, it is mandatory to make the patient comfortable, and to place the muscle in a position between full contraction or relaxation. It is well known that the presence of anxiety may greatly enhance the deep tendon reflex, as may hyperthyroidism. In hypothyroidism, there is a diminished response with increased latency.

## Examination of the Cranial Nerves

A full examination of the cranial nerves should be performed, especially when the painful syndrome involves the head. Only the most salient aspects of the cranial nerve examination are included below.

The olfactory nerve is tested by using a volatile oil, or mint. Each nostril is tested separately. A unilateral anosmia may indicate a basal frontal tumor.

The second cranial nerve is the optic nerve. Like the olfactory nerve, it is not truly a peripheral nerve, but rather an extension of the optic tract. The examination of the optic nerve should include a measure of visual acuity, visual fields, and funduscopic appearance. When abnormal, the visual field examination in particular is quite localizing; a homonymous hemianopia indicates disease posterior to the optic chiasm, whereas a bitemporal or binasal hemianopia indicates an anterior lesion. The presence of a Marcus-Gunn pupil (a paradoxically dilating pupil in the presence of light) may be discovered if the pin light is rapidly alternated from side to side. This sign also indicates disease anterior to the chiasm, and may be seen as an early sign of multiple sclerosis. The presence of optic atrophy or papilledema will also prompt a search for an intracranial lesion.

The third, fourth, and sixth nerves are named the oculomotor, trochlear, and abducens nerves, respectively. These are tested in conjunction with the optic nerve. Both pupils are examined for size, shape, position, and reaction to light and accommodation. The presence or absence of Horner's syndrome (unilateral ptosis, miosis, and anhydrosis) should be specifically determined in cases involving the brachial plexus, thoracic outlet, cervical spine, neck, or cranium. The ocular movements are tested in all directions, and the presence of any diplopia noted.

The trigeminal nerve is a motor and sensory nerve. The function of its motor root is verified as the patient bites down. Any weakness or deviation should be noted. The sensory division carries afferent fibers for the face, tongue, and mucous membranes and should be examined for pain, touch, and temperature. The only part of the face not innervated by the trigeminal nerve is the posterior angle of the mandible. The corneal reflex may be affected quite early in trigeminal nerve disease, and should be examined in all cases by touching the cornea with a small wisp of cotton. Any deficit of the trigeminal nerve in cases of trigeminal neuralgia should raise the question of intracranial disease. Examination of the seventh, or facial nerve, is readily done by having the patient display the range of expressions. The examiner should remember the bilateral innervation of the muscles of the forehead, which allow ready differentiation of upper-motor neuron from lower-motor neuron weakness.

The acoustic division of the eighth nerve is tested by having the patient listen to a tickling watch or lightly rubbed fingers in front of the ear. It should be ascertained whether the vibrating tuning fork is better heard by air or bone conduction. The vestibular division is generally not tested unless dizziness or vertigo is part of the complaint.

The ninth, tenth, eleventh, and twelfth cranial nerves are examined by testing palatal movement, tongue, pharyngeal sensation, and the pharyngeal reflex. Dysfunction of the vagus nerve will be reflected in a nasal or hoarse quality of the voice. An inspection of the vocal cords may reveal paralysis. The spinal accessory nerve is tested in head rotation and shrugging of the shoulders. The hypoglossal nerve is examined by having the patient protrude the tongue of which time any asymmetry, atrophy, or fibrillations may be seen.

## Examination of the Nonorganic Complaint

While bearing in mind that bizarre symptoms and signs may occur as a part of organic disease, the question of hysteria, hypochondriasis, depression, or other psychogenic disorder often arises early in the evaluation of chronic pain. Often the amount of symptoms is out of proportion to the physical findings. Caution must be exercised in reaching such a diagnosis, since organic disease may exist in the absence of the physical signs. Additionally, organic disease and psychogenic disorders may co-exist. Particular caution must be exercised not to quickly dismiss the patient with multiple, so-called psychosomatic complaints. Even if the physician is not able to provide treatment for these patients, he or she can be instrumental in referring the patient to the appropriate clinician for treatment.

It is well known that the individual with hysterical tendencies often reacts to all painful stimuli, sometimes with an exaggerated motor response. Indeed, there seems to be a group of patients who will feel pain at any level of stimulation.[14] Hyperesthesia and tenderness may be found. Again, the symptoms may be totally out of proportion to the amount of pressure exerted by the examiner. While distracted, the patient may actually be able to tolerate a greater stimulus without showing any sign of suffering. The distribution of claimed sensory loss may fail to correspond to any known nerve distribution. A frequent pattern of sensory loss is the "glove and stocking" distribution, with complete loss of all modalities below the wrist or elbow in the arm and below either the ankle or knee in the leg. While the glove and stocking anesthesia of true peripheral neuropathy shows a gradual transition of sensation at its border, the anesthesia of nonorganic causes often ends abruptly at joint level. Such a patient may be confused by examining the hands while they are crossed behind his or her back while the palms and dorsal surfaces of the hands are alternately stimulated. The patient may also demonstrate inconsistent reporting if the hands are crossed and pronated with the fingers interlocked, following which the hands are rotated toward the chest. With this maneuver, the fingertips are on the same side as the respective arms, but the thumbs are not interlocked and are therefore on the side opposite the fingers. The patient with nonorganic sensory loss might either make mistakes, or show signs of anxiety or hesitation when a testing is carried out alternately in this position.

In both consciously and unconsciously motivated anesthesia, a relatively meticulous midline distribution is common. In this pattern, there is complete loss of sensation over one half of the body which may include the penis, vagina, and rectum. This differs from the pattern of organic lesions in which sensation begins to return slightly before the midline is reached by the examiner. In addition, a midline sensory loss is distinctly uncommon in the perineum. The midline sensory loss may even persist on testing vibratory[4] sensation at the sternum, even though the entire sternum should be stimulated by the tuning fork. Again, midline sensory change found in the presence of symmetric cutaneous reflexes on the abdomen rules out anesthesia.

Brainstem, thalamic, and subcortical lesions may on occasion produce confusing patterns of pain, sensory loss, and dyesthesia that must not be mistakenly attributed to nonorganic disease. These lesions are typically vascular in origin, and therefore are seen predominantly in the older population. Lateral medullary lesions (Wallenberg's syndrome) lead to pain and dyesthesia in an alternating distribution; the face is affected on the same side, the body on the other. Medullary lesions can cause bilateral facial pain if both the descending root of the trigeminal nerve and the crossed quintothalamic fibers are involved.[4] Thalamic lesions usually cause contralateral pain, but may lead to a peculiar cheiro-oral distribution of dyesthesia.[11] In some cases, multiple subcortical infarctions may produce confusing bilateral sensory disturbances.

Regarding the motor system, nonorganic weakness again is usually atypical. There may be a degree of diffuse atrophy present, but never the true atrophy seen with lower motor neuron lesions. In the event of feigned weakness, the muscles must be tested in detail. The characteristics of the nonorganic response are sudden "giving-way" of the effort, or an absence of "follow-through" when the examiner withdraws his or her effort. Testing done with the patient on the examining table may indicate weakness of dorsiflexion or plantar flexion of the foot that is totally absent when the patient is standing upright and is asked to walk on the heels or toes.

The reflexes should also be closely examined in this situation. In some cases the deep tendon reflex response may be greatly exaggerated in the absence of clonus. Generally, the superficial reflexes listed above are not characteristically affected in nonorganic weakness. The pyramidal tract responses are particularly crucial in the diagnosis of psychogenic disorders. A positive Babinski sign is not seen in purely nonorganic disorders.

It is also important to note any abnormal responses to maneuvers during the physical examination such as straight-leg raising. Straight-leg raising in general should not produce sciatic radiation at angles of five or ten degrees. A full Lasegue's maneuver (straight-leg raising test followed by dorsiflexion of the foot) may lead to a paradoxical relief of pain in these patients. Similarly, Patrick's hip sign (flexion, abduction, and external rotation at the hip) may also provoke an exaggerated complaint of sciatic pain, which, in the absence of hip disease, is quite significant. In extremely severe cases of nonorganic pain and weakness, there may be trophic changes seen in the skin and nails, vasomotor changes with cyanosis and edema, abnormalities of sweating, and even some osteoperosis. Such severe cases may closely resemble reflex sympathetic dystrophy.

Almost any neurologic or somatic complaint may be of psychogenic origin. Common examples are dramatic visual changes, deafness, bizarre tremors, and dysphonia. The reader is referred to the extensive discussion in DeJong's textbook.[5] Special diagnostic procedures may be necessary in the final differentiation between organic and nonorganic disease. These tests, depending on the complaint, may include radiologic imaging procedures, electromyography and nerve conduction studies, and evaluations of autonomic nervous system function. A psychological assessment (Chapter 4) and psychometric (Chapter 5) testing can help determine psychological factors affecting the patients pain, but only with conversion disorder can organic etiology be confidently ruled out by these examinations. It is more often the case that causative factors are impossible to determine. Treatment, therefore, may require both medical and psychological management.

## Ancillary Tests

### Radiologic Testing

The past decade has seen computerized tomography (CT) become widely available, and the fairly recent introduction of magnetic resonance imaging (MRI) has furthered this technological explosion. It is now possible to study almost every sector of the body in remarkable detail via noninvasive imaging. Rather than replacing CT, MRI has become complementary to CT in the diagnosis of many problems. The best example of this is the field of spinal canal diseases. CT scanning is capable of providing very detailed information regarding facet hypertrophy, the shape of the lateral recesses, foraminal stenosis, and the presence or absence of vertebral fracture. When performed in conjunction with myelography, the CT technique is capable of resolving small disc herniations, even those herniations that are located far laterally and otherwise would have been missed in the time prior to the introduction to CT. MRI, while it does not resolve bony detail well, is particularly suited to visualization of the spinal cord. Thus, MRI has become the definitive test in the evaluation for possible intramedullary tumor or syrinx. Infusion techniques using CT or MRI may aid in the differentiation of recurrent disc herniation from postoperative scarring in the spinal canal. Because of the noninvasive nature of these tests, and the minimal toxicity associated with the more recently introduced contrast agents, one should not hesitate to radiologically evaluate any chronic pain problem in which a structural lesion is at all suspected.

The resolution and sensitivity of MRI is such that it has become the screening evaluation of choice for suspected cases of multiple sclerosis or small subcortical infarctions. When used in concert, CT scanning and MRI approach the 100% sensitivity level in detection of intracranial mass lesions.

### Laboratory Tests

In this application, blood tests are generally used to provide confirmatory information regarding the presence of inflammation and infection, or to rule out the presence of metabolic or neoplastic disease. In general, a hemoglobin, hematocrit, differential white-cell count, and sedimentation rate will confirm the presence of chronic infection or inflammation. A kidney and liver profile should be obtained to test for the presence of systemic disease. A serum glucose level is of particular importance in cases of painful peripheral neuropathy and plexopathy, because of the prevalence of diabetes mellitus. Hypothyroidism may result in a myxedematous compression of the median nerve in the carpal tunnel or may produce a sensory ataxia with hyperalgesia. Thyroid function tests should be obtained if this condition is suspected. An elevated sedimentation rate in the case of mononeuropathy or polyneuropathy raises the possibility of collagen vascular disease which may be then characterized serologically. In some cases of neuropathy, peripheral nerve biopsy can usually provide information regarding which fiber populations are most severely affected, whether regeneration is occurring, and other specific diagnostic features. Nerve biopsy may in fact provide diagnostic information in cases of amyloidosis, necrotizing angiopathic neuropathy, leprosy, sarcoidosis, and in vasculitis. Subacute combined degeneration may present with burning paresthesias in the feet or hands, and is diagnosed on the finding of vitamin B12 deficiency. Thiamine deficiency in the alcoholic also may produce a peripheral neuropathy that mimics that caused by vitamin B12 deficiency.

Examination of the cerebrospinal fluid (CSF) may be valuable in several conditions. Elevated protein may be seen in chronic infection, tumor, or arachnoiditis. An elevated white-cell count may raise the possibility of chronic inflammation as well. In syndromes consistent with early multiple sclerosis, the presence of oligoclonal bands may be confirmatory of the diagnosis. CSF, if obtained, should also be sent to the serology laboratory to rule out syphilis.

## Pharmacologic Blockade

There is a definite role for local nerve blockade in the evaluation of chronic pain. Therapeutic blockade will be discussed in detail in a later chapter. A good response to sympathetic blockade may finalize the diagnosis of causalgia and predict a good long-term result of sympathectomy. It should be noted that anesthetizing a painful region will usually result in temporary abolition of the pain, whether or not the pain is caused by nociception or deafferentation. With the exception of sympathetic pain, therefore, nerve blocks do not reliably predict the outcome of ablative or stimulation procedures, although they may be quite helpful in describing the anatomy of the pain syndrome.

The patient may also be tested with small intravenous doses of morphine, given every minute until a total of 30 mg is given.[19] This is usually preceded by a test saline injection, with an attempt made to reverse the morphine effect by giving Naloxone at the end of the test. Those with nonorganic pains often obtain total pain relief out of proportion to very small doses of morphine, or demonstrate other idiosyncratic responses.

Morphine does not suppress the pain of deafferentation, but should provide good relief in nociceptive pain unless the patient has developed narcotic tolerance.

Pentothal has also been used as an intravenous test agent. There is some disagreement in the literature as to the meaning of a response, with many feeling that dramatic relief following a small dose of Pentothal is indicative of a conversion reaction. However, Tasker demonstrated a good response to short-acting barbituate in 16 of 36 patients with deafferentation pain. He felt that a response predicted a good outcome following epidural stimulation.[27]

## Tests of Autonomic Function

Although the special tests of autonomic function are not commonly done, the examiner should be familiar with them, since these tests may also yield helpful information in the diagnosis of lower brain stem and spinal cord lesions, lesions of the sympathetic system, or interruption of fiber pathways at the peripheral nerve level. The completeness of nerve section after sympathectomy may be verified by using these tests.

The sweating test is probably the most important objective test of autonomic function. Perspiration is a sympathetic function. Various methods have been developed, the most common of which involves painting the skin with iodine in oil after which the skin is dusted with starch powder. The starch turns dark blue in the presence of iodine and moisture, and therefore will temporarily stain those areas in which sweating function is intact. Alternatively, the examiner may simply examine the papillary ridges of the fingers for sweat droplets on the skin with the use of the ophthalmoscope. The thermoregulatory sweating pattern is quite diffuse, whereas the spontaneous or emotion sweating pattern typically involves the palms.[5]

As piloerection is a function of the sympathetic division of the autonomic nervous system, this response may be elicited by gentle stroking of the skin, tickling, or the application of cold. A convenient method is to spray ethyl chloride at the nape of the neck. This reaction appears slowly, generally following a latent period of approximately five seconds. It spreads gradually from the sight of stimulation.

Reflex erythema may be induced by stroking the skin firmly with a blunt point, inducing the formation of a red line and a welt. This response disappears after interruption of cutaneous nerves and below complete spinal cord lesions. An exaggeration of this response is termed dermatographia. This response may be indicative of autonomic imbalance with parasympathetic predominance.

A related test is the histamine flare test in which an intradermal injection of 0.1cc 1:1000 solution of histamine phosphate is normally followed by thc immediate development of redness and pain at the injection site, followed by the appearance of a spreading flush and wheal at the sight of injection. Generally, bilateral injections are performed for comparison purposes. The histamine flare test will be abnormal in peripheral nerve lesions, but is only reliable if the blood supply is intact.[5] In hysterical anesthesia the reaction is present, but is painless.

The lesion of the sympathetic division is followed by temporary vasodilatation, redness, and an increase in skin temperature. This hyperthermic state is soon replaced by coolness and pallor of the skin that may progress to cyanosis. The cutaneous muscles in the affected area fail to respond to stimuli from other parts of the body; therefore, warming and cooling fail to cause any flushing, pallor, sweating, or other changes in skin temperature. This provides the basis for using thermography in evaluation of sympathetic or peripheral nerve lesions.

Autonomic vasodilatation and sweating act to decrease skin resistance; areas deprived of autonomic supply will show a greatly increased resistance, which is easily measured by means of a microammeter. This test is most useful in the diagnosis of peripheral nerve lesions. In these lesions, one can differentiate between partial and complete involvement and also detect early signs of regeneration. This apparatus also provides a convenient way to distinguish between primarily psychogenic factors and organic disease.[5]

## Electrophysiological Tests

Electromyography (EMG) in conjunction with the neurological examination may prove invaluable in documenting radiculopathy in the context of disc disease and in those cases where neuropathy must be distinguished from myopathy. In conjunction with nerve conduction and velocity studies (NCV), the electrophysiologist is able to quantify functional impairment due to entrapment syndromes of the median, ulnar, radial, peroneal, and sciatic nerves. In patients with functional weakness, nerve condition velocities will be normal. During electromyography, insertional activity will be normal, and no abnormal spontaneous activity will be seen in the patient with nonorganic disease. The recruitment pattern may be subnormal, which may correlate with poor voluntary effort seen at physical examination. Repetitive studies may demonstrate either regeneration, or progression of disease.

Recurrent disc disease poses problems for the electromyographer in that the paraspinal musculature is altered by the prior laminectomy. If at least twelve months have elapsed between the first disc problems and the recurrence, however, the ratio of fibrillations to positive waves seen on the EMG may allow the examiner to strongly suspect an acute problem.

Evoked potential monitoring may be of use in ascertaining the presence of a central nervous system lesion. The visual system (visual evoked response, or VER), auditory system (brainstem and auditory evoked response, or BEAR), and somatosensory pathways (SER) may be studied by this technique, which involves computer-generated averaging of the electroencephalogram after repetitive stimulation. Motor-evoked responses are now measured clinically, although the technique is relatively difficult. Somatosensory evoked potentials in patients with pain have been studied, with the hope that an electrophysiological correlate of the pain experience could be ascertained. Another possible application would be the identification of components of the evoked potential that could predict response to stimulation or ablative therapy.[1,3,17,27] As of yet, however, evoked potentials have little to add to the evaluation or management of the chronic pain patient, and remain investigational in this application.

## References


1. Blair, R.D.G., Lee, R.G., & Vanderlinden, G. (1975). Dorsal column stimulation: Its effect on the somatosensory evoked response. *Archives of Neurology* 32:826–829.
2. Brodal, A. (1969). *Neurological Anatomy in Relation to Clinical Medicine.* Oxford: Oxford University Press.
3. Chapman, C.R., Chen, A.C.N., & Harkins, S.W., et al. (1979). Brain evoked potentials as correlates of laboratory pain: A review and perspective. In: *Advances in Pain Research and Therapy.* Vol. 3. (Ed.) J.J. Bonica. New York: Raven Press.
4. Crawford, A.S., & Knighton, R.S. (1953). Further observations on medullary spinothalamic tractotomy. *Journal of Neurosurgery* 10:113–121.
5. DeJong, R.N. (1970). *The Neurologic Examination.* New York: Hoeber.
6. Devor, M., & Janig, W. (1981). Activation of myelinated afferents ending in neuroma by stimulation of the sympathetic supply in the rat. *Neuroscience Letters.* 24:43–47.
7. Finneson, B.E. (1962). *Diagnosis and Management of Pain Syndromes.* Philadelphia: W.B. Saunders.
8. Fishbain, A.A., Goldberg, M., Meagher, B.R., et al. (1986). Male and female chronic pain patients categorized by OSM-III psychiatric diagnostic criteria. *Pain* 26:181–197.
9. Foerster, I. (1927). *Die Leitungsbahnen des Schmerzgefuhls.* Vienna: Urban and Schwarzenberg.
10. Fricton, J.R., Kroening, R., & Haley, D., et al. (1985). Myofascial pain syndromes of the head and neck: A review of clinical characteristics of 164 patients. *Oral Surgery* 60:615–623.
11. Garein, R., & Lapresle, J. (1954). Syndrome sensitif de type thalamique et a topographic cheiro-orale par lesion localisee du thalamus. *Revue Neurologique* 90:124–129.
12. Haymaker, W., & Woodhall, B. (1953). *Peripheral Nerve Injuries.* Philadelphia: W.B. Saunders.
13. Kellgren, J.H. (1938). Observations on referred pain arising from muscle. *Clinical Science* 3:175–190.

14. Loesser, J.D. (1983). Definition, etiology, and neurological assessment of pain originating in the nervous system following deafferentation. In: *Advances in Pain Research and Therapy*. Vol. 5. (Eds.) J.J. Bonica et al. New York: Raven Press.
15. Loh, L., & Nathan, P.W. (1978). Painful peripheral states and sympathetic blocks. *Journal of Neurology, Neurosurgery, and Psychiatry* 41:664–671.
16. Melzack, R., & Loesser, J.D. (1978). Phantom body pain in paraplegics: Evidence for a central pain generating mechanism for pain. *Pain* 4:195–210.
17. Namerow, N.S. (1969). Somatosensory evoked responses following cervical cordotomy. *Bulletin of Los Angeles Neurological Society* 34:184–188.
18. Noordenbos, W. (1979). Sensory findings in painful traumatic nerve lesions. In: *Advances in Pain Research and Therapy*. Vol. 3. (Eds.) J.J. Bonica et al. New York: Raven Pres.
19. Plotkin, R. (1982). Results in 60 cases of deep brain stimulation for chronic intractable pain. *Applied Neurophysiology* 45:173–178.
20. Rasminsky, M., Kearney, R.E., Aguayo, A.J., et al. (1978). Conduction of nervous impulses in spinal roots and peripheral nerves in dystrophic mice. *Brain Research* 143:71–81.
21. Seltzer, Z., & Devor, M. (1979). Ephaptic transmission in chronically damaged peripheral nerves. *Neurology* 29:1061–1065.
22. Simons, D.G. (1975). Muscle pain syndromes, Part 1. *American Journal of Physical Medicine* 54:289–311.
23. Simons, D.G. (1975). Muscle pain syndrome, Part 2. *American Journal of Physical Medicine* 54:289–311.
24. Simons, D.G. (1987). Myofascial pain syndromes due to trigger points. In: *Pain and Disability*. (Eds.) M. Osterweis et al. Washington, D.C.: National Academy Press.
25. Steinbrocker, O. (1949). Some simple diagnostic measures in neuromuscular and articular pain. *American Practitioner* 3:723.
26. Sweet, W.H. (1980). Central mechanisms of chronic pain. In: *Pain*. Vol. 58. (Ed.) J.J. Bonica. New York: Raven Press.
27. Tasker, R.R., Tsuda, T., & Hawrylyshyn, P. (1983). Clinical neurophysiological investigation of deafferentation pain. In: *Advances in Pain Research and Therapy*. Vol. 5. (Eds.) J.J. Bonica et al. New York: Raven Press.
28. Travell, J.G., & Rinzler, S.H. (1952). The myofascial genesis of pain. *Postgraduate Medicine* 11:425–434.
29. Travell, J.G., & Simons, D.G. (1983). *Myofascial Pain and Dysfunction: The Trigger Point Manual*. Baltimore: Williams and Wilkins.
30. Yates, A., & Smith, M.A. (1984). Musculoskeletal pain after trauma. In: *Textbook of Pain*. Eds.) P.D. Wall & R. Melzack. New York: Churchill Livingstone.

# 4

# Psychological Assessment of the Chronic Pain Patient: Behaviors, Cognitions, and Dynamics

*Paul M. Camic*

A good deal has been written about psychological assessment and treatment of chronic pain.[1–5] It is not the aim of this chapter to review these studies but rather to draw from them in presenting a systematic approach to psychological evaluation of the individual presenting with chronic pain of a nonmalignant etiology. Several studies are cited, however, as they pertain to the process and method of psychological evaluation of chronic pain. Recent research findings in assessment and evaluation are introduced in the context of their clinical utility and applicability in the assessment process.

Until recently, psychological assessment was seen as something to be requested after the medical and surgical evaluation was completed and physical etiology ruled out. This method of requesting psychological assessment was based on the belief that pain was either a physical or psychological problem and not an interaction of emotional, physical, and environmental factors. The conceptualization of chronic pain as either a physical or psychological problem is inaccurate, although still employed by many individuals in both health care and insurance industries. The persistence of this dichotomous conceptualization is problematic for the patient, clinician, and insurance compensation board. While it may seem clinically justifiable to categorize the patient as having a psychological disturbance when medical treatment fails, clinical evidence does not support this categorization. It is simply not useful, nor accurate, to tell the patient with chronic pain, "It's all in your head."

The chapter's primary focus is to present the psychological evaluation within a multidisciplinary clinic as a replicable model of psychological assessment. This chapter will be useful for physicians, dentists, physical therapists, and insurance and workmen's compensation professionals to increase their understanding of the psychologist's role in a multidisciplinary clinic. It aids psychologists by first reviewing different assessment concepts and, second, presenting a comprehensive assessment process found to be effective in an active, multidisciplinary pain service. One of the essential tenets of a psychological assessment for chronic pain is its incorporation within a larger, multidisciplinary evaluation model. A psychological assessment or psychiatric diagnosis is meaningless unless it is a part of a comprehensive evaluation that includes physical examination, medical tests when indicated, laboratory work-up as needed, and physical therapy evaluation. Likewise, an individual suffering from chronic pain who receives only a medical evaluation prior to treatment determination is also not being adequately assessed.

Although this chapter presents the "nuts and bolts" of the assessment process, its goal is not to recommend a standardized assessment that is identical for each patient in a cookbook fashion. In our experience, a standardized approach of psychological tests, behavioral analysis, clinical interview, psychiatric diagnostic work-up, and biofeedback evaluation is not necessary for all patients seen in a pain clinic. In addition, it is extremely time consuming and costly.

The purpose of the psychological assessment is to determine what psychological and behavioral factors are interacting with the patient's pain, disability status, and mood. The question of psychological etiology in relation to pain is not truly answerable, but as a working hypothesis should not be discarded. In determining what psychological factors interact with the patient in pain a thorough understanding of premorbid functioning is crucial. This includes personality style, social and family relations, vocational history, and medical history. Particular attention to childhood experiences with medical problems and psychiatric illness is important.

Preexisting psychological problems, such as marital disharmony, character disorders, lack of assertiveness, and internalization of anger, to name a few, may or may not interact negatively with the patient's pain problem. The psychological evaluation seeks to evaluate this interaction and plan treatment accordingly.

Another purpose of the psychological assessment is the part it can play in a presurgical evaluation. A psychological evaluation or psychometric testing cannot determine organic or psychogenic etiology, nor can it as of yet predict surgical outcome. The evaluation can be useful, however, in determining behavioral factors and psychopathology that may negatively impact the postsurgical recovery period. This may vary from noncompliance to risk of major depressive reaction to a psychotic reaction from surgery.

## Clinic Milieu and Training Preparation

The clinic setting where all members of the treatment team are present, or readily available, is an essential component to the multidisciplinary clinic approach. In this setting, discussion on a formal and informal basis occurs among team members between meetings with the patient. These discussions among team members lead to a better understanding of the physical, psychological, and vocational aspects of the pain problem. Questions about assessment procedures and treatment recommendations often surface during these discussions. These questions, rather than becoming potential turf battles between disciplines, can lead to a greater understanding about the complexities of the patient's pain. It is during these discussions between members of the multidisciplinary team that a further exchange of ideas and opinions about the patient takes place, leading to a coherent and organized recommendation about treatment.

In addition to actually being present in the pain clinic, a multidisciplinary clinic approach to the evaluation of chronic pain requires the psychologist to integrate his or her *assessment* methodology with that of a neurologist, neurosurgeon, anesthesiologist, physical therapist, and/or dentist. Although this does not require an additional graduate degree in one or all of the above areas, it does necessitate the psychologist's becoming familiar with the evaluation and decision-making processes of the other members of the multidisciplinary clinic. The direct observation of dental, neurological, and physical examinations, in addition to participating in treatment planning conferences, while not essential, adds to the training of the psychologist working with chronic pain patients.

After the psychological assessment of a chronic pain patient is complete, it is necessary to be knowledgeable about dental, anesthesiological, neurosurgical, neurological, and physical therapy *treatments* in order to foster an integrative treatment plan. The level of understanding of these treatment approaches need not be at the cellular level, but should encompass basic neurologic, anatomical, and physiological knowledge. Knowing the possible hazards of these treatments is also helpful in formulating treatment recommendations. Stated another way, the assessment of pain for a presurgical evaluation, for example, is different from assessing appropriateness for a rehabilitation program. While the psychologist is not determining whether surgery is warranted, he or she may be asked to assess the likelihood of emotional problems developing during the recuperative postsurgery period. Being knowledgeable about a particular surgical procedure and the recuperative time anticipated after surgery is therefore essential. If psychologists are to provide useful input into the decision-making process, they must be informed and knowledgeable about physical mechanisms and somatic treatments in addition to being skillful and knowledgeable clinicians within their own discipline of psychology.

The multidisciplinary approach of the clinic with physicians of different specialties, dentists, surgeons, and physical therapists necessitates that the clinical psychologist is familiar with several theoretical perspectives. These perspectives include a knowledge basis about normal human development and psychopathology, in addition to psychodynamics,[47] family systems theory, behavioral analysis, cognitive therapy,[38,39,45] biofeedback,[16,37] and pharmacology as related to a chronic pain population. The ability to treat patients in all the above areas is not necessary—and probably impossible—but an understanding and appreciation of these areas is necessary for adequate assessment of the highly complex problem of pain. Knowledge of only behavioral approaches to assessment and treatment, such as contingency management or classical conditioning, is as undesirable as only evaluating the patient's pain as an intrapsychic conflict utilizing drive theory. As we break down the barriers erected by mind-body dualism[9,46] in our understanding of the mechanisms of chronic pain, we also must end the separateness of intrapsychic and behavioral perspectives if an effective and valuable assessment is to occur. The perspective of the psychological examination should therefore be multitheoretical to determine adequate treatment planning.

## Theoretical Considerations for Assessment

The operant approach to the assessment of pain is an approach that has been written about extensively and is almost synonymous with pain assessment.[4,6-8] Fordyce,[6] a leading proponent of operant therapy, defines pain behaviors as behaviors that are observable and are capable of being maintained by reinforcement contingencies. He identifies several aspects of pain behaviors: (1) verbal complaints of pain and suffering and nonlanguage sounds such as moans and sighs; (2) body posturing and gesturing such as limping and rubbing a body part; (3) display of functional limitations such as reclining for excessive periods of time; and (4) pain reduction behavior such as medication use and use of the health care system. These measurable behaviors make up the pain behavior construct.

According to Fordyce and others,[1,6,7] while these behaviors are seen as operants of pain, they are also viewed as possibly eliciting reinforcing responses from family, friends, co-workers, and insurance companies. After the originating organic problem has healed, it is postulated that pain behaviors on the part of the patient continue to maintain the actual pain symptom. The reinforcing effects by family and friends, such as assisting and taking care of the patient in pain, decreased work responsibilities, etc., are powerful determinants in maintaining pain behavior. More recently, Fordyce[48] has urged a redefining of pain as specific and distinct from suffering. By separating these two concepts, Fordyce has added an additional evaluative benchmark that contributes to understanding our patients. Helping patients differentiate between pain, suffering, the meaning of inactivity, and disability status is a crucial part of the treatment process.

The work of Fordyce and his colleagues is nothing short of a dramatic breakthrough in the evaluation and treatment of chronic pain. They refocused the chronic pain problem away from a strictly psychoanalytical understanding to one with an operant and respondent behavioral basis.[9-12] They took what was previously believed to be an internal mental phenomena (a psychosomatic illness) and introduced an approach that involves observation and analysis of behaviors and associated this with dysfunctional and functional management of chronic pain. This approach involves the patient as an active participant in both the evaluation process and the patient's treatment. The patient is seen as a data collector and collaborator in determining treatment decisions. The removal of the patient from a passive and dependent role, as fostered in both psychoanalysis and traditional medicine, further advances the concept of engaging the patient in managing his or her response to the symptoms of pain. The findings generated from their research have significantly contributed to additional clinical research endeavors throughout the world. Several reports in the clinical research literature support the operant and respondent behavioral construct as a clinically useful tool in both assessment and treatment of pain.[13-18] It is beyond the scope of this chapter to detail the specifics of the operant approach. The reader is referred to these sources to gain a deeper understanding of operant and other behavioral approaches to pain management.

There are, however, several problems with an operant approach as the singular psychological assessment perspective toward chronic pain. Favorable treatment results reported by operant pain programs cannot be used conclusively to determine operant factors as etiological. Schmidt[19] states that chronic pain behavior is a function of disturbed proprioceptive processing, not operant conditioning. This process, he continues, is more than simply a response to pain signals. He postulates that pain patients have a shorter endurance to pain-relevant situations. The proprioceptive stimuli, while encompassing pain stimuli, can also encompass feelings of anxiety, tension, or depression. It is therefore possible that some pain patients, through a shorter endurance to situations that increase pain, tend to exhibit illness behavior as a coping response. If this were true, then some pain behaviors may be useful or even necessary for the patient. Each pain behavior therefore must be carefully analyzed to determine whether it reduces pain or serves another purpose, such as a way to compensate for psychological deficits or as a clue to the fragility of the patient's character structure. When patients rub an area of their body or stand during part of or all an interview, it is important not to assume this is an attention-gaining behavior with reinforcing properties. If the behavior leads to a reduction in pain, it may not be advisable to reduce this behavior nor to label it abnormal pain behavior.[33] Pain behavior can also be an expression of emotional pain that unconsciously seeks out a physical symptom as both a psychologically safe and socially conforming way to seek help. Psychic dynamics are altered and pain may become symbolic of anger, dependency, sexual gratification, and/or aggression.[9,47]

Another problem with the operant approach is the paucity of long term follow-up studies of the effectiveness of operant treatment programs. While end-of-treatment data are impressive, data collected past 12 months after treatment is largely unavailable.[23,28,40,44] If the psychological assessment is limited to an operant analysis, it seems clear that treatment options will also be limited to operant approaches and will fail to examine pain as a symbolic or intrapsychic phenomenon. Limiting psychological assessment to a behavioral analysis and psychological treatment to operant interventions detracts from the range of expertise a psychologist has been trained to offer. It serves to make psychological intervention a packaged technology and not the interactive therapy that it needs to be. While it is tempting to go from research findings with rats in the experimental laboratory to the human who exhibits inadequate coping strategies in a behavioral analysis, this reductionist approach ultimately fails our responsibility to the patient.

These concerns call into question the near exclusive use of patient observation,[32] an operant procedure. Observations are typically made when the patient is in the waiting room, inpatient unit, or during an interview with the spouse and patient. In a clinic setting, careful recording of these observations is both time consuming, potentially inaccurate, and of questionable clinical utility.[20] Like the use of the MMPI to differentiae organic from psychogenic pain, directly observing pain behaviors in the clinic as the sole classification procedure for abnormal or dysfunctional coping may be overstated. In most clinic settings there are time and staff limitations. Unlike the inpatient unit or research laboratory, the outpatient clinic's mission is to formulate a diagnosis and treatment plan in the most cost-effective manner possible. The multidisciplinary clinic has the additional task of a medical and functional (physical therapy) evaluation to undertake, as well as the psychological assessment. Considering these factors and reviewing the data on observational methods of pain behaviors, there is not significant evidence to support an elaborate pain behavior observation rating scale for patients' diagnostic clinic visits.

The construct of pain behaviors, though, continues to remain important, if not central, to psychological assessment. The etiological significance of operants for the development and maintenance of the construct, *for all chronic pain patients*, is questionable, however. Treatment results certainly support an operant approach as helpful for *some* patients. Other pain patients do well with an integrative cognitive-behavioral approach while others respond well to psychodynamic treatment.[34] The theoretical orientation of a psychologist or psychiatrist, as an assessing clinician, to decide what patient will benefit from what treatment is also an important evaluation variable. The multitheoretically trained clinician is therefore ideally suited for this endeavor.

Turk and Rudy[21] at the University of Pittsburgh Medical School have taken a different route from only analyzing and assessing pain behaviors.

In what is an exciting advance in pain assessment, they have attempted to classify physical, behavioral, and psychosocial information into a multiaxial paradigm. They are working to establish profiles of pain groups using the classification system of Dysfunctional, Interpersonally Distressed, and Adaptive Coper obtained from the Multidimensional Pain Inventory (MPI). This research is a continuation of the earlier work of Kerns and associates[22,23] at Yale in an attempt to develop a psychometric instrument able to assess pain behaviors from a cognitive-behavioral basis. Rather than seek out personality abnormalities as much of the MMPI research has done, the Pittsburgh and Yale groups are working in the direction of a multidimensional measurement instrument specifically designed for a chronic pain population. The research takes on a further multidisciplinary approach in attempting to systematically integrate medical findings with the MPI profiles[21] mentioned above. This research has produced the Multiaxial Assessment of Pain (MAP) based upon the taxonomy of chronic pain syndromes developed by the International Association For the Study of Pain.[25] It is this and similar integrative approaches to pain assessment involving the disciplines of medicine, surgery, psychology, vocational rehabilitation, and physical therapy that leads to development of a comprehensive treatment plan. Assessment of chronic pain that does not take this integrative and multidisciplinary approach can no longer be justified and can be considered antiquated and out of step with developments of the last decade.

A further advance in the psychological assessment of the chronic pain patient comes from a Dutch and Belgian group who have critically examined the Three Systems Model of Emotions and found it to be highly applicable to chronic pain patients.[24] This model examines the overt-motoric, verbal-cognitive, and physiologic response systems and proposes psychological treatments based upon the system that, during the assessment, appears most disrupted. While this conceptualization is not new per se, these researchers have more clearly refined the decision-making process that occurs after the assessment data are collected. This approach allows the determination of treatment to become more systematic and is more likely to be based upon specific diagnostic criteria. This data can then be included with information from the physical examination and laboratory tests to form a comprehensive evaluation.[24] Further discussion about the process of assessment is detailed in the next section of the chapter.

Before outlining a step-by-step approach to psychological assessment, I would like to further review the myriad of assessment strategies and approaches in the current literature. Some of these are included in the clinic assessment process I will describe but others are not. The most common and probably most widely used strategy is a structure or semi-structured clinical interview.[17,26,29,30,42] Each patient is interviewed with specific questions presented in a predetermined order. It is possible to probe for additional information if it appears this will be useful to the assessment. The order of the questions and their content always remain unchanged. A semistructured interview generally occurs during the patient's first meeting with the psychologist. This interview is discussed at length in the next section.

The second most prevalent assessment procedure is the pain diary.[5] Pain diaries take many different sizes and shapes. Their content varies from rating pain intensity on an hourly basis to including more detailed data such as time, place, medication use, activity level, antecedents, responses of others, and cognitions during a pain episode.[18,23] Pain diaries are most commonly used in cognitive and behavioral treatment programs and less commonly in psychodynamic and medically based approaches.

The third most common assessment procedure is the observation and recording of pain behaviors by someone other than the patient.[4,8,14,30–32] The settings for observing pain behaviors vary. Both inpatient pain units and outpatient pain clinics are frequently cited as locations for observing pain behavior. The patient is observed during physical examination, physical therapy, in the waiting room, walking down the hall, in a therapy session, during group therapy, etc. The observer is frequently a nurse, social worker, physical therapist, psychologist, or physician. Through behavioral analysis, these behaviors are then determined to be abnormal or adaptive illness/pain behaviors.[33–35] Treatment success is sometimes determined by a reduction in these illness/pain behaviors.[3,28,31]

Vlaeyen and associates, utilizing an inpatient setting, have classified pain behavior along three dimensions: Withdrawal-Approach, High Arousal-Low Arousal, and Visible-Audible.[31] They suggest an observation scale can be developed based upon this classification system that could then be related to treatment. For example, those patients with a High Arousal score might receive biofeedback while those with high scores in Withdrawal might best be served with operant therapy. Chronic pain behavior in this study was considered as the overt-motoric factor of the chronic pain syndrome and defined as the interaction between the patient and his or her environment.[31,72]

This approach to pain assessment and treatment as previously discussed in this chapter is problematic.[36] Analysis of pain behaviors as the exclusive psychological assessment tool limits the ability of the psychologist to adequately and fully assess the patient. Many factors influence pain behaviors other than those that are observable. Factors such as cognitive abilities, depression, unconscious motivation, chronicity of pain, degree of relief of pain, etc., also act to influence pain behaviors. These factors cannot be addressed through observation of behaviors alone and need to be considered when interviewing the patient. This expansion of the interview to factors not necessarily viewed as operants strengthens the formulation and resulting treatment recommendations. Observing pain behaviors is seen as one component, of the evaluation process, and not the sole task of the psychologist. Limiting the formal observation of pain behaviors to the physical examination, the physical therapy assessment, as well as the psychological interview, in our experience, is sufficient for treatment planning. This has the added benefit of no additional time involvement on the part of the treatment team and allows physician, physical therapist, and psychologist a common evaluation tool.

Another factor to consider is the cost of inpatient behavioral assessment. Funding for inpatient programs is becoming limited as insurance companies and governmental sources encourage outpatient evaluation and treatment of chronic pain. Rather than depend upon inpatient observation of chronic pain patients as part of the assessment process, an outpatient semistructured psychological interview, physical examination, biofeedback, and physical therapy evaluations would provide essentially the same information at less cost and in a shorter period of time.

Psychophysiologic evaluation is another psychological strategy utilized with chronic pain patients. Stress from threatened or actual job loss, marital problems, reduced social and physical activity, and financial insecurity can induce heightened muscle activity or autonomic arousal. Increased muscle activity and autonomic arousal lead to nociceptive stimulation in central and peripheral locations thereby increasing the sensation of pain.[16,19,46] Psychophysiologic monitoring of these increases in muscle and autonomic activity can be accomplished easily with electromyograph biofeedback (EMG-biofeedback) and peripheral temperature biofeedback (thermal).[16] Patients who show responsivity to this assessment have benefited from biofeedback-assisted relaxation training to help manage pain symptoms.[37] Emotional reactions to pain such as depression, somatization, obsessive-compulsive behavior, and anxiety also contribute to further increases in pain symptoms.[2,16] With the exception of anxiety, biofeedback training cannot directly decrease these emotional reactions. Biofeedback can, however, help in breaking the pain cycle if psychophysiologic arousal is a component of an emotional reaction: pain → emotional response → increased pain → increased muscle contraction → further emotional deterioration.

Pain associated with muscle spasms and limitation of movement, taken together with positive physical findings, is another area where psychophysiologic evaluation is useful. Over a period of time patients typically reduce their physical activity because of the pain related to muscle spasm. Decreased physical activity may lead to muscle atrophy. When this occurs the muscle group affected may tire more easily. This in turn increases the likelihood of additional spasms and increased pain. The cycle continues as the patient further reduces physical activity levels.[37] Psychological assessment of these patients typically reveals a reactive depression triggered by the pain problem[38] as well as cognitive distortion around increased spasmodic activity.[39]

## The Clinical Assessment

The primary purpose of the clinical psychology assessment is to ascertain whether behavioral, cognitive, psychodynamic, and psychophysiologic factors are affecting the patient's pain, physical functioning, and disability status. Once this is determined, a treatment plan is developed concurrently with other members of the health care team. Although the psychological assessment cannot be used to differentially diagnose organic from psychological etiology, it can lend vital information to overall treatment planning, including decisions about medical and surgical interventions.

### Patient Preparation

Most patients referred to a psychologist as part of a multidisciplinary evaluation become quickly concerned that their physician no longer believes their pain "to be real" but rather "only in my head, in my imagination." A struggle then develops between the patient, the referring physician, and the psychologist as to why the patient is being seen. It is clear that this is not an ideal footing in which to begin the psychological assessment. Careful preparation of the patient for *all* components of the multidisciplinary assessment leads to better patient cooperation through which more accurate information can be gathered.

All new patients, at the time of their *first* call to the pain clinic, either to seek information or request an appointment, are informed about the multidisciplinary approach to pain evaluation and treatment. At this time they are told "you will see one or more physicians during the assessment, a health psychologist and physical therapist." After their initial visit with one of our physicians, the patient is once again told he or she will see a health psychologist.

The physician then explains to the patient "chronic pain is a complex problem involving different systems within your body. As part of our evaluation we ask each patient to see Dr. Camic, our clinical health psychologist." Depending upon the patient's response to this statement, the physician (neurologist, neurosurgeon, anesthesiologist, or dentist) may need to explain about the multidisciplinary approach. The patient then schedules the next appointment. This matter-of-fact but informative approach results in a very high degree of patient compliance in cooperating with the psychological assessment and, when necessary, a psychiatric evaluation (see Chapter 8 by Dr. Benca). The dichotomy of "real versus mental" pain is quickly diffused and put to rest at an early point in the assessment process.

### The Patient Interview

The psychological assessment is usually scheduled over a three-week period, one visit per week. Occasionally the distance from the patient's home to the hospital, difficulty in securing transportation for all three visits, or weather conditions make three trips to the hospital over a three-week period not feasible. Adjustments in this interview schedule are certainly possible and may even be necessary for some pain clinics.

The rationale for this three-session/three-week evaluation period is (1) to see the patient and members of his or her family at different points in time (2) to collect pain diary data for two complete weeks, (3) to administer psychological tests, score and interpret them by the third visit for inclusion in the feedback and treatment recommendation portion of the evaluation, and (4) to allow time for concurrent medical diagnostic tests, when indicated, to be performed and analyzed. Hence, by the end of a three-week period the psychological, medical, and physical therapy evaluations are complete in a cost-effective and relatively time-conserving manner.

### First Assessment Interview

The first interview with the clinic psychologist may or may not take place after a pain clinic physician has seen the patient. If the latter is true, a screening visit with a clinic physician, usually a neurologist or anesthesiologist, is concurrently scheduled during this first week. The patient is instructed by telephone to bring all X rays and reports of previous tests and treatments with him or her for this visit. Prior to seeing the patient for the first time the psychologist and clinic physician review these records.

If the psychologist is the first clinician to see the patient, he or she thoroughly explains the multidisciplinary assessment process and answers any initial questions the patient may have. This is an important period in the assessment. It serves to personally introduce the patient to the clinic and sets the tone about the investigative and multidisciplinary aspect of the evaluation. This brief introductory period also invites the patient to fully participate in the assessment and begins to educate the chronic pain patient about pain management rather than pain cure. While this explanation about the assessment process may disappoint or anger some patients, it outlines the work to be done and begins to change patients' expectations about treatment and their resulting rehabilitation.

Rather than utilizing the traditional open-ended, exploratory interview commonly used by psychologists in mental health clinics and psychiatric settings, a semistructured interview is preferred when pain is the presenting problem. A preprinted semistructured interview allows the clinician to obtain specific data about each patient in an organized format without interfering with the clinical assessment needs of the psychologist. It further insures that the interview will be completed in a timely fashion and that relevant information about each patient is easily accessible to all members of the clinical team. Lengthy narrative reports are discouraged, except when required for insurance reports or as legal opinion.

At the end of this chapter is an example of the interview form employed at the University of Chicago Hospitals. Although primarily used on an outpatient basis, the semistructured interview can also be easily adapted for an inpatient consultation. The interview is designed for completion within sixty to seventy-five minutes. Completion of this interview is the primary goal of the first assessment session with the psychologist. Each patient is also requested to complete the Beck Depression Inventory[27,45] and West Haven-Yale Pain Inventory[22] at this first visit. The Beck is an efficient and reliable screening instrument for depression. The West Haven-Yale Pain Inventory, which takes ten to fifteen minutes to complete, is an instrument that quickly assesses patients' coping style, activity level, cognitions relative to pain, and the response of a significant other to the patient's pain behavior.

In addition the completion of the above semistructured interview, the psychologist also introduces the pain diary at this time. The pain diary is given to the patient for a two-week period. Data from the diary is reviewed with the patient and significant other (spouse, roommate, close friend) on the second and third assessment visits. Keeping a diary and reviewing data with the clinician involves the patient as an active participant in treatment and begins the task of rehabilitation and patient-focused pain management. The diary includes: (1) reporting levels of pain intensity, (2) medication use, (3) activity level, (4) cognitions relating to pain, and (5) responses by others to the patient's pain behaviors.

After the pain diary is explained to the patient, a recap of this first interview with the psychologist occurs. The recap, lasting between two and seven minutes, reviews the multidisciplinary approach once again, outlines what will occur during the next two visits, and allows time for the patient to ask questions.

## Second Assessment Session

The second assessment session generally occurs about one week after the first visit and takes about two hours to complete. This allows the patient to keep the first week of a two-week long diary. This is not the same diary format that is recommended for use during treatment, however. During treatment of chronic pain the patient is not requested to report pain intensity on an hourly basis. One of the goals of treatment is to help the patient begin to attend less to pain intensity. The assessment requires understanding of hourly pain intensity levels so as to better analyze the pain and generate working hypotheses about the nature of the pain and the effect it has on each patient.

The goals of the second assessment session are: (1) complete (if needed) the semistructured interview began in the first session; (2) review in detail, day by day, the first week's pain diary; (3) administer psychometric tests *as necessary*; (4) meet with the spouse or significant other of the patient, alone, for a half-hour interview; and (5) remind the patient to keep the second-week pain dairy. A review of how to record the pain diary may be necessary if the patient has not kept accurate or thorough records for the previous week.

At this time in the assessment process the psychologist should be developing several hypotheses about the nature of the patient's pain. These hypotheses should be oriented toward developing a behavioral, cognitive, and psychodynamic understanding of the patient. Important questions that need to be answered as hypotheses are formulated include:

Behavioral

Does the patient report pain intensity greater than what the physician expects for this medical condition?
What activities is the patient no longer able to engage in because of pain?
Do reports of pain intensity and decreased physical activity affect disability status and/or financial compensation?
Instead of complaining of pain, what else could the patient be doing? Does the patient receive social support that reinforces non-pain related activity?

Cognitive

How does the patient label his or her pain? What adjectives are used?
What language does the patient use to tell about other aspects of his or her life? Is the tone and style different from when pain is described? Has the pain affected the patient's cognitions about other aspects of his or her life?
How does the patient understand the pain? Is such understanding accurate?

Psychodynamic

Has the patient experienced a significant loss in childhood? (loss of a parent, close friend, pet, physical functioning) How did they cope with that loss?
How does the patient express anger and disappointment?
Does the patient have access to a full range of emotional expression?
Does the pain have symbolic meaning?
What is the quality of the patient's interpersonal relationships? Is there object constancy? Are there deficits in self object choice?

Data from psychometric tests can also substantiate or refute hypotheses generated in the interest of clinical decision making. Psychometric tests can represent different theoretical perspectives and may add to further understanding the patient. For example, the MMPI has an empirical-psychoanalytic orientation; the Beck, a cognitive; the West Haven-Yale, a cognitive-behavioral, etc. See chapter 5 by Dr. Eggebrecht and associates for a detailed discussion of psychometric testing.

## Third Assessment Sessions

By the third assessment session the psychologist should have a good working history of the patient. This data has been obtained through interviews with both the patient and his or her significant others, by reviewing the patient's medical chart, and by speaking directly with the referring physician. In addition to a history of the problem, the psychologist should now have an understanding of how the pain affects the patient's physical and social activities, interpersonal relationships, emotional state, and vocational status. The goals for this third assessment session are: (1) perform a psychophysiologic evaluation, (2) review and analyze the second-week pain diary with the patient, and (3) obtain additional interview data from the patient to further support or reject your working hypotheses. After the completion of this session, the data obtained from the complete psychological assessment is reviewed and presented at a staff meeting, together with assessment data from the physical therapist and physician(s) who have seen the patient in the pain clinic. The referring physician, if not a member of the clinic staff, is personally invited to attend the staffing.

The final component of the psychological assessment—a psychophysiological evaluation—is performed during the third assessment visit. This part of the evaluation takes approximately thirty minutes and involves electromyographic biofeedback (EMG-biofeedback), thermal biofeedback, and pulse velocity biofeedback. The EMG-biofeedback electrodes are attached in two locations: at the primary site of pain and on the frontalis muscle three-quarters of an inch above each eye. A thermal electrode is placed on the index finger of the dominant hand while pulse velocity is measured from the index finger of the nondominant hand. The rationale in using these three instruments is to ascertain striated muscle sympathetic nervous system, and cardiovascular involvement in the patient's response to pain, respectively. While positive findings in any of these three areas cannot be taken as causative in relation to the pain symptom, they can add or detract support for the clinician's hypotheses about what exacerbates and maintains pain.

## Patient Feedback

At the conclusion of the three interviews two tasks face the psychologist. The first is integrating the data and developing a coherent treatment plan with the other members of the multidisciplinary team. The second task is presenting the treatment plan to the patient and the patient's family. Whether the treatment consists of only one modality, such as physical therapy, or multimodalities, such as cognitive-behavioral treatment, biofeedback, and medication, the patient should be presented with a *clear* rationale for treatment and allowed to participate in the decision-making process. If psychological testing is part of the evaluation, the interpretation of those tests should also be presented to the patient. After completing what may be hours of psychometric tests and interviews, a patient is more likely to participate in treatment if the findings of each step of the assessment are reviewed. Integrating the data obtained in the psychology evaluation, and presenting this data to the patient as a rationale for treatment recommendations, complete the assessment process. An effective psychology assessment serves to educate patients about chronic pain, to engage their interest as active participants in treatment, and to formulate a theoretically grounded treatment plan.

## References


1. Melzack, R. (Ed.) (1983). *Pain Measurement and Assessment.* New York: Raven Press.
2. Craig, K. (1984). Emotional aspects of pain. In: *Textbook of Pain.* (Eds.) P. Wall and R. Melzack. Edinburgh: Churchill Livingstone, pp. 153–161.
3. Holzman, A., Turk, D.E. (1986). *Pain Management: A Handbook of Psychological Treatment Approaches.* New York: Pergamon.
4. Fordyce, W. (1976). *Behavioral Methods for Chronic Pain and Illness.* St. Louis: C.V. Mosby.
5. Turk, D.E., Meichenbaum, D., & Genest, M. (1983). *Pain and Behavioral Medicine: A Cognitive-Behavioral Perspective.* New York: Guilford.
6. Fordyce, W. (1974). Pain as a learned behavior. *Advances in Neurology* 4:415–422.
7. Keefe, F. (1982). Behavioral assessment and treatment of chronic pain: Current status and future directions. *Journal of Consulting and Clinical Psychology* 50:896–911.
8. Keefe, F., & Gil, K. (1985). Recent advances in the behavioral assessment and treatment of chronic pain. *Annals of Behavioral Medicine* 7(3):11–16.
9. Engel, G. (1959). Psychogenic pain and the pain-prone patient. *American Journal of Medicine* June:899–918.
10. Sternbach, R. (1974). Varieties of pain games. *Advances in Neurology* 4:423–430.
11. Beecher, H. (1956). Limiting factors in experimental pain. *Journal of Chronic Disease* 4:11.
12. Schilder, P. (1935). *The Image and Appearance of the Human Body.* London: Kegan Paul, Trench, Trobner.
13. Fordyce, W. (1983). The validity of pain behavior measurement. In: *Pain Measurement and Assessment.* New York: Raven Press.
14. Keefe, F., & Block, A. (1982). Development of an observation method for assessing pain behavior in chronic low back pain patients. *Behavior Therapy* 13:363–375.
15. Fordyce, W., Lansky, D., Calsyn, D., Shelton, J., Stovlov, W., & Rock, D. (1984). Pain measurement and pain behavior. *Pain* 18:53–69.
16. Keefe, F., & Gil, K. (1986). Behavioral concepts in the analysis of chronic pain syndrome. *Journal of Consulting and Clinical Psychology* 54(6):776–783.
17. Follick, M., Smith, T., & Ahern, D. (1985). The sickness impact profile: A global measure of disability in chronic back pain patients. *Pain* 21:67–76.
18. Follick, M., & Ahern, D., Laser-Walston, N. (1984). Evaluation of a daily activity diary for chronic pain patients. *Pain* 19:373–382.

19. Schmidt, A. (1987). The behavioral management of pain: A criticism of a response. *Pain* 30:285–291.
20. Turk, D., & Flor, H. (1987). Pain > pain behaviors: The utility and limitations of the pain behavior construct. *Pain* 31:277–295.
21. Turk, D., & Rudy, T. (1987). Toward a comprehensive assessment of chronic pain patients: A multiaxial approach. *Behavior Research and Therapy* 25(4):237–249.
22. Kerns, R., Turk, D., & Rudy, T. (1985). The West Haven Yale Multidimensional Pain Inventory. *Pain* 23:345–356.
23. Kerns, R., Turk, D., Holzman, A., & Rudy, T. (1986). Comparison of cognitive-behavioral and behavioral approaches to the outpatient treatment of chronic pain. *Clinical Journal of Pain* 4:195–206.
24. Vlaeyen, J., Snijders, A., Schuerman, J. Van Eek, H., Groenman, N., and Bremer, J. Chronic pain and the three systems model of emotions. A critical examination. In Press.
25. International Association for the Study of Pain Subcommittee on Taxonomy. (1986). Classification of chronic pain: Description of chronic pain syndromes and definitions of pain terms. *Pain* 53:1–225.
26. Melzack, R. (1975). The McGill Pain Questionnaire, major properties and scoring methods. *Pain* 1:277–299.
27. American Psychiatric Association. (1987). *Diagnostic and Statistical Manual of Mental Disorders—Revised* Washington, D.C.: APA Press.
28. Camic, P.M., & Brown, F.D. (1987). Evaluation of change in psychologic pain management treatment. *Pain* S(4):S174.
29. Heaton, R., Lehman, R., & Getto, C. (1980). *Psychosocial Pain Inventory*. Odessa, Florida: Psychological Assessment Resources, Inc.
30. Richards, J., Nepomuceno, C., Riles, M., & Suer, Z. (1982). Assessing pain behavior: The UAB pain behavior scale. *Pain* 14:393–398.
31. Vlaeyen, J., Van Eek, H., Groenman, N., & Schuerman, J. (1987). Dimensions and components of observed chronic pain behavior. *Pain* 31:65–75.
32. Ignelzi, R., Kramer, E., & Atkinson, J. (1980). Patient pain intensity report to different health professionals. Paper presented at the Association for the Advancement of Behavior Therapy. New York, November 25–27.
33. Pilowsky, I. (1969). Abnormal illness behavior. *British Journal of Medical Psychology* 42:347–351.
34. Pilowsky, I. (1978). A general classification of abnormal illness behaviors. *British Journal of Medical Psychology* 51:131–137.
35. Pilowsky, I. (1985). Pain and illness behavior: Assessment and management. In: *Textbook of Pain*. (Eds.) P. Wall and R. Melzack. Edinburgh: Churchill Livingstone, pp. 767–775.
36. Kramer, E., Block, A., & Atkinson, J. (1983). Assessment of pain behavior: Factors that distort self-report. In: *Pain Measurement and Assessment*. (Ed.) R. Melzack. New York: Raven Press.
37. Kravitz, E., Moore, M., & Glaros, A. (1981). Paralumbar muscle activity in chronic low back pain. *Archives of Physical Medicine and Rehabilitation* 62:172–176.
38. LeFebore, M.F. (1984). Cognitive distortion and cognitive errors in depressed psychiatric and low back pain patients. *Journal of Consulting and Clinical Psychology* 49:517–525.
39. Smith, T., Ahern, D.K., Follick, M.J. (1985). Cognitive distortion and disability in chronic low back pain patients. *Cognitive Therapy and Research*.

40. Kores, M., Murphy, W.D., Rosenthal, T., Elias, D., & Rosenthal, R. (1985). A self-efficacy scale to predict outcome in chronic pain treatment. Society of Behavioral Medicine Annual Meeting, New Orleans.
41. Wallston, K.A., Wallston, B.S., & DeVellis, R. (1978). Development of the Multidimensional Health Locus of Control (MHLC) Scales. *Health Education Monograph* 6:160–170.
42. Brown, G.K., & Nicassio, P.M. (1987). Development of a questionnaire for the assessment of active and passive coping strategies in chronic pain patients. *Pain* 31:53–64.
43. Roberts, N., Smith, R., Bennett, S., Cape, J., Norton, R., & Kilbum, D. (1984). Health beliefs and rehabilitation after lumbar disc surgery. *Journal of Psychosomatic Research* 28:139–144.
44. Camic, P.M. (1987). Measurement of treatment efficacy in chronic non-malignant pain: Initial indication of change. Paper presented at Department of Psychiatry Grand Rounds Seminar, University of Chicago, April.
45. Beck, A.T. (1976). *Cognitive Therapy and Emotional Disorders*. New York: International Universities Press.
46. Sternback, R. (Ed.) (1978). *The Psychology of Pain*. New York: Raven Press.
47. Pilowsky, I. (1978). Psychodynamic aspects of the pain experience. In: *The Psychology of Pain*. (Ed.) R. Sternbach. New York: Raven Press, pp. 203–217.
48. Fordyce W. (1988). Pain and suffering: A reappraisal. *American Psychologist* 43(4):276–283.

**PAIN CLINIC PSYCHOLOGIC EVALUATION**

Medical Hx#________________

Date:________________

Name:________________________Telephone(H)____________________

Address:______________________________(W)____________________

___________________________________________________

Marital Status:________________# of children____ # at home______

Date of Birth:_________________Age:__________________________

Current Occupation:__________________________________________

How is yearly income presently obtained:_________________________

Referring Provider (name, address, telephone): ____________________

__________________________________________________________

Ask patient to describe current pain (when does it occur, changes in intensity, time of day, etc.)

__________________________________________________________

__________________________________________________________

__________________________________________________________

History of pain problem (origin, changes over time in intensity, location, sensation, etc.)

__________________________________________________________

__________________________________________________________

__________________________________________________________

__________________________________________________________

__________________________________________________________

Current Medication (all, including over the counter with dose):

__________________________________________________________

__________________________________________________________

__________________________________________________________

Previous treatment:Surgeries__________________________________

__________________________________________________________

__________________________________________________________

Nerve Blocks_______________________________________________

Phy. Ther._________________________________________________

TENS______________Neuroprobe__________Biofdbk (type)__________

Acupt.________Psychotherapy_________Pain Mgmt Prog____________

**Figure 4.1.** Pain clinic psychologic evaluation.

Other:____________________________________________________________

Have the patient point to the area(s) of the pain and trace where she/he experiences it (record this below). Then ask the patient about the intensity of the pain. Record this as follows: 1 = Low, 2 = moderate, 3 = intense, 4 = worse (if patient has multiple locations of pain, rate each area).

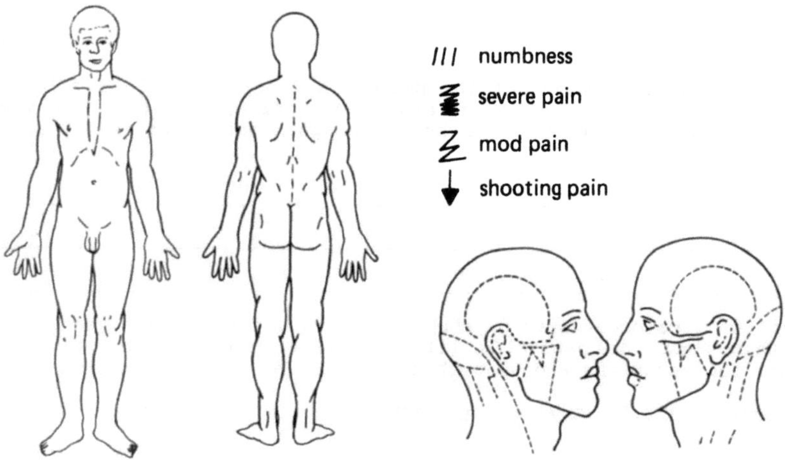


(It may be useful to have the patient shade the exact areas of pain)

Of the previous treatments the patient has had, what treatments helped the most?

____________________________________________________________

____________________________________________________________

Currently, is there anything that makes the pain better or less intense? (probe for specifics e.g. meds, laying down, warm bath, exercise, etc.)

____________________________________________________________

____________________________________________________________

____________________________________________________________

What makes the pain worse? __________________________________

(if not volunteered, ask specifically about the following):

loud noises______anger_______anxiety_______physical activity__________

marital difficulties___________other worries__________________________

____________________________________________________________

Do you have any other medical problems (e.g. high BP, G-I disturb., headaches)

____________________________________________________________

____________________________________________________________

____________________________________________________________

**Figure 4.1.** *Continued.*

As a child or teen-ager did you have any medical problems? (wait for the patient to reply then ask specifically about allergies and asthma).

______________________________________________________________

______________________________________________________________

Where you ever physically or sexually abused as a child or teen-ager?

______________________________________________________________

Now inquire about members of the patient's family and close friends; Did anyone in your family or among your friends, when you were younger, have any medical problems? Once again ask specifically about allergies or asthma.

______________________________________________________________

______________________________________________________________

______________________________________________________________

As part of a comprehensive psychological evaluation it is important to ascertain what the patient's life was like prior to the onset of his/her pain symptoms and what it has been like since the onset.

**BE SPECIFIC THIS IS VITAL INFORMATION**

Now I would like to ask you a few questions about yourself prior to the beginning of the pain symptoms we have been talking about:

Occupational: Was the patient working? Doing what? On a scale of 1 to 10 how much did the patient like his/her job? (1 = very little) Where there any financial concerns?

______________________________________________________________

______________________________________________________________

______________________________________________________________

How has this changed since the beginning of the pain?

______________________________________________________________

______________________________________________________________

______________________________________________________________

Recreation/leisure: Prior to the onset of the pain what did the patient do for exercise and leisure? Ask specifically about sports, movies, dinning out visiting friends and relatives, vacations, how she/he spent weekends, etc.

______________________________________________________________

______________________________________________________________

______________________________________________________________

______________________________________________________________

______________________________________________________________

**Figure 4.1.** *Continued.*

How has this changed since the onset of the pain? (Be specific)

______________________________________________________________________

______________________________________________________________________

______________________________________________________________________

______________________________________________________________________

<u>Marital/family</u>: If the patient is married or living as married, ask her/him to describe the relationship prior to the onset of the pain. It might be helpful to use the 1 to 10 scale here where 1 = very problematic and 10 = perfect. Try to determine how satisfied/dissatisfied the patient was with the relationship prior to the onset of the pain. Ask about time spent together, sexual satisfaction, companionship, etc.

______________________________________________________________________

______________________________________________________________________

______________________________________________________________________

______________________________________________________________________

______________________________________________________________________

How has this changed since the onset of the pain? (Be specific as to the information obtained in the above question)

______________________________________________________________________

______________________________________________________________________

______________________________________________________________________

______________________________________________________________________

______________________________________________________________________

```
*******************************************************************
*  At this time  note the patient's pain behaviors during         *
*  the interview:                                                 *
*                                                                 *
*  Complains of pain_____Grasps area of pain___Grasps other       *
*                                                                 *
*  area(s)______Moans_____Cringes_______Winces________Gets up     *
*                                                                 *
*  to pace____Leaves room_____Frequently changes position______   *
*                                                                 *
*  Lies down_____Becomes angry_________Anxious_________________   *
*                                                                 *
*  Other observations__________________________________________   *
*                                                                 *
*    __________________________________________________________   *
*                                                                 *
*    __________________________________________________________   *
*                                                                 *
*******************************************************************
```

**Figure 4.1.** *Continued.*

Ask the patient: "If you did not have a pain problem, what would you do that you are unable to do at the present time?"

______________________________________________________________

______________________________________________________________

______________________________________________________________

______________________________________________________________

"How much relief of the pain is necessary for you to engage in the above activities?" Interviewer: Now go back to the above and in parenthesis put in the amount of relief required in percent from e.g (30%).

As the patient to describe a typical day for him/her at this time:

______________________________________________________________

______________________________________________________________

______________________________________________________________

______________________________________________________________

Approximately how many hours per day do you spend lying down because of the pain:

______________________________________________________________

Prior to the onset of the pain problem, did you engage in any of the following activities?

Dusting____________ Vacuuming______________ Dish washing_______________

Shopping_________ Cloths washing____________ Cloths ironing____________

Cooking_____________ Errands_____________ Repair work__________________

Yard work____________________________ Bill paying________________________

Of the above activities you did prior to the onset of the pain, which ones are you unable to do presently?

______________________________________________________________

______________________________________________________________

Are you presently receiving workman's compensation___________________

unemployment_______________________ social security______________________

Is litigation pending in regards to your pain problem?

______________________________________________________________

^^^^^^^^^^^^^^^^^^^^^^^^^^^^^^^^^^^^^^^^^^^^^^^^^^^^^^^^^^^^^^^^^^^^^^^^^^^^^^

**Figure 4.1.** *Continued.*

Interviewer Notes:

Sometimes people who experience pain, as you have described to me today, have emotional "side effects" from the pain such as depression, anger, anxiety and other feelings. Since the onset of your pain problem, have you noticed changes in the way you feel? [probe for subclinical depression as well as premorbid functioning. Determine if the patient is depressed]

<<<<<<<<<<<<<<<<<<<<<<<<<<<<<<<<<<<<<<<<<<<<<<<<<<<<<<<<<<<<<<<<

**END OF STRUCTURED INTERVIEW**

Formulation:

Recommendations:

**Figure 4.1.** *Continued.*

Diagnosis: Axis I_____________________________#______________________

Axis II_____________________________#______________________

Axis III__________________________________________________________

(If tests have been requested and results are not yet available, do not issue a diagnosis)

Psychometric Evaluation:_____Yes_____No (if yes, what tests were administered:)

_____________________________________________________________________

Biofeedback Evaluation:____Yes____No____ (if yes, summarize results)

_____________________________________________________________________

_____________________________________________________________________

_____________________________________________________________________

SIGNED:______________________________________________________________
[degree]

**Figure 4.1.** *Continued.*

# 5

# Psychometric Evaluation

*Dirk B. Eggebrecht, Michael T. Bautz, Margit I.D. Brenig, Michael Pfingsten, and Carmen Franz*

As shown by everyday experience and by the results of experimental investigations, individuals have differing reactions to pain. According to a summary of the findings of recent neurophysiological and psychological research, the experience of pain in humans is a complex system of interrelated physiological and psychological processes. Pain may be understood as a product of the factors that contribute to pain sensitivity. Pain is at once a sense perception, a response to specific peripheral stimulation, and an interaction of this response with a complicated network of psychological factors difficult to describe.[100]

Psychic factors may contribute to pain which even has clearly organic causes, as in the case of cancer, and they may influence decisively the perception of symptoms and ways of coping with them. It often happens that the instance and description of pain cannot be explained solely by the actual results of somatic examination. The psychic component of the pain may become so great, regardless of an original diagnosis of clearly organic causes, that a psychosomatic concept of therapy is indicated. Instead of linear cause and effect connections, other complex interacting effects in accordance with "diathesis stress models"[40,90] may be assumed. These insights imply that the physicians who work as pain therapists in their role as initial investigators should not assume a one-sidedly somatic cause of pain, but instead should consider the patients' psychological picture. Psychologists or their trained colleagues should proceed with psychological exploration and testing of patients.

In this context psychological testing has gained increasing significance.[53] These procedures supposedly help to address three major aspects important in the diagnosis of chronic pain: (1) delineation of an "objectifiable" pain personality, (2) separation of functional from organic causes of pain, and (3) prediction of success for a specific somatic therapy.

This chapter presents an evaluation of the degree to which psychological tests may provide evidence concerning perception of and coping with pain, typical pain-specific problems, personality characteristics, criteria for therapeutic indications, and perspectives of success for relevant therapeutic methods.

## Measurement and Assessment of the Pain Experience

Generally, measurement can be defined as assignment of numbers to objects or events to represent quantities of attributes according to rules. But considering that pain is a totally private object that cannot be felt by any other person than the individual in pain it appears difficult to quantify this complex and subjective phenomenon. It is obvious that some operational definition is needed to relate the concept of pain to observable reactions or physical objects that can be measured.

In the case of clinical pain the most frequent verbal reactions are complaining, moaning, crying, and requests for pain relievers. Nonverbal reactions include gestures, rubbing of the painful body part, taking medication, and protecting oneself.[20] All these behaviors are more or less reliable and specific indicators for the experience of pain.[105] The measurement of the subjective experience of pain goes beyond simply establishing the presence or absence of a painful sensation by attempting to quantify the basic dimensions of pain, such as intensity, quality, extent, and length.

### Measurement of Pain Intensity

Studies show that, of the many different types of scales used to assess the intensity of pain, most of these yield similar results.[36] The two most frequently used scale types are represented here.

#### *Verbal Rating Scale (VRS)*

Beecher[4] determined that patients were best able to classify the intensity of their pain if they were presented with scales that provided behavioral descriptions, preferably with a limited number of categories, rather than scales of the linear, numerical variety on which, for example, the patient rates intensity on a one to ten scale. The former type of verbal rating scale[37] is widespread in clinical practice. This scale includes usually five or seven degrees, each of which is given a description, such as "no pain," "light pain," etc., up to "very strong pain." One disadvantage of the VRS is that it allows only a fairly crude estimation of pain intensity. An extension of this scale to more than seven gradations does not lead to a greater differentiation of the subjective experience of pain.[28,105]

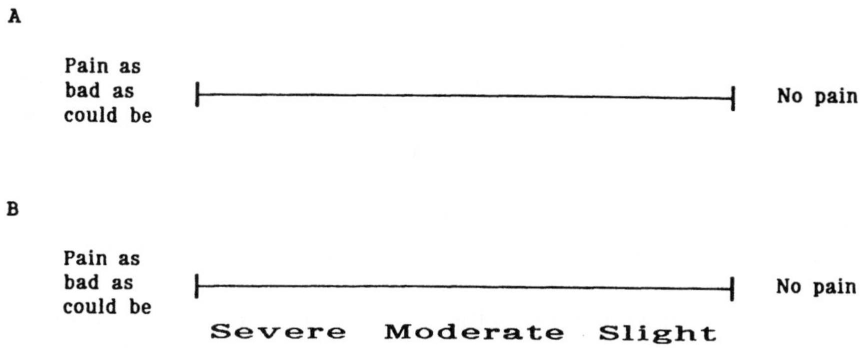


**Figure 5.1.** Visual analogue (A) and graphic rating scale (B) providing uniform distributions of results.

Another disadvantage of the VRS is that measurement remains only at an ordinal scale level, i.e., these measures are only rank ordered, thereby making calculation of scale means or standard deviations empirically meaningless. Often the data from such a scale are interpreted and applied statistically, as if they were derived from an interval scale.[10] This higher level of measurement requires that numbers with equal intervals are assigned to objects separated by equal intervals so that differences are empirically meaningful.

*Visual Analogue Scale (VAS)*

With this type of scale, which is widespread in clinical and experimental measurement, the intensity of pain sensitivity is marked at a point on the length of a line. Less often the intensity of emotions accompanying pain is measured in the same manner, e.g., in pain diaries. A VAS consists of one straight vertical or horizontal line (usually 10 cm long) which is given a limit at each end with a description of the extremes, such as "no pain at all" versus "worst pain possible." The patient is supposed to mark a certain length of this line that is equivalent to the intensity of pain experienced. The distance of this mark from the "no pain" end of the scale, measured in millimeters, is taken as a numerical expression of the patient's pain intensity. One decisive advantage of the VAS over the VRS is that this scale is not bound to a fixed number of categories and therefore permits a greater measurement sensitivity.

The graphic rating scale is a variation of the VAS, on which several descriptive concepts (as on the VRS) are placed at equal intervals along the scale. Scott and Huskisson[79] found that this modification leads easily to a cluster of responses around the descriptors. The authors found that out of six scales researched, only the VAS and one particular graphic rating scale (see Fig. 5.1) provided useful measurements. Only these two types of scale showed a uniform distribution of responses over the entire scale, thereby permitting greater sensitivity.

The validity of this measuring instrument (VAS) is questionable because an outer criterion is lacking in most cases. A number of studies showed high positive correlation of the VAS with other pain scales.[36,79,106] In one clinical study[63] it was shown that the VAS gave the most sensitive measurement of the effects of analgesics. Using experimental measurement of subjective pain experience, Price and colleagues[69] supported the validity of the VAS.

Determining the reliability of the VAS is also problematic. The findings of several researchers[36,69,79] show that, although in experimental research consistent measurement with the VAS is possible, the determining of the reliability according to traditional testing theory is not applicable to measuring clinical pain. To produce a test-retest reliability, it must be assumed that the subjective intensity of pain remains consistent over a certain period of time. With repeated measurements within a short time span the reliability appears adequately high.[34] It is generally considered that the reliability of a scale varies with its sensitivity.

These theoretical measurement problems have a subordinate role in daily clinical practice, in which the VAS has been proven to be a simple, sensitive, and reproducible method for quantifying patients' pain intensity. It can be used to measure the same patient's responses at different points in time during an ongoing course of therapy, plus it can be used to compare different groups of patients in clinical trials. A limitation also common to other types of scales is a result of the extremes of the VAS. A patient giving a rating of "worst pain possible" cannot reach a higher score if the pain then gets even worse. Therefore, we recommend the initial use of the common VAS, followed by the repeated application of "pain relief scales" on which the extremes have been defined as "no pain relief" and "complete pain relief."

Another problem is that older pain patients may have trouble understanding the VAS instructions. In this case the VRS appears to be the more appropriate measure for clinical pain intensity.

## Assessing the Dimensions of Pain

Subjective descriptions of pain are always the first clues for diagnosis, differential diagnosis, decision about the necessity of therapy, and planning and carrying out of therapeutic procedures. In the course of the entire treatment the patients' expression of pain is a necessary criterion along with objective medical criteria such as X-ray results. In the final analysis the subjective experience of pain as related to the psychic condition provides the main criterion of treatment success or failure.

> Describing pain solely in terms of intensity is like specifying the visual world only in terms light flux, without regard to pattern, color, texture, and the many other dimensions of visual experience. (Melzack, 1983, p. 2)

Verbal pain description scales are intended to assess not only intensity, but also type and quality of subjective pain.

The development of such scales had its theoretical basis in the gate control theory.[61] Extending the same concept, Melzack and Casey[59] described a three-dimensional model of pain perception that included motivational-affective, sensory-discriminative, and cognitive-evaluate components. This model led to more comprehensive approaches in current methods for measuring pain in either a clinical or experimental context (see Fig. 5.2). The fact that physiological substrates of various perceptual pathways are localized in different structures of the central nervous system explains why there can be a lack of connection between the sensory and the affective components of pain perception. Clinical and experimental findings show that it is possible to influence purposely the affective component of pain sensation by using neurosurgery (leucotomy) or medications (tranquilizers, such as diazepam). The same is true for the sensory component by using narcotics (such as Fentanyl).[25,26] Price and colleagues[68] also demonstrated the importance of using separate measures for the affective and sensory dimensions of pain. Painful affect was considerably alleviated when women in labor focused on the birth of their child rather than on their own pain.

While several factor analytic studies tend to support a three-dimensional model of subjective pain,[70,9] others take the position that the distinction between motivational-affective and cognitive-evaluative components appears superfluous[8,14,44,74,75] and they favor the two component model of Beecher.[5] Beecher[4,5] emphasizes the meaning of the distinction between a sensory and a reactive pain component (which includes cognitive and emotional factors). In general, these studies make it clear that for the experience of pain there is not simply a one-dimensional issue at stake that can be understood exhaustively by examining pain intensity.

The psychologists Melzack and Torgerson[60] initiated the analysis and clinical usefulness of pain language. In order to expand the work of the adjective list invented by these authors, Melzack[56] developed the first standardized pain scale (McGill Pain Questionnaire, MPQ). Also available for this instrument are a short form (SF-MPQ),[58] a number of translated forms of the test,[39,46,51,71,91] plus various modifications for specific pain syndromes.[33,43] Translations are fraught with difficulties, because for every different language the connotations and intensity of adjectives must be assessed carefully to reach a sound basis comparable to that of the MPQ. To avoid this problem there are various pain scales that have been developed and applied in the original language and are more or less empiri-

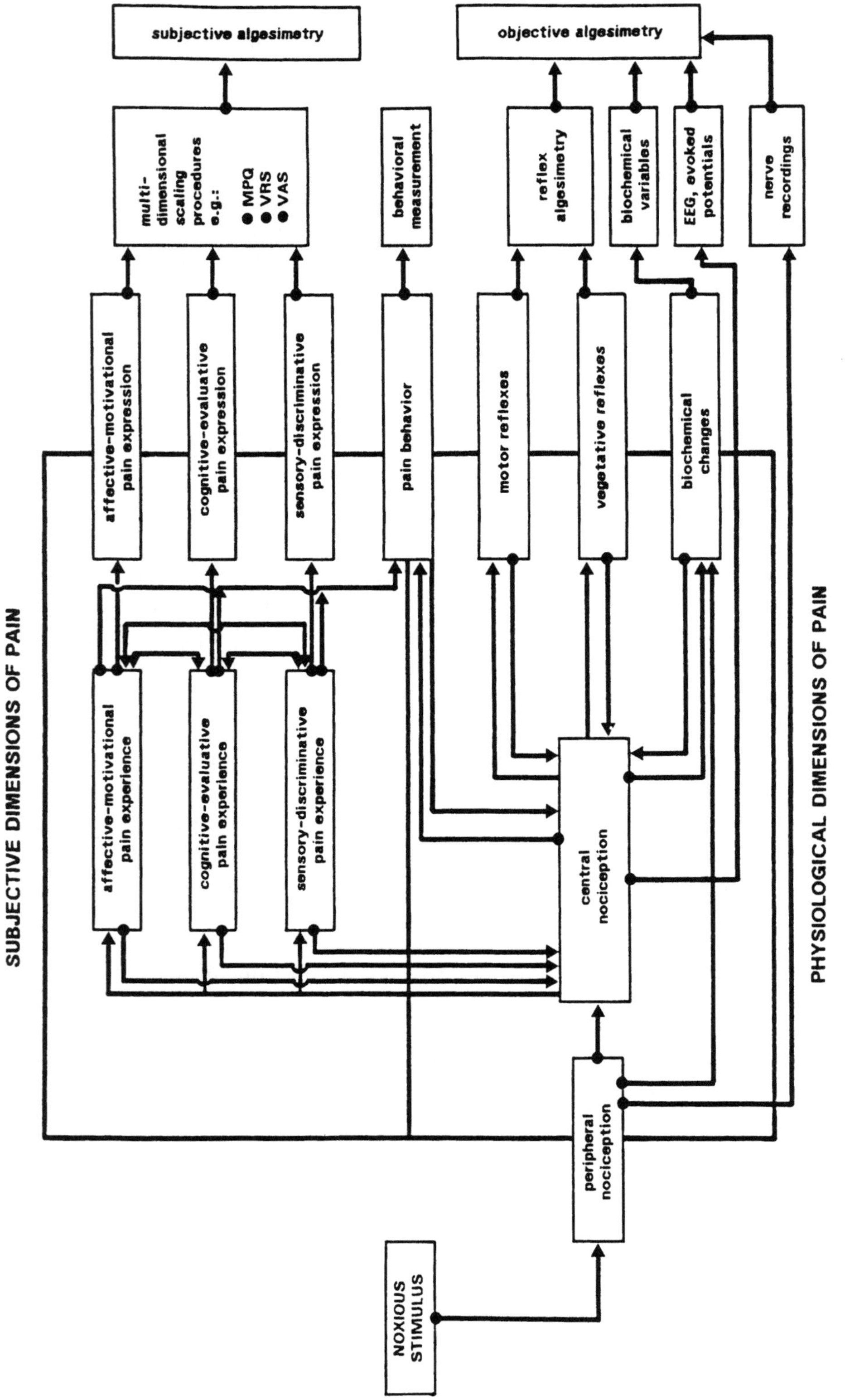
subjective algesimetry
objective algesimetry
multi-dimensional scaling procedures e.g.: ● MPQ ● VRS ● VAS
behavioral measurement
reflex algesimetry
biochemical variables
EEG, evoked potentials
nerve recordings
affective-motivational pain expression
cognitive-evaluative pain expression
sensory-discriminative pain expression
pain behavior
motor reflexes
vegetative reflexes
biochemical changes
SUBJECTIVE DIMENSIONS OF PAIN
affective-motivational pain experience
cognitive-evaluative pain experience
sensory-discriminative pain experience
central nociception
PHYSIOLOGICAL DIMENSIONS OF PAIN
peripheral nociception
NOXIOUS STIMULUS

cally supported. These adjective lists are comparable in their relevance with the MPQ.[14,17,32]

Pain scales may be applied in the following areas:

1. As a screening procedure for exploring the extent of emotional damage to patients with chronic pain. Studies using discriminant analyses and correlational procedures confirm the close association between the results of psychometric testing[3,29,76] and the single scores of the pain scales that assess non-sensory pain experience.[31,41,52,87]
2. As a method of checking the course of therapy in which particular interventions have been carried out, especially in pain research.
3. In the context of a test battery to supplement a medical differential diagnosis, in which certain acute, narrowly defined pain syndromes, such as acute radicular low back pain, may be more precisely distinguished as chronic pain illnesses, such as various types of chronic headaches. An application in computer-assisted diagnosis, using artificial intelligence systems, may be possible for well-defined pain syndromes.

The indicators of validity introduced above show support that the pain description scales provide high sensitivity for understanding the emotional disturbance connected with pain. However, the "meaning of the pain," grasped in this way, does not allow for any concrete classification in a psychodiagnostic category system.

## Pain and Personality

The most frequently used instrument in research concerned with chronic pain is the Minnesota Multiphasic Personality Inventory (MMPI).[29] The advantages of this test, when compared to projective and other personality testing procedures, include its ease of application and the objectivity of its scoring criteria.

In investigations with chronic pain patients, particular scales of the MMPI emerge as relevant. The scales "Hs" (hypochondriasis), "D" (depression), and "Hy" (hysteria) appear to indicate a psychic participation in the experience of pain. These three scales form a graphic configuration that has been labeled as "psychosomatic V" or "conversion V", in which the T scores for "Hs" and "Hy" lie above those for "D." In the case of T values above 70 points, this configuration is supposed to help identify patients

◄

**Figure 5.2.** Model of the complex central nervous processing of noxious stimulation with different pain expressions. Possible starting points for subjective and objective pain measurement and appropriate algesimetric methods are indicated on the right.

likely to somaticize under stress or to show symptoms of conversion hysteria or hypochondria.

A large number of investigations have examined the validity of MMPI results, especially those concerned with the so-called pain personality, as well as those dealing with the prognostic value of this instrument. However, among the various studies there is little agreement over conclusions.[7,12,16,24,48,65,101,102]

The question of whether or not it is possible to clarify this configuration as a functional pain experience was quickly abandoned for lack of a clear definition of psychogenic pain. Therefore, the dichotomy of psychogenic versus somatic pain also must be doubted in principle. Moreover, recent studies suggest that pain patients show more similarities than differences in psychic structure, whether or not clearly organic causes for pain have been found.[20]

A further aspect of the problem is the extent to which conclusions about the scale configuration "psychosomatic V" may be applied to actual experience and behavior of patients with chronic back pain. This issue involves the construction of the test itself. According to Lienert,[45] test profiles may be considered reliable only if the single subscales can display high reliability coefficients as well as low intercorrelations among one another. Neither condition has been met for the MMPI. It is our purpose in the following to give a brief sketch of why MMPI profiles for chronic pain patients do not represent their "reality," but instead present specious profiles based on an obsolete system of psychiatric classification.

It is recognized that scales "Hs" and "Hy" contain 15 common items, so that common variation of the two scales must follow, as long as the patient completes the questionnaire without missing any items. Indeed 15 items compose over two thirds of the "Hs" scale. The Depression scale has seven items in common with the "Hy" scale and four items in common with the "Hs" scale. It is also very likely that the "D" values share common variation with at least the "Hy" scale, as seven items compose approximately a third of the "D" scale. The "V configuration" is, therefore, a product of the high intercorrelations of the single subscales. A precise inspection of the items reveals, furthermore, that in both the "Hs" and the "Hy" scales one-third of the items are related to general health, working ability, and possible consequences of pain. Because the patients are in pain their responses will be slanted necessarily toward one extreme. A response set is unavoidable.

The interpretation of this scale configuration must be seen as an artifact of the construction of the concept "conversation V," i.e., conversion hysteria or hypochondria. The interpretation of the test results has been influenced by clinical observations for this particular group of patients. For example, it has been observed in some cases that chronic pain arises and is maintained via the mechanism of conversion. In this manner, a similarity of content between test and observation has been construed artificially. In our view it is not legitimate, therefore, to apply psychiatric concepts, such as those reflected in MMPI scales, to explain the psychosocial component of the experience of pain.[96]

If the MMPI items are subjected first to an item analysis and then to a factor analysis, factors may be extracted that help in understanding more accurately the contents of test results already found.[22] If this basis is taken to interpret test results, then it must be ascertained, as Waddell and colleagues[98] have stated, that "these patients were neither personality deficient, neurotic, hypochondriac, hysterical, nor mad but simply distressed by their physical problem and presented that distress to the physician" (p. 212).

According to the available evidence it seems untenable, on the basis of the MMPI, to postulate a generally premorbid personality typing in cases of organic or nonorganic pain. Other personality testing procedures may be taken to demonstrate the same problem. It is safer—and more useful clinically—to suggest that the effects of pain and personality are interrelated and that personality changes occur because of chronically experienced pain.

The prognostic value of the MMPI has been supported in part by several studies.[30,42,47,54,55,65,80] It must be noted critically that these studies are carried out by assessing *group* differences, rendering questionable their prognostic value for individuals.

One review[49] calls attention to the continued widespread use of the MMPI. Numerous publications with this test have shown, in our opinion, that from the use of the MMPI and other personality tests there has been no answer to the question of a pain personality or to the question of organic versus psychogenic pain. Moreover, these tests fail to provide reliable prognostic information for individuals.

To summarize, we firmly believe that in this instance the value of an obsolete test procedure has been overestimated. Generally, early hopes that psychometric personality tests would predict individual response to illness or outcome of specific treatments have not been realized but have prompted the development of different psychologic questionnaires giving a more comprehensive description of the patient including aspects such as pain history, illness behavior, and personal distress (see Chapters 4 and 8).

## Pain and Anxiety

Numerous studies report the association of fear and pain.[81] While pain is a frequent symptom in fear syndromes it can be also the cause of anxiety states[86] and can amplify somatic complaints especially in acute pain. Schmidt and Struppler[78] point out that in states of anxiety the same vegetative reactions occur as in cases of acute pain, and that anxiety states appear most often when the cause of the pain remains unclear.

Woodforde and Merskey,[106] who described reactive and illness intensifying anxiety states, agree with these views. Price and Blackwell[67] measured significantly higher anxiety scores for migraine headache patients than for normal subjects.

In one investigation,[14] a positive linear covariation between anxiety and acute pain could be confirmed for low and average degrees of anxiety. For high anxiety the data showed a tendency toward reduced pain. The latter phenomenon has been described as "stress induced analgesia." According to Sternbach,[84] chronic pain patients show a low level of anxiety, because the surprise effect of the pain has been overcome. Exceptions are the case of patients who suffer from a life-threatening disease such as cancer, or patients who remain undiagnosed, or those who are in extreme chronic pain.

There is undoubtedly a close relationship among pain, fear, and individual reactions to pain; however, the specific response combination in any one case cannot be predicted in advance. Higher levels of anxiety may be associated with increased pain levels, but a decrease in anxiety does not lead necessarily to a decrease in pain. The multiplicity of "pain-anxiety" relationships demands a differentiated exploration of anxiety phenomena in connection with history of pain, during which process test procedures may be introduced as screening instruments. The following questions should be in the foreground:

Is the anxiety associated with social factors (such as fear of losing employment)?
Is the anxiety a personality state or trait (STAI)[83]?
Is it fear or is it a form of neurosis?

According to this assessment, an appropriate treatment plan can follow, which takes anxiety into consideration.

## Pain and Depression

Depression and depressive moods, independent of the cause of illness, are often part of the diagnosis for patients with chronic pain.[84] Although in the literature there is no agreement on the degree and frequency of depression in the context of chronic pain diseases, there is no denying that strong connections exist between pain and depression.[76]

According to Kielholz,[38] every second depressed patient has headaches as a secondary symptom. Walcher[99] points out that when physical symptoms are in the foreground they may mask the recognition of depression. Merskey and Spears'[62] pain studies with psychiatric patients showed a simultaneous appearance of depression and pain behavior. Magni and Bertolini[50] point out that for pain patients the depressive symptoms often appear before the physical symptoms begin. They cite the work of

Schneider—"depression without depression"—to support this view. The diagnosis becomes even less clear when it is assumed that there can be a shifting back and forth between the occurrence of psychic and somatic symptoms.[82] Neuroendocrinologic research findings[2,88,93] suggest that chronic pain and depression emerge under common precipitating conditions. For example, a positive correlation could be shown between the level of endorphin measurement and the experimental pain threshold and tolerance. Patients with a clearly somatic diagnosis showed a lower endorphin level than did those with pain that seemed more psychogenic in origin.

Blumer and Heilbronn[6] view both pain and depression as the simultaneous expression of a particular mood state. In their opinion, the patients who suffer chronic pain experience their symptoms more as physical than as psychic. They consider that their feelings of hopelessness are a result of pain rather than a result of depression. Our explanation, following Sternbach,[85] is that depression is a reaction to pain and may be also masked by the pain. The patients often described that they feel uncomfortable in a psychological sense, while they maintain a thoroughly somatic view of their symptoms. Our clinical experience shows that depression frequently becomes chronic along with a lasting painful illness, even though the pain remains as a central problem and the patient claims "My only problem is my pain"[6] (p. 390).

In summary, it may be asserted that a depression or depressive mood does not provide an appropriate differential diagnostic criterion for chronic pain syndromes. The chronicity of the complaints can be a decisive or precipitating factor in the development of depression accompanying chronic pain. It is just as often the case that chronic pain patients show *no* unusual emotional changes. Perhaps these patients possess better pain coping mechanisms or they experience a lower intensity of pain.

The best procedure in the diagnosis of depression is first to provide a psychometric clarification, followed by clinical interviews in order to make the diagnosis more precise.

In the first step (psychometric) the following instruments have proven useful in the area of pain diagnosis.

Beck Depression Inventory[3]
Self-Rating Depression Scale[108]
Depressivity-Scale[94]

Such instruments provide the appropriate information for the therapist about which patients are in a critical emotional state and need further clarification as to the psychic component of their pain. In addition to taking a thorough history of the pain, further investigation uses the leading motives of the standardized interview to gain insight into the psychopathological aspects of depression. Appropriate instruments for the second step are the following:

Present State Examination[103]
Schedule for Assessment of Depressive Disorders[35]
Standardized Clinical Interview DSM/R[104]

In concluding the issue of pain and depression, the following may be maintained: It would be desirable to attain greater understanding of the conditions under which chronic pain and depression arise by using controlled clinical trials accompanied by epidemiological studies, thus combining somatic and psychological assessment and interventions. This information could provide clues as to the interactive associations between chronic pain and depression. Also it could be used to clarify by what means and to what degree the physical and the emotional aspects of suffering could be changed or influenced.

## Pain Drawings and "Physical Impairment"

In order to delimit the so-called psychogenic aspect of pain, multifaceted anamnestic parameters and psychological procedures have been used. Adler[1] suggested, as nonorganic pain indicators, a vague and diffuse pain localization, the inadequacy of described complaints and morphologic findings, the constant presence of the same degree of pain, the lack of dependence upon arbitrary motion, inadequate reactions to medication, and the patient's emphasis upon the organic causes of pain. However, to distinguish psychogenic pain e.g. from central pain, which can also be constant and not generally responsive to analgesics, the presence of one or two of these indicators is not sufficient to diagnose psychogenic pain.

These experiences form a background for the introduction of procedures focusing upon particular aspects of the pain description. Strian[86] found that, in contrast to organically caused pain, which despite greater variability exhibited typical organ-specific appearance, the presentation of more psychogenically conditioned pain is more vague and uncertain; moreover, description of the latter seems to include more regions of the body and invites generalizations to other uncomfortable feelings. The same conclusions have been reached by Leavitt and Garron[43] in investigating patients with chronic back pain.

Clinical observation should distinguish the symptoms and signs of physical disease from those of distress and illness behavior. This is mostly illustrated by the pain drawing. The *way* that patients draw their pain is influenced by distress, and the patient's apparently straightforward description of pain provides both physical information about the pain and psychologic information about their response to it. Similarly, the adjectives that patients use to describe pain fall into two distinct patterns: those that describe the sensory qualities of pain and other adjectives that are mainly about the emotional qualities of the pain experience.

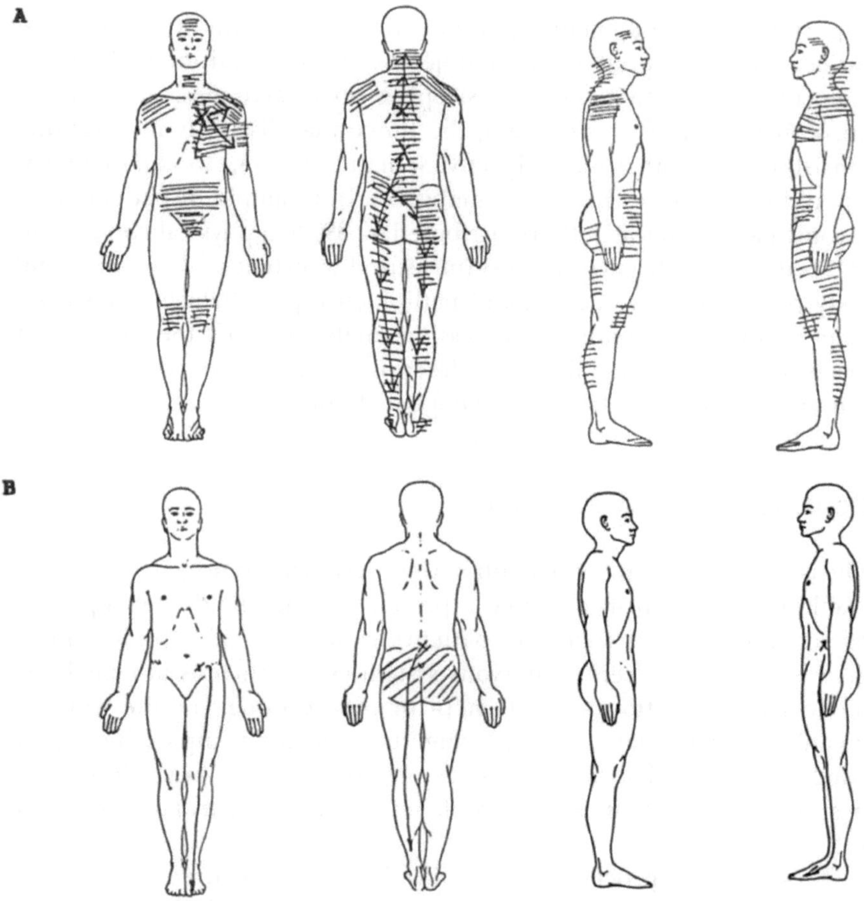


**Figure 5.3.** (A) Pain drawing of a male patient, 57 years old, describing nonanatomic pattern of pain. Diagnosis: disc prolapse $L_5/S_1$. This drawing suggests possible influence of psychologic distress on the pain complaints. (B) Pain drawing of female patient, 54 years old, describing low-back pain caused by degenerative disc disease $L_5/S_1$ and irritation of facet joints.

Inappropriate descriptions of symptoms and inappropriate responses to examination have also been described and provide a clinical measure of distress and illness behavior (see Fig. 5.3).

Evaluation takes into consideration the possible physiological extension of pain in comparison with the drawing and the application of various symbols to describe the complaints. A system of coding these drawings has been developed by Ransford and colleagues.[72] Attempts at validation yielded differing findings;[14,72,92] however, a study of Dzioba and Doxey[16] confirmed the basic validity of pain drawings for prognostic purposes.

In Waddell and Main's[97] study, the concepts of "psychic component" and "functional disability" are borrowed from Fairbank and colleagues.[19]

Important to this judgment is not the estimation of pain intensity by the patients themselves, but instead a subjective, illness-conditioned disability in normal, daily activities such as sleeping, sexual activities, and relationships. According to this concept, the functional disability or invalidity consists of a combination of objective somatic changes, stress, pain behavior, and disturbances in social interaction. In a sample of patients with chronic back pain the authors attributed 40.3% to a physical component of "invalidity," while psychic stress (measured by extent of depression and body perception) was 22.5%, and pathological pain behavior was 8.4% (data according to multiple regression analysis). Thus the use of this procedure gives a general picture describing the event of pain on a continuum between somatic and psychogenic limits.

## Routine of Pain Assessment

The proof for a linear connection in time between psychogenic cause and resulting pain is hardly available at present.[62,85] Independent of a psychic or somatic cause of pain, the patient's experience of chronic pain is greatly affected by central nervous system events such as affectual and mood states, attention, suggestion, prior conditioning, and the symbolic meanings of the pain and suffering state. In this complex biological, psychological, and social factors are involved. For the practitioner it is useful to consider that psychic problems appear in *combination* with physical complaints.

Questionnaire procedures for collecting a standardized history have been used for a long time in medical practice.[23,27,77,86] Various studies show that an interview of the patient by the doctor could be equally valuable and even more productive of information on particular questions.[11,107]

Because chronic pain presents such a complex phenomenon, including psychological and social aspects in addition to somatic factors, it is important for the diagnosis of pain patients to operationalize these numerous aspects as objectively as possible. This serves the purpose of maintaining a broad clinical picture of the patient in order to facilitate a multifaceted plan for therapy.

In a first step it is useful to select those patients whose pain experience may be influenced by psychological factors. For this purpose complex questionnaires such as the Göttingen Inventory for Patients may be used. This questionnaire, in addition to the Depressivity-Scale and the Complaint-List of von Zerssen[94,95] and the Göttingen Pain Scale[17] includes also sociobiographical variables, parameters of clinical pain experience (topography, intensity, duration, quality, psychic correlates), causal attributes, sleep disturbance and use of medication. The intensity of pain is measured by both a visual analogue scale and a verbal rating scale. These questionnaires may be sent to the patients before the first contact in the pain clinic. Data from these questionnaires will be discussed in the regular staff meeting to decide which patients need a further psychological investigation. If further psychological evaluation is warranted, these patients are then requested to complete a personality inventory, e.g., the "Freiburger Presonlichkeits-Inventar" (FPI)[18] or the Picture Frustration Test (PFT),[73] the State-Trait Anxiety Inventory (STAI),[83] and the Illness Behavior Questionnaire (IBQ).[66]

Similar inventories are in no case substitutes for a detailed somatic or psychological interview. Their purpose is to supplement physician's reports and current X-ray results, etc., so that a thorough field of brief information is available, often before the initial session with the patient. This method serves, therefore, to economize and specify the diagnostic process. According to our experience, the data obtained by using such questionnaires facilitates a multidisciplinary approach to a complicated phenomenon.

One further advantage of standardized data collection is that it makes possible the comparison of clinical work between hospitals or replication of scientific investigations. It is worth mentioning that the routine application of such procedures leads to an improvement in the daily organization within the pain unit of either an inpatient or outpatient setting.

## References


1. Adler, R. (1979). *Schmerz*. In: *Lehrbuch der Psychosomatischen Medizin*. Th. v. Uexkuell (Ed.). München: Urban & Schwarzenberg.
2. Almay, B.G.L., Johansson, F., v. Knorring, L., Terenius, L.Y., & Aström, M. (1978). Endorphines and chronic pain. *Pain* 5:153–162.
3. Beck, A.T., Ward, C.H., Mendelson, M., Mock, J., & Erbaugh, J. (1961). An inventory for measuring depression. *Arch Gen. Psychiat.* 4:561–571.
4. Beecher, H.K. (1956). Relationship of significance of wound to the pain experienced. *Journal of the American Medical Association* 161:1609–1613.
5. Beecher, H.K. (1959). *Measurement of subjective responses. Quantitative effects of drugs*. New York: Oxford University Press.
6. Blumer, D., & Heilbronn, M. (1982). Chronic pain as a variant of depressive disease: The pain-prone disorder. *Journal of Nervous Mental Disease* 170(7): 381–406.
7. Blumetti, A.E., & Modesti, L.M. (1976). Psychological predictors of success or failure of surgical intervention for intractable back pain. In: *Advances in Pain Research and Therapy*. Vol. 1. J.J. Bonica and D.G. Albe-Fessard (Eds.). New York: Raven Press.
8. Brenig, M., Eggebrecht, D., Hildebrandt, J., Pfingsten, M., & Bautz, M. (in press). Eine faktorenanalytische Untersuchung zur Erfassung der Dimensionaltät klinischer Schmerzbeschreibungen. *Diagnostica*.
9. Byrne, M., Troy, A., Bradley, L.A., Marchisello, P.J., Geisinger, K.F., van der Heide, L.H., & Prieto, F.J. (1982). Cross-validation of the factor structure of the McGill Pain Questionnaire. *Pain* 13:193–201.

10. Chapman, C.R. (1976). Measurement of pain. In: Advances in Pain Research and Therapy. (Eds.) J.J. Bonica and D.G. Fessard. Vol. 1. New York: Raven Press.
11. Collen, M.F., Cutler, J.L., Siegelaub, A.B., & Cella, R.L. (1969). Reliability of a self-administered medical questionnaire. *Archives of Internal Medicine* 123: 664–668.
12. Cummings, C., Evanski, C.M., DeBenedetti, M.J., Anderson, E.E., & Waugh, T.R. (1979). *Use of the MMPI to predict outcome of treatment for chronic pain*. In: *Advances in Pain Research and Therapy*. J.J. Bonica, J.C. Liebeskind, & D.G. Albe-Fessard (Eds.). New York: Raven Press.
13. Cziske, R. (1980). Kurzspeicher und Interozeption – einige Zusammenhänge. *Kybernetische Forschungsberichte* 21(3):88–92.
14. Cziske, R. (1983). Faktoren des Schmerzleidens und ihre Messung: Revidierte Mehrdimensionale Schmerzskala. *Diagnostica* 29:61–74.
15. Dennis, M.D., Rocchio, P.O., & Wiltse, L.L. (1981). The topographical pain representation and its correlation with MMPI scores. *Orthopedics* 9(6):614–623.
16. Dzioba, R.B., & Doxey, N.C. (1984). A prospective investigation into the orthopaedic and psychologic predictors of outcome of first lumbar surgery following industrial injury. *Spine* 9:614–623.
17. Eggebrecht, D., Hildebrandt, J., & Franz, C. (1987). *Vorläufiges Manual zum Göttinger Schmerzfragebogen*. Göttingen: Schmerzambulanz Universitätsklinik.
18. Fahrenberg, J., Hampel, R., & Selg, H. (1984). *Das Freiburger Persönlichkeitsinventar (FPI)*. Göttingen: Hogrefe.
19. Fairbank, C.J., Davies, J.B., Couper, J., & O'Brien, J.P. (1980). The Oswestry low back pain disability questionnaire. *Physiotherapy* 66:271–273.
20. Fordyce, W.E. (1976). *Behavioral methods for chronic pain and illness*. St. Louis: C.V. Mosby.
21. Fordyce, W.E., & Steger, J.C. (1982). Chronischer Schmerz. In: W. Keeser, E. Pöppel, and P. Mitterhusen (Hrsg.) *Schmerz. Fortschritte der klinischen Psychologie* 27. München: Urban & Schwarzenberg.
22. Franz, C., Paul, R., Bautz, M., Choroba, B., & Hildebrant, J. (1986). Psychosomatic aspects of chronic pain: A new way of description based on MMPI item analysis. *Pain* 26(1):33–43.
23. Garrat, J., & Bennett, A.E. (1971). A validated interview schedule for use in population surveys of chronic disease and disability. *British J. Prev. Soc. Med.* 25:97–104.
24. Gentry, W.D., Shows, W.D., & Thomas, M. (1974). Chronic low back pain: A psychological profile. *Psychosomatics* 15:174–177.
25. Gracely, R.H., McGrath, P., & Dubner, R. (1978). Ratio scales of sensory and affective verbal pain descriptors: Manipulation of affect by diazepam. *Pain* 5:19–29.
26. Gracely, R.H., McGrath, P., & Dubner, R. (1979). Fentanyl reduces the intensity but not the unpleasantness of painful tooth pulp sensations. *Science* 203: 1261–1263.
27. Grüntzig, A., & Galla, J. (1970). Die Ergebnisse eines Fragebogens im Vergleich mit der ärztlichen Diagnose. *Methods Inf. Med.* 9:21–27.
28. Handwerker, H.O. (1984). Experimentelle Schmerzanalyse beim Menschen. In: M. Zimmerman and H.O. Handwerker (Hrsg.). *Schmerz. Konzepte und ärztliches Handeln*. New York and Berlin: Springer.

29. Hathaway, S.R., & McKinley, J.C. (1951). *The Minnesota Multiphasic Personality Inventory.* New York: The Psychological Corporation.
30. Herron, L.D., & Pheasant, H.C. (1982). Changes in MMPI profiles after low back surgery. *Spine* 7:591–597.
31. Hildebrandt, J., Brenig, M., & Eggebrecht, D. (1987). Schmerzbeschreibung, Beschwerden und Depressivität bei Patienten mit chronischen Kopfschmerz-syndromen. *Z. Psychother. Psychosom. Med. Psychol.* 37(9/10):337–342.
32. Hoppe, F. (1985). Zur Faktorenstruktur bon Schmerzerleben und Schmerz-verhalten bei chronischen Schmerzpatienten. *Diagnostica* 31(1):70–78.
33. Hunter, M. (1983): The headache scale: A new approach to the assessment of headache pain based on pain descriptions. *Pain* 16:361–373.
34. Huskisson, E.C. (1983). Visual analogue scales. In: R.D. Melzack (Ed.) *Pain Measurement and Assessment.* New York: Raven Press.
35. Jablensky, A., Sartorius, N., Gulbinat, W., & Ernberg, G. (1986). The WHO instruments for the assessment of depressive disorders. In: N. Sartorius and T.A. Ban (Eds.) *Assessment of Depression.* Berlin: Springer.
36. Jensen, M.P., Karoly, P., & Braver, S. (1986). The measurement of clinical pain intensity: A comparison of six methods. *Pain* 27(1):117–126.
37. Keele, C.A. (1966). Measurement of pain and analgesia. Proceedings of the Royal Society of Medicine (Suppl.) 59:73–78.
38. Kielholz, P. (1971). *Diagnose und Therapie für den Praktiker.* München: Lehmann.
39. Kiss, I., Müller, H., & Abel, M. (1987). The McGill Pain Questionnaire—German Version. A study on cancer pain. *Pain* 29:195–207.
40. Knapp, T.W. (1983). *Migräne I: Symptomatologie und Ätiologie.* Weinheim: Beltz.
41. Kremer, E., & Atkinson, J.H. (1981). Pain measurement: Construct validity of the affective dimension of the McGill Pain Questionnaire with chronic benign pain patients. *Pain* 11:93–100.
42. Kuperman, S.K., Golden, C.J., & Blume, H.G. (1979). Predicting pain treatment results by personality variables in organic and functional patients. *Journal of Clinical Psychology* 35(4):832–836.
43. Leavitt, F., & Garron, D.C. (1979). Validity of back pain classification scale among patients with low back pain not associated with demonstrable organic disease. *Journal of Psychosomatic Research* 23:301–306.
44. Leavitt, F., Garron, D.C., & Bieliauskas, A. (1978). Stressing life events and the experience of low back pain. *Journal of Psychosomatic Research* 23:49–55.
45. Lienert, G.A. (1969). *Testaufbau und Testanalyse.* Weinheim: Beltz.
46. Ljunggren, A.E. (1983). Descriptions of pain and other sensory modalities in patients with lumbago-sciatica and herniated intervertebral discs. Interview administration of an adapted McGill Pain Questionnaire. *Pain* 16:265–276.
47. Long, C. (1981). The relationship between surgical outcome and MMPI profiles in chronic pain patients. *Journal of Clinical Psychology* 37:744–749.
48. Long, C.J., Brown, D.A., & Engelberg, J. (1980). Intervertebral disc surgery. *Journal of Neurosurgery* 52:818–824.
49. Love, A.W., & Peck, C.L. (1987). The MMPI and psychological factors in chronic low back pain: A review. *Pain* 28:1–12.
50. Magni, G., & Bertolini, C. (1983). Chronic pain as a depressive equivalent. *Postgraduate Medicine* 73:79–90.
51. Maiani, G., & Sanavio, E. (1985). Semantics of pain in Italy: The Italian version of the McGill Pain Questionnaire. *Pain* 22:399–405.

52. McCreary, C. (1983). Pain descriptions and personality disturbance. In: R.D. Melzack (Ed.). *Pain Measurement and Assessment*. New York: Raven Press.
53. McCreary, C., & Janison, K. (1975). The chronic pain patient. *Cons.-liasion Psychiat.* 35:205–218.
54. McCreary, C., Turner, J., & Dawson, E. (1979). The MMPI as a predictor of response to conservative treatment for low back pain. *Journal of Clinical Psychology* 35:278–284.
55. McCreary, C. (1983). Pain description and personality disturbance. In: R.D. Melzack (Ed.) *Pain Measurement and Assessment*. New York: Raven Press.
56. Melazck, R.D. (1975). The McGill Pain Questionnaire: Major properties and scoring methods. *Pain* 1:277–299.
57. Melzack, R.D. (Ed.) (1983). *Pain Measurement and Assessment*. New York: Raven Press.
58. Melzack, R.D. (1987). The short form McGill Pain Questionnaire. *Pain* 30: 191–197.
59. Melzack, R.D., & Casey, K.L. (1968). Sensory, motivational, and central control determinants of pain: A new conceptual model. In: D. Kenshalo (Ed.) *The Skin Senses*. Springfield: Charles C Thomas.
60. Melzack, R.D., & Torgerson, W.S. (1971). On the language of pain. *Anesthesiology* 34:50–59.
61. Melzack, R.D., & Wall, P.D. (1965). Pain mechanisms: A new theory. *Science* 150:971–979.
62. Merskey, H., & Spear, F.G. (1967). *Pain: Psychological and Psychiatric Aspects*. Baltimore: The Williams and Wilkins Co.
63. Ohnhaus, E.E., & Adler, R. (1975). Methodological problems in the measurement of pain: A comparison between the verbal rating scale and the visual analogue scale. *Pain*. 1:379–384.
64. Pheasant, H.C. (1975). Sources of failure in laminectomies. *Orthop. Clin. North Am.* 6:319–325.
65. Pheasant, H.C., Gilbert, D., Goldfarb, J., & Herron, L. (1979). The MMPI as a predictor of outcome in low-back surgery. *Spine* 4:78–84.
66. Pilowsky, I., & Spence, N.D. (1981). *Manual for the Illness Behaviour Questionnaire (IBQ)*. Adelaide: University of Adelaide.
67. Price, K.P., & Blackwell, S. (1980). Trait levels of anxiety and psychological responses to stress in migraineurs and normal controls. *Journal of Clinical Psychology* 36:658–660.
68. Price, D.D., Harkins, S.W., & Baker, C. (1987). Sensory-affective relationships among different types of clinical and experimental pain. *Pain* 28:297–307.
69. Price, D.D., McGrath, P.A., Rafii, A., & Buckingham, B. (1983). The validation of visual analogue scales as ratio measures for chronic and experimental pain. *Pain* 17:45–56.
70. Prieto, E.J., Hopson, L., Bradley, L.A., Byrne, M., Geisinger, K.F., Midax, D., & Marchisello, P.J. (1980). The language of low back pain: Factor structure of the McGill pain questionnaire. *Pain* 8:11–19.
71. Radvilla, A., Adler, R.H., Galeazzi, R.L., & Vorkauf, H. (1987). The development of a German language (Berne) pain questionnaire and its application in a situation causing acute pain. *Pain* 28:185–197.
72. Ransford, A.O., Cairns, D., & Mooney, V. (1976). The pain drawing as an aid to the psychologic evaluation of patients with low-back pain. *Spine* 1:127–134.

73. Rauchfleisch, U. (1979). *Handbuch zum Rosenzweig Picture-Frustration Test (PFT).* Bern: Huber.
74. Reading, A.E. (1979). The internal structure of the McGill Pain Questionnaire. *Pain* 7:353–358.
75. Reading, A.E. (1982). An analysis of the language of pain in chronic and acute patient groups. *Pain* 13:185–192.
76. Romano, J.M., & Turner, J.A. (1985). Chronic pain and depression: Does the evidence support a relationship? *Psychological Bulletin* 97(1):18–34.
77. Rose, G.A. (1965). Chest pain questionnaire. *Milbank mem. Fd. Quart.* 43:32–39.
78. Schmidt, R.F., & Struppler, A. (1982). *Der Schmerz. Ursachen—Diagnose—Therapie.* München: Piper.
79. Scott, J., & Huskisson, E.C. (1976). Graphic representation of pain. *Pain* 2:175–184.
80. Smith, W.L., & Duerksen, D.L. (1979). Personality and the relief of chronic pain: predicting surgical outcome. *Clin. Neuropsychol* 1:35–38.
81. Spear, F.G. (1967). Pain in psychiatric patients. *Journal of Psychosomatic Research* 11:187–193.
82. Spiegelberg, U., Schirg, B., & Betz, B. (1970). Syndromwechsel (syndrome shift) und Verstimmung. *Nervenarzt* 40:73–77.
83. Spielberger, C.D., Gorsuch, R.L., & Lushene, R.E. (1970). *Manual for the State-Trait Anxiety Inventory.* Palo Alto, Calif.: Consulting Psychologists Press.
84. Sternbach R.A. (1974). *Pain-patients—Traits and Treatment.* New York: Academic Press.
85. Sternbach, R.A. (1978). *The Psychology of Pain.* New York: Raven Press.
86. Strian, F. (1983). *Angst—Grundlagen und Klinik.* New York and Berlin: Springer.
87. Taenzer, P. (1983). Postoperative pain: Relationships among measures of pain, mood, and narcotic requirements. In: R. Melzack (Ed.). *Pain Measurement and Assessment.* New York: Raven Press.
88. Terenius, L.Y. (1980). Biochemical assessment of chronic pain. In: H.B. Kosterlitz and L.Y. Terenius (Eds.) *Pain and Society.* Dahlem Konferenzen. Weinheim: Chemie.
89. Thorner, R.M., & Remein, Q.P. (1961). Principles and procedures in the evaluation of screening for disease. *Public Health Monograph* 67:1–24.
90. Turk, D.C., & Flor, H. (1984). Etiological theories and treatments for chronic back pain. II. Psychological models and interventions. *Pain* 19:209–233.
91. Vanderiet, K., Adriaensen, A., Carton, H., & Vertommen, H. (1987). The McGill Pain Questionnaire constructed for the Dutch language (MPQ-DV). Preliminary data concerning reliability and validity. *Pain* 30:395–408.
92. v.Bayer, C.L., Bergstrom, K.G., Brodwin, M.G., & Brodwin, S.K. (1983). Invalid use of pain drawings in psychological screening of back pain patients. *Pain* 16:103–107.
93. v.Knorring, L., Almay, B.G.L., Johannsson, F., & Terenius, L.Y. (1978). Pain perception and endorphin levels in cerebrospinal fluid. *Pain* 5:359–365.
94. v.Zerssen, D. (1976a). *Klinische Selbstbeurteilungs-Skalen (KSb-S) aus dem Münchener Psychiatrischen Informations-System (PSYCHIS München): Die Paranoid-Depressivitäts-Skala.* Weinheim: Beltz.
95. v.Zerssen, D. (1976b). *Klinische Selbstbeurteilungs-Skalen (KSb-S) aus dem Münchener Psychiatrischen Informations-System (PSYCHIS München): Die Beschwerden-Liste.* Weinheim: Beltz.

96. Waddell, G., McCulloch, J.A., Kummel, E.G., Venner, R.M. (1980). Non organic physical sign in low back pain. *Spine* 5:117–125.
97. Waddell, G., & Main, C.J. (1984). Assessment of severity in low-back disorders. *Spine* 9:204–208.
98. Waddell, G., Main, C.J., Morris, E.W., DiPaoba, M., & Gray, I.C. (1984). Chronic low back pain, psychologic distress, and illness behavior. *Spine* 9:209–213.
99. Walcher, W. (1969). *Die larvierte Depression.* Wien: Hollinek.
100. Wall, P.D. (1984). Introduction. In: P.D. Wall and R.D. Melzack (Eds.) *Textbook of Pain.* London: Churchill Livingston.
101. Watkins, R.G., O'Brien, J.P., Draugelis, R., & Jones, D. (1986). Comparisons of preoperative and postoperative MMPI data in chronic back patients. *Spine* 11:385–390.
102. Wiltse, L.L., & Rocchio, P.D. (1975). Preoperative psychological tests as predictors of success of chemonucleolysis in the treatment of the low-back syndrome. *Journal of Bone Joint Surgery* 57-A:478–483.
103. Wing, J.K., Cooper, J.E., & Sartorius, N. (1973). *Present State Examination.* Weinheim: Beltz Test.
104. Wittchen, H.U. (1985). *Standardisiertes klinisches Interview für DSM III (SKID).* München: Max-Planck-Institut für Psychiatrie.
105. Wolff, B.B. (1982). Die Messung von Schmerz beim Menschen. In: W. Keeser, E. Pöppel, and P. Mitterhusen (Hrsg.) *Schmerz. Fortschritte der klinischen Psychologie* 27. München: Urban & Schwarzenberg.
106. Woodforde, J.M., & Merskey, H. (1972). Some relationships between subjective measures of pain. *Journal of Psychosomatic Research* 16:173–178.
107. Young, D.W. (1972). Comparison of information collected by a questionnary with that in a patient hospital record. *Methods Inf. Med.* 11:20–22.
108. Zung, W.W.K. (1965). A self rating depression scale. *Archives of General Psychiatry* 12:63–70.

# 6

# Role of the Anesthesiologist in the Treatment of Pain

*Terri L. Dallas and Richard S. Finn*

Once hidden behind the mask and surgical garb of the operating room, in the past decade anesthesiologists have become more and more involved in the assessment and management of pain. They are increasingly consulted because of the growing awareness that anesthesiologists are familiar with the extensive anatomy/neuroanatomy of pain, appreciate the drugs available for treatment, supply specific regional anesthetic techniques for the evaluation and treatment sequence, and have long acknowledged that physical pain is influenced by innumerable nonphysical factors.[1]

Pain is one of the most complex human experiences. Acute pain is a biologically useful signal that reflects impending or ongoing tissue damage. If acute pain is not effectively treated, it becomes a chronic condition. As a chronic condition, pain loses much of its warning function and induces variable degrees of physical, emotional, and psychosocial devastation in patients afflicted with it. Such problems are so remarkably resistant to conventional medical therapies that chronic pain is the most frequent cause of disability in the United States today.[2]

Many physicians have wondered why certain patients respond poorly to surgical or medical interventions that are usually efficacious for others. Often, they blame these patients for their bad response to good therapy. Yet, to treat all pain in the same way in every patient is an overly simplistic approach. If a complaint of "pain" is reevaluated as an expression of "suffering," and a comprehensive attempt is made to find the cause of the "suffering," it often becomes apparent that inappropriate and even harmful therapy has been done by early, sometimes routine, surgical or medical interventions.[3] At times, the therapeutic relationship has been so badly frayed that the patient presents as a hostile, mistrusting, and angry individual who feels abused.[4]

The pain evaluation process *must* result in an accurate physical and psychological diagnosis, for only then will appropriate therapy follow.

## Evaluation of Chronic Pain

After initial evaluation, the anesthesiologist should decide whether the patient needs further diagnostic workup, which may include differential nerve blocking. The aims of the diagnostic nerve block are as follows: (1) to identify pain as central or peripheral, (2) to identify pain as somatic or autonomically mediated, (3) to predict the efficacy and potential side effects of chemical or surgical neuroablation, and (4) to diagnose specific nerve root or peripheral nerve involvement in the pain complaint. Examples of useful diagnostic nerve blocks for benign pain include differential spinal or epidural blocks, sympathetic nerve blocks, paravertebral somatic nerve blocks, facet nerve blocks, and trigger point injections.

Of these tools, the differential spinal block has become a routine test. Winnie[5] reported that in the majority of patients in whom symptoms were either bizarre or seemingly unrelated to any precipitating factor, without differential nerve blocking to aid diagnosis, pain would have been dismissed as psychogenic. Generally, if these patients are not properly diagnosed and treated, they frequently become addictive, psychotic, and even suicidal.

## The Conventional "Sequential" Differential Spinal

To perform a differential spinal block, one prepares four solutions in four separate syringes (Table 6.1)—normal saline, 0.25% procaine, 0.5% procaine, and 1% procaine—all in normal saline. Tell the patient that after the placement of a single needle in the back, each of the solutions will be injected sequentially. Instruct the patient further to tell which, if any, of the solutions—referred to as Solution A, Solution B, Solution C, and Solution D—relieves the pain.

Solution A (Table 6.2) is normal saline, which serves as a placebo. Solution B, 0.25% procaine, is the mean sympatholytic concentration of procaine, i.e., one sufficient to block B fibers, but insufficient to block A delta and C fibers. Solution C, 0.5% procaine, the mean sensory blocking concentration of procaine, is sufficient to block A delta, B fibers, and C fibers, but insufficient to block A alpha, beta, and gamma fibers. And, finally, Solution D, 1% procaine, provides complete blockade of all fibers. If the concentration in Solution D is insufficient to produce complete motor, sensory, and sympathetic block, it should be increased to 5% to achieve this.

It is extremely important that the administration of each injection is identical to and indistinguishable from the rest; in addition, it is equally

**Table 6.1.** Solution Preparation for Conventional "Sequential" Differential Spinal

| 10 cc Solution | Preparation | |
|---|---|---|
| | To Procaine | Add Normal Saline |
| Solution A: 0% procaine | | 10 cc |
| Solution B: 0.25% procaine | 5 cc 0.5% | 5 cc |
| Solution C: 0.5% procaine | 5 cc 1% | 5 cc |
| Solution D: 1% procaine | 1 cc 10% | 9 cc |

Note: This will be a hypotonic solution.

important that the observations the physician makes following each injection are made in an identical manner. In order to determine the presence or absence of sympathetic, sensory, and/or motor blockade (Table 6.2), the physician must question the patient about subjective changes in the level of pain, both when the patient is at rest and during the physician's attempts to mechanically reproduce the pain. Obviously, if the less experienced physician were to check blood pressure only after injection of the sympatholytic concentration, ascertain the response to pinprick only after the sensory blocking concentration, and assess motor function only after the motor blocking concentration, he or she would be clearly indicating to the patient an expectation that each injection is expected to produce specific effects.

The results of a differential spinal block are interpreted as follows: If the patient's pain is relieved following the first injection, the mechanism underlying the patient's pain is classified as "psychogenic." It is well established that 30 to 35% of all patients who have true organic pain will obtain

**Table 6.2.** Injection Sequence: Conventional Differential Spinal

| Sequence 5 cc Injected at 10-min Intervals | | Blockade |
|---|---|---|
| Solution A | Saline (placebo)[a] | |
| Solution B | 0.25% procaine[a] | Sympathetic B fibers |
| Solution C | 0.5% procaine[a] | Sensory A delta and C fibers |
| Solution D | 1% procaine | Motor[b] A alpha and B gamma |

[a] Following each injection observe:
1. Blood pressure
2. Pulse rate
3. Patient's evaluation of pain at rest
4. Patient's response to mechanic reproduction of pain
5. Signs of sympathetic block: temperature change, psychogalvanic reflex
6. Signs of sensory block: response to pinprick
7. Signs of motor block: ability to move toes, feet

[b] If complete motor blockade does not result, use 1 cc of 5% procaine.

relief from an inactive agent, so relief following the injection of normal saline *may* simply represent a placebo reaction (technically, a psychogenic response). However, this can usually be differentiated clinically from true psychogenic pain since the placebo reaction is usually of rather short duration and is self-limiting, whereas pain relief provided by a placebo in a patient suffering from true psychogenic pain is usually extremely long lasting, if not permanent. The possibility that the pain is entirely psychogenic will be substantiated or refuted by the results of the psychological evaluation.

If the patient does not obtain relief from the placebo injection and does obtain relief following the injection of 0.25% procaine, a sympathetic mechanism is indicated, provided that with the onset of pain relief there are signs of sympathetic blockade and no signs of sensory blockade. Although 0.25% procaine is the mean or usual sympatholytic concentration, a few patients who may have a decreased critical sensory blocking threshold will get relief from this concentration of procaine because it is actually producing analgesia, i.e., sensory block. However, that response is the exception and not the rule. Establishing the diagnosis of a sympathetic mechanism for pain is extremely fortuitous for the patient; this pain can usually be completely and permanently relieved by a series of sympathetic blocks. Furthermore, it is the predominant pain mechanism in patients whose referring physicians could find "no cause whatsoever for their pain." Traditionally, these pain syndromes have been called "causalgias," but "reflex sympathetic dystrophy" is a better term since it indicates the mechanism as well as the symptom complex.

If the 0.25% procaine solution does not provide pain relief but 0.5% procaine does, relief is the result of a sensory block, i.e., blockade of the A delta and/or C fibers, indicating a somatic or organic basis for the patient's pain. But the patient must exhibit signs of sympathetic blockade following the injection of 0.25% procaine and show signs of sensory blockade following 0.5% procaine. Again, 0.5% procaine is the mean or usual sensory blocking concentration. It is conceivable that an individual with an *elevated* critical sympatholytic threshold might require 0.5% procaine to produce a sympathetic (rather than sensory) block. In this case, the mechanism indicated is sympathetic and not somatic, even though the pain relief was produced by 0.5% procaine.

If the patient does not obtain relief with 0.25% or 0.5% procaine, 1% procaine (or if necessary, 5% procaine) is injected to produce blockade of all modalities. If this increase in concentration relieves the pain, the pain mechanism is considered somatic, assuming that the patient has an elevated critical sensory blocking threshold. But if the patient fails to obtain relief in spite of complete sympathetic, sensory, and motor blockade, a "central mechanism" is indicated as the cause of pain. Possible "central mechanisms" include a lesion higher in the nervous system than the level of spinal anesthesia, true psychogenic pain, the phenomenon known as encephalization, and psychogenic pain or malingering. If the patient were anticipating financial benefit from pending litigation, it would not be to his or her advantage to state that anything removed the pain, and for this reason many pain clinics refuse to accept patients involved in litigation. Although it is difficult to rule out pain or malingering, our experience with a differential spinal produced useful information about the pain in several patients with pending litigation.

Although the conventional technique of differential spinal blockade has been extremely effective in pinpointing neural mechanisms of pain syndromes in many patients and has been particularly effective in identifying the mechanism in pain syndromes of questionable or unknown etiology, it is quite time consuming. The physician must wait for a sufficient interval after each injection to allow for the various responses, and in cases where the 1% concentration of procaine does not provide complete blockade of all modalities (an absolute requirement in many cases for accurate diagnosis), an additional injection of 5% procaine is necessary. Following blockade of all modalities, a considerable period of time is necessary for full recovery. Not only does the time required to perform the differential spinal test limit its utility for the physician in a busy pain clinic, but for the patient, the necessity of lying on one side for a prolonged period may cause great discomfort or even exaggeration of pain.[6,7]

## The Anatomic Approach

Differential nerve blocks to determine mechanisms of pain in different parts of the body are summarized in Table 6.3.

The techniques utilized to relieve pain in the different regions of the body are as follows: If a placebo injection does not produce relief for pain in the head, neck, and arm, any local anesthetic agent can be used for a stellate ganglion block. If the sympathetic block can be achieved without spillover onto somatic nerves in the painful area (e.g., head pain), then the concentration of local anesthetic is unimportant; however, it may be possible to reduce some of the local anesthetic injected at the stellate ganglion, or to induce sequential blocks on two separate occasions, allowing the sympathetic block to wear off before proceeding with the somatic block. In any case, if the patient does not obtain relief following the stellate ganglion block, then the somatic nerves to the painful area should be blocked.

For pain in the thorax, following a placebo injection, a differential segmental epidural injection is safest, using the same local anesthesia concentrations described for the differential spinal. It must be remembered, however, that with thoracic pain, relief following an extensive sympathetic block, in addition to indicating a possible sympathetic mechanism, *may* indicate visceral (rather than somatic) pain mediated by sympathetic fibers. This can be confirmed if the patient's pain is relieved (on

**Table 6.3.** Procedural Sequence: Differential Diagnostic Nerve Blocks[5]

| Site of Pain | Saline | Local Anesthetic | Local Anesthetic |
|---|---|---|---|
| Head | Placebo block | Stellate ganglion block | Block C2<br>Block of trigeminal I, II, III (or branches) |
| Neck | Placebo block | Stellate ganglion block (or individual nerve) | Cervical plexus block |
| Arm | Placebo block | Stellate ganglion block (or individual nerve) | Brachial plexus block |
| Thorax | Placebo block | Dilute thoracic epidural<br>Paravertebral block<br>Intercostal block | Concentrated thoracic epidural<br>Paravertebral block<br>Intercostal block |
| Abdomen | Placebo block | Celiac plexus block | Paravertebral block<br>Intercostal block |
| Leg | Placebo block | Lumbar paravertebral<br>Sympathetic block | Lumbar paravertebral<br>Somatic block |

a different occasion) by a stellate ganglion block. If it is unwise to use a differential thoracic epidural injection in a particular patient because of cachexia, hypovolemia, etc., an alternative procedure is to block appropriate paravertebral or intercostal dermatomes. If this fails to provide relief, the origin of the patient's pain is visceral; complete temporary relief of pain with return of pain following recovery from anesthesia indicates a peripheral, somatic mechanism; and complete relief that persists long after recovery of sensation indicates a peripheral, but reflex, sympathetic mechanism.

For abdominal pain, if a placebo injection fails to provide relief, blocking appropriate paravertebral or intercostal dermatomes should be attempted to make certain that the pain is not somatic (body wall) in origin. Since patients have great difficulty localizing "abdominal pain," and cannot differentiate between body wall and true visceral involvement of a lesion, if the paravertebral or intercostal blocks fail to provide relief, a celiac plexus block should establish that the pain is truly visceral in origin.

For pain in the leg, differential nerve blocks are preferred when the pharmacologic approach is contraindicated or undesirable. Following a placebo block, lumbar paravertebral sympathetic blocks at the level of L2, 3, and 4, or, if unsuccessful, lumbar paravertebral somatic blocks of the appropriate peripheral nerve blocks, are used to provide relief. Interpretation of results from differential nerve blocks for head, neck, arm, and leg pain are virtually self-evident: Relief following a placebo injection indicates a "psychogenic mechanism," that is, a placebo reaction or true psychogenic pain. Relief following sympathetic blocks indicates a sympathetic mechanism, usually a sympathetic dystrophy, and relief following the blockade of somatic nerves indicates an organic somatic mechanism. Failure to obtain relief in spite of complete anesthesia in any of these areas would tend to indicate a "central mechanism," any of four possibilities mentioned above as the cause of pain.[7] The interpretation of the results of differential blocks for thoracic and abdominal pain have already been discussed.

## Treatment Strategies

When surgery is not a definitive therapy for the control of pain, or the workup fails to reveal the need for surgery, nonsurgical approaches for pain control must be sought.

## Medication

Chronic pain patients are often referred to the pain clinic because their physicians can no longer handle the polypharmacy that is a common problem in this group. Some physicians continue to treat chronic pain as if it were acute, or patients visit many physicians who liberally prescribe analgesics as a stopgap measure.[8] Although narcotic analgesics are useful in the treatment of acute pain and the pain of advanced cancer, they are not appropriate for treatment of chronic pain.

Good pharmacologic control of chronic pain is often achieved by using nonanalgesic drugs. For example, anticonvulsant agents have been used successfully to treat certain types of orofacial pain such as tic douloureux. Tricyclic antidepressants have helped restore disturbed sleep cycles in patients with persisting pain. These drugs work by blocking the uptake of norepinephrine at postsynaptic receptors and the reuptake of serotonin and norepinephrine, thereby increasing their availability.

Steroids and nonsteroidal antiinflammatory agents are effective with chronic pain patients when inflammation is a critical factor; it may also be necessary to coordinate pharmacologic and psychologic management to speed rehabilitation.[9] If a patient comes to the pain center with complicated polypharmacy, immediate inpatient detoxification is necessary before any pain program can be effective.

## Nerve Blocks

Nerve blocks can be utilized as the pain therapeutic modality for two types of pain. In organic pain syndromes where pain is localized and the cause cannot be removed (malignancy, chronic pancreatitis, etc.), pain relief can be provided by neurolytic blocks utilizing alcohol or phenol. When neurolytic blocks are performed on peripheral nerves to preserve motor function, a subarachnoid alcohol block must be utilized since very hypobaric alcohol may produce selective dorsal rhizotomy. In our practice, cranial nerve blocks and subarachnoid blocks are done with absolute alcohol, and peripheral somatic blocks are done with 6% phenol. If this concentration of phenol is not effective, up to 12% phenol may be dissolved in an aqueous solution by the addition of glycerol. When performing therapeutic celiac plexus block, we utilize 6% phenol, although 50% alcohol is employed in many other centers.

In sympathetically mediated pain (reflex sympathetic dystrophies, causalgia, etc.) the performance of the sympathetic block that establishes the diagnosis actually begins the therapy.

## Reflex Sympathetic Dystrophy

The term "reflex sympathetic dystrophy" was first used by Evans in 1947 and continues to be used to describe pain not related to the partial nerve damage associated with causalgia.[10] Precipitating events for reflex sympathetic dystrophy may include fractures, infections, lacerations, operations, injuries to muscle and ligaments, tumors, osteoporosis, vasculitis, injections, angina, myocardial infarctions, and psychological disorders.

Many other terms have also been used to describe this disease: posttraumatic sympathetic dystrophy, Sudeck's atrophy, posttraumatic dystrophy, shoulder/hand syndrome, traumatic edema, posttraumatic pain syndrome, sympathetic neurovascular dystrophy, causalgiastate, posttraumatic vasomitral disorder, painful osteoporosis, chronic segmental arterial spasms, posttraumatic sympathetic dysfunction, posttraumatic painful osteoporosis, posttraumatic spreading neuralgia, sympathalgia, acute atrophy of bone, traumatic angiospasm, chronic traumatic edema, and peripheral trophoneurosis. These confusing terms all relate to similar syndromes that may be grouped together under a single heading: Reflex sympathetic dystrophy (RSD).

## Assessment of Pain

Necessary information for making an accurate diagnosis of sympathetic dystrophies comes from understanding the mechanism of injury, eliciting the history of pain, and performing a physical examination. The psychological status of the patient must also be assessed to allow for complete diagnosis and implementation of an effective treatment program. When chronic pain persists, problems with drug dependence, pain behavior,

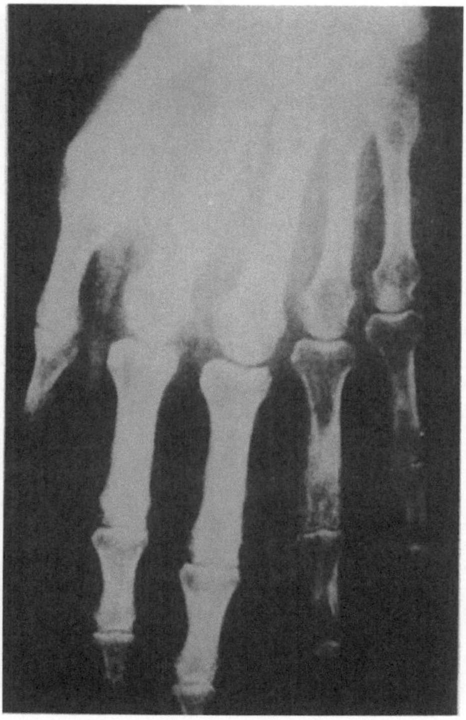

**Figure 6.1.** Patient with stage III RSD shows signs of patchy osteoporosis and demineralization in the subepiphyseal, periarticular, and distal joints.

and the development of central pain mechanisms may add to the physical problems.[11]

X-ray films and electrophysiological studies have proven to be of little value in the assessment of pain from reflex sympathetic dystrophy. A simple method is to measure skin temperature difference on the affected limb and compare it to the temperature of a nonaffected extremity by using surface electrodes or by simple palpation of the skin. One can usually palpate differences of more than 2°C.[11]

More definitive temperature changes may be seen by using thermography. It displays the variation of color in the cholesteric class of liquid crystals that results from temperature change. The greater the severity of RSD, the more pronounced is the temperature difference (and the color variation) between the affected and nonaffected side.[12,13]

In people with chronic pain, X-ray examinations often show patchy osteoporosis, demineralization in the subepiphyseal, periarticular, and distal joints. (Fig. 6.1) Such an X-ray should be taken with patient's both hands or feet on the same X-ray plate to eliminate the problems associated with differences in penetration, angle, or exposure.[11] Plethysmograms, bone scanning using $^{99}$Tc pyrophosphate, and Doppler techniques are other methods by which blood flow in extremities may be assessed.[11,14,15]

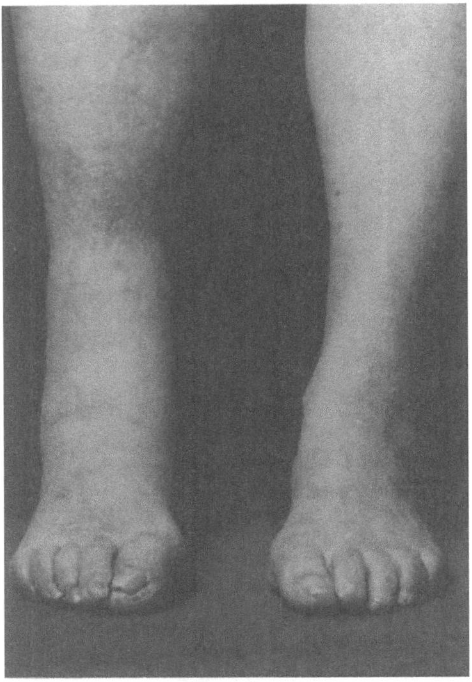

**Figure 6.2.** Stage II RSD. Note brittle nails, brawny edema, and differences in skin texture.

## Clinical Features

Reflex sympathetic dystrophy affects blood vessels, skin, muscles, and ultimately, bone. Symptoms depend on the stage of the disease—acute, dystrophic, or atrophic. However, not all patients will exhibit all the classical aspects of the syndrome. The common denominators are the presence of burning pain (dysesthesia), increased sensitivity to stimulation (hyperesthesia), and a painful syndrome characterized by overreaction to stimuli followed by sensations to stimuli (hyperpathia) in their absence.[16] Reflex sympathetic dystrophy can be described in three stages. Stage I is the acute or denervation phase characterized by the following:

Hyperpathia and burning pain
Increased blood flow, thus increased temperature in affected area
Accelerated hair and nail growth
Increased or decreased sweating, although skin usually feels dry
Localized soft edema
Rubor
Reduced range of motion secondary to pain

This state has been reported to last anywhere from 0 to 3 months; however, some patients may remain in this stage for several years.

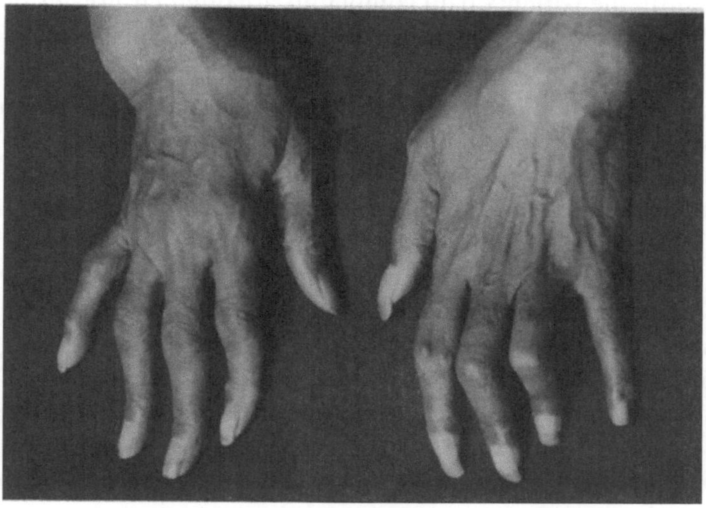

**Figure 6.3.** Atrophic phase of RSD: irreversible structural changes are seen in pericapsular fibrosis in the bones with tendon contracture leading to a frozen, useless extremity; thin, smooth, glossy skin; and muscle wasting.

Stage II begins as sympathetic hyperactivity manifests itself (Fig. 6.2) in the following signs and symptoms:

Hyperpathia and burning pain
Decreased blood flow, thus decreased temperature to affected area
Decreased hair growth and brittle nails
Markedly increased sweating (hyperhydrosis)
Spreading brawny edema
Pale, cyanotic color
Greatly limited range of motion leading to decreased muscle usage
Causalgic personality (constant attention to protection of affected extremity, withdrawal, desire for seclusion, dramatic reactions to painful stimuli)[11]

As the disease process progresses, either secondary to lack of treatment or lack of favorable response to persistent therapy, an atrophic stage begins. This stage fluctuates between the two previous stages (Fig. 6.3):

Less hyperpathia and burning pain
Fewer blood flow alterations, leading to less temperature difference
Increased or decreased sweating
Muscle wasting
Irreversible structural changes (i.e., pericapsular fibrosis in the bones with tendon contracture leading to a frozen, useless extremity)
Thin, smooth, glossy skin
Psychoneurosis, the personality characteristic of chronic pain syndrome

Significantly, the patient's pain complaints are often far greater than the injury. When severe, the pain always spreads to involve adjacent territories.

A great variety of stimuli may intensify the pain or provoke severe attacks, but the stimuli commonly fall into two classes: (1) anything that increases the activity of the limb, such as mechanical stimuli, cold, heat, muscular activity and movement, or even touching the affected area and (2) anything that increases the activity of the central nervous system or disturbs the status quo in the sensory neuronal pool may intensify pain. These incidents fall into several categories: (1) somatosensory, i.e., responses to temperature changes (many patients complain that heat increases and cold eases the pain; others claim that warmth gives greater relief; in other groups, both warm and cold intensify pain; (2) auditory stimuli in which the pain may be exacerbated by loud and unexpected noises, (3) visual disturbances, i.e., a sudden burst of sunlight, and (4) emotional disturbances, that may include witnessing a mishap, fear, anxiety, fatigue, and so on.[16]

Audrey Thomas, R.N., and associates, founders of the Reflex Sympathetic Dystrophy Syndrome Association, reported statistics of a survey of 271 reflex sympathetic dystrophy patients as follows:[18]

Incidence: males—22%; females—78%
Avg age onset: 33 yr
Age youngest: 4 yr
Avg time between onset and diagnosis: 1.1 yr
Avg time with RSD: 4.6 yr
Area of body first affected: upper extremity—42%, lower extremity—58%
Multiple areas involved: 69%
Most common precipitating factor: unknown—70%; injury—23%
Frequent muscle spasms: 82.7%
Formation of fibrous tissue: 59.9%
Most common medical disorder before onset of RSD: allergies—42%, headaches—31%
Most common medical disorder after onset of RSD: fatigue—55%, tension headache—29%
Still have RSD: 94%

## Etiology

The cause of RSD is not fully understood. For this reason finding a cure is difficult. Therapy is, therefore, directed toward treating the symptoms. Many authors support various views of the etiology of these symptoms, such as immunodeficiencies, i.e., reduced IgG or phytohaematagglutin (PHA); viruses, i.e., Epstein-Barr, coxsackie, herpes zoster; and genetic disorders such as human leukocyte antigen (HLA). Much study is still needed to support these theories.[19-21]

## Mechanism of Reflex Sympathetic Dystrophy

Debate about the mechanism of pain continues. Three possible sites have been suggested for the pain impulses: (1) the peripheral tissues where pain is felt, (2) the damaged segment of the nerve, and (3) the central nervous system.

The classical explanation is that a reflex increase in segmental sympathetic activity occurs, producing ischemia and increasing pain because of inadequate blood flow.[22] Vasodilation—producing warmth—and erythema may at times result from ischemia, with tissue hypoxia and accumulation of $CO_2$ and lactate causing dilatation of microvasculate through autoregulatory mechanisms (Fig. 6.4).[23]

Doupe and associates postulated that trauma or nerve damage caused a synapse between sympathetic efferent fibers and sympathetic afferent sensory fibers, forming a kind of short circuit. Thus, when the sympathetic impulse is generated, it creates physiological consequences (e.g., vasomotor and sudomotor changes) and depolarizes the somatic nerve, thus producing pain. This further contributes to the release of chemical substances in the periphery.[24]

In 1965, Melzack and Wall proposed the gate control theory to explain the interaction of multiple factors in the production of the sensory and emotional experience. They proposed that the balance of large- and small-fiber input to the central nervous system (CNS) is disrupted by injury to a body area. Whenever fast-conducting large fibers are proportionally reduced in number, a state of imbalance results. The spinal cord, receiving an excess of slowly conducted, unopposed impulses, now "opens the gate."

Small-fiber traffic through the system is thereby increased and pain results. Conversely, stimulating large fibers "closes the gate" and reduces the pain. This is the basis of the therapeutic use of large-fiber stimulation TENS (transcutaneous electrical nerve stimulator) for the relief of intractable pain (Fig. 6.5).[25,26]

## Sympathetic Blockade

Historically, sympathetic blockade has been the mainstay of RSD treatment.[27,28] Traditionally, sympathetic blockade of the upper extremity has been accomplished via the stellate ganglion, whereas lower extremity blockade has been performed through the lumbar sympathetic plexus.

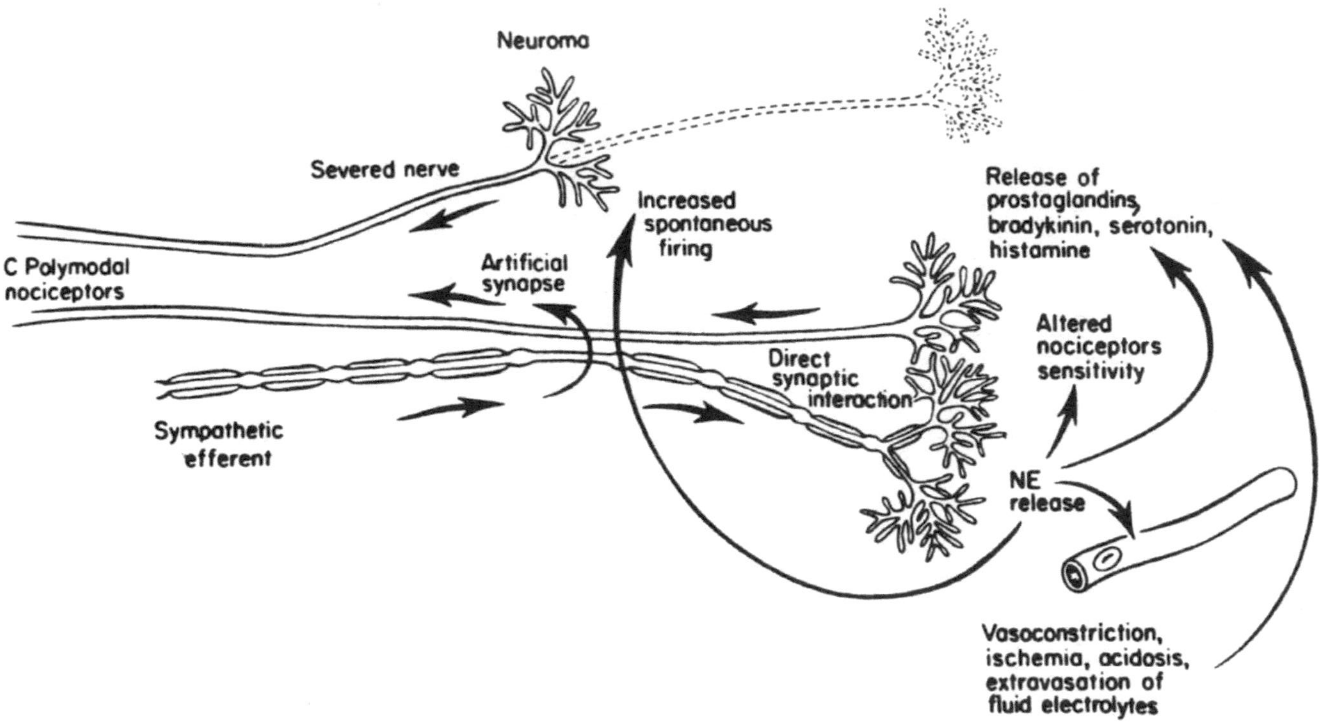


**Figure 6.4.** Possible interaction between the sympathetic nervous system and peripheral nociceptors. From Abram, S.E., "Sympathetic Pain," in Raj, PP (1986), *Practical Management of Pain*. Chicago: Year Book Medical Publishers, p. 211. Reproduced with permission.

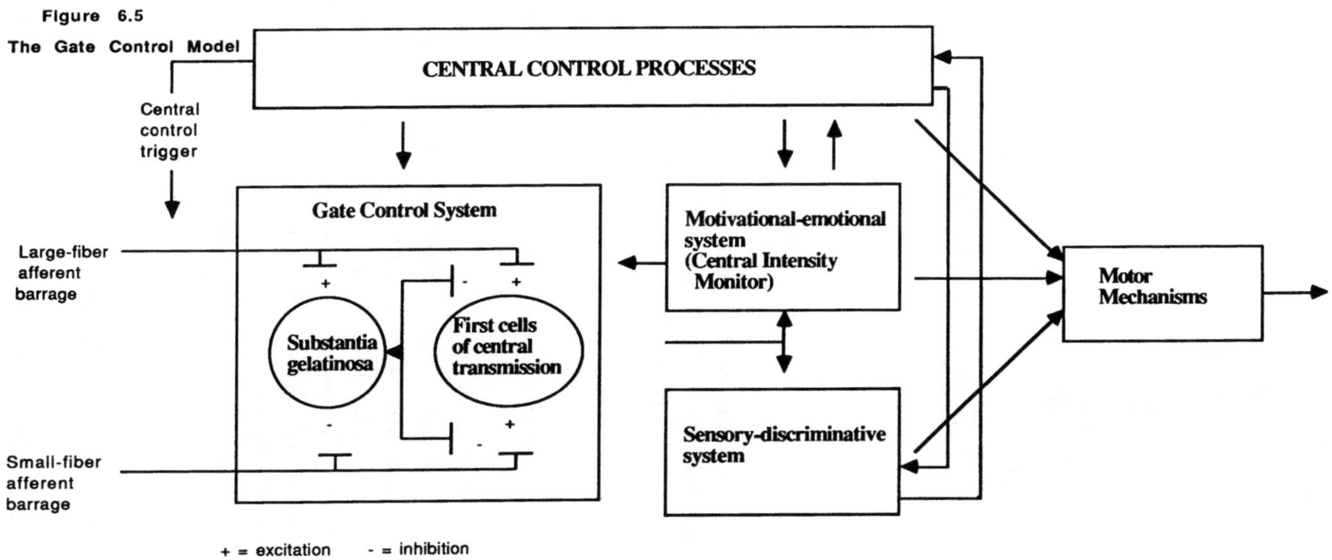


**Figure 6.5.** The gate control model. From Melzack, R. and Wall, P. (1968). Used with permission.

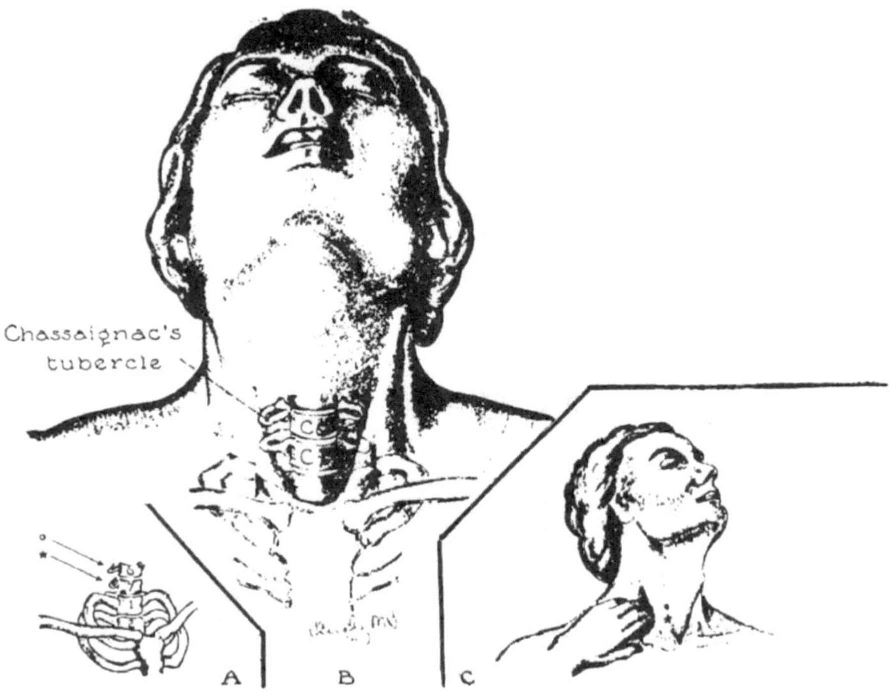


**Figure 6.6.** Anterior paracervical approach for stellate ganglion blockade at the level of C6. Method of palpating Chassaignac's tubercle of transverse process of $C_6$ vertebra. From Moore, D.C. (1981), *Regional Block. A Handbook for Use in the Clinical Practice of Medicine & Surgery*, 4th ed. Springfield, IL: Charles C Thomas, p. 130.

Before these techniques became standard, sympathectomy was accomplished by surgical destruction.[29]

In a review of 113 cases, Patman and co-workers had 93 patients obtain good-to-excellent pain relief after either blockade or destruction of appropriate sympathetic ganglion. They reported 20% of their patients with residual symptoms.[29] Similar results were reported in a followup study of 156 patients.[30] In a series of 140 cases, 92% of the patients received good-to-excellent relief of symptoms, which persisted to followup 9.2 months after treatment.[31] We use two methods of sympathetic blockade in our clinic: direct blockade of sympathetic ganglion and intravenous regional blockade of postganglionic sympathetic fibers.

## Upper-Extremity Sympathetic Blockade

Stellate ganglion blockade is the standard technique for upper-extremity sympathectomy. We use 5 to 10 cc of 0.25 to 0.5% bupivicaine and occasionally add 20 to 40 mg of depomedrol. The block is accomplished using an anterior paracervical approach at C6 (Figs. 6.6 and 6.7). A detailed

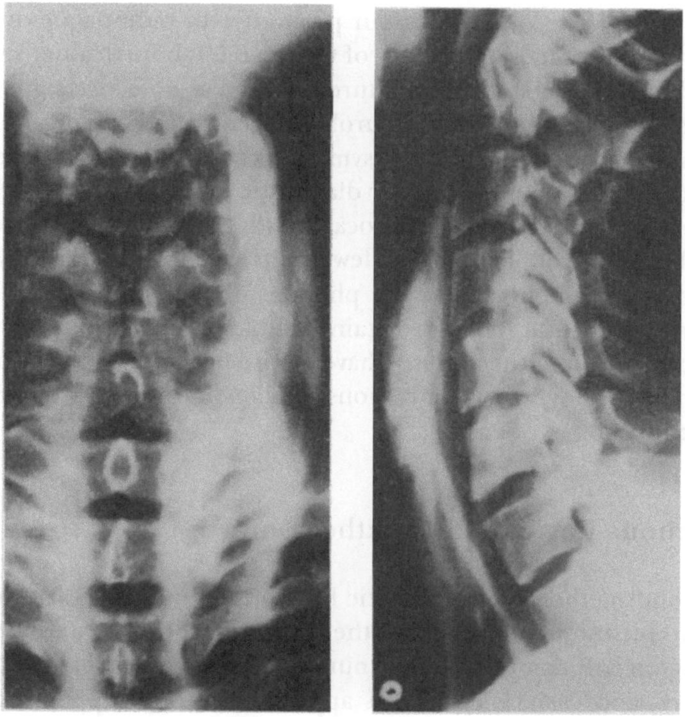

**Figure 6.7.** Verification of needle placement by using contrast medium prior to local anesthetic. (A) AP view, (B) lateral view. From Cousins, M. and Bridenbaugh, P. (1988). Sympathetic neural blockade of the upper and lower extremity. *Neurol Blockade in Clinical Anesthesia and Management of Pain*, 2nd ed., p. 481.

description of this technique as well as associated morbidity can be found in Moore's excellent monograph.[32] The appearance of Horner's syndrome may be associated with blockade of only the most cephalad fibers in this ganglion, so we also look for vasodilation and increase in temperature in the ipsilateral extremity as demonstration of an adequate block. We initially plan to do a series of three blocks over a one-week period. We continue to perform stellate blocks after the third block for recurrence of symptoms as long as the time period between block and recurrence of symptoms continues to expand. When that time period plateaus, we try another technique (see below). Because of the high morbidity associated with permanent neurolytic agents, we do not employ them for stellate blockade. Instead, we have tried both steroids and morphine.

## Lower-Extremity Sympathetic Blockade

Sympathetic blockade of the lower extremity is accomplished under fluoroscopic guidance. The patient is placed in a prone position and a 7-in. 22 gauge needle is placed at the ventrolateral border of the spinal bodies at the L2-3 interspace. We confirm our position with radiopaque dye (Figs. 6.8 and 6.9), and then inject 10 cc of 0.25 to 0.5% bupivicaine. Vasodilation and increase in skin temperature are used as objective signs of successful blocks. We then use a neurolytic agent for a chemical ablative sympathectomy with resolution of symptoms by temporary blockade. The same technique is employed as for diagnostic block, but 3 cc of a neurolytic agent is injected instead of a local anesthetic. Initially, we were using 3 cc of absolute alcohol, but after a few occurrences of L1 neuritis, we have switched to 8% phenol. With 8% phenol we have found that we must occasionally repeat a block to obtain complete destruction of the sympathetic ganglion. Other groups have informed us that they avoid this problem by employing concentrations of phenol up to 12% (Raj's written communication).

## Intravenous Regional Sympathectomy

The second method of sympathetic blockade we use is the intravenous regional technique with guanethedine, a technique developed by Hannington-Kiff and validated by numerous other investigators.[33–40] Simple, quick, and easy to learn, it is applicable to both upper and lower extremities. During the procedure, guanethedine acts at sympathetic postganglionic nerve endings causing a depletion in noradrenaline (NA). Initially, guanethedine causes NA release from nerve endings and also inhibits reuptake of NA from the sympathetic cleft into the neurosecretory granules. The result of these actions is a profound decrease in sympathetic function in the blocked limb. At very high concentrations, guanethidine has also been shown to cause retraction of the nerve axon, which is essential in a chemical sympathectomy.[41]

The intravenous regional technique is performed on an outpatient basis. An IV is started in the affected limb, with 20 cc of 0.5% lidocaine with 20 mg guanethedine for upper extremities, or 30 cc of 0.5% lidocaine with 40 mg guanethedine for lower extremities. The tourniquet is inflated before the drug is instilled and is kept inflated for 20 minutes. Afterward, the tourniquet is gradually released, and skin temperature and vasodilation are monitored, although they may not be a useful indication of the efficacy of the block. The patient receives a series of three blocks within a one-week period.

The results of at least two studies show equal efficacy of both IV regional (IVR) and stellate ganglion blockade.[28,37] Currently, there are no studies directly comparing IVR to lower extremity sympathetic blockade. Other techniques of sympathetic blockade, such as continuous block utilizing an indwelling catheter or continuous IV infusion, have been described by other groups.[42–44] We rarely employ these techniques because they require that the patient be admitted to the hospital. However, we occasionally use these techniques for inpatients with good results.

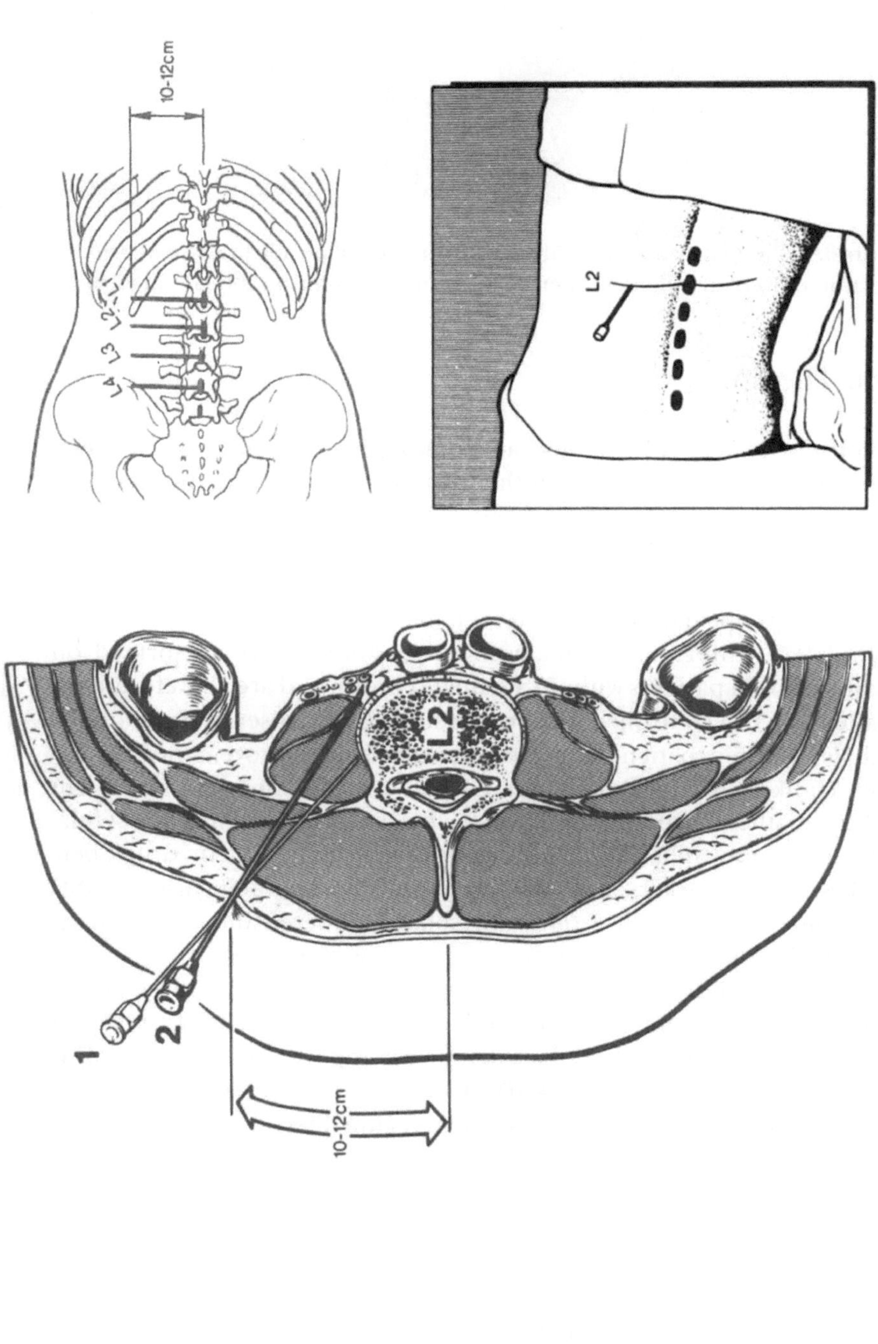


**Figure 6.8.** Lumbar sympathetic block. Needle placement is ventrolateral to the vertebral body of L2.

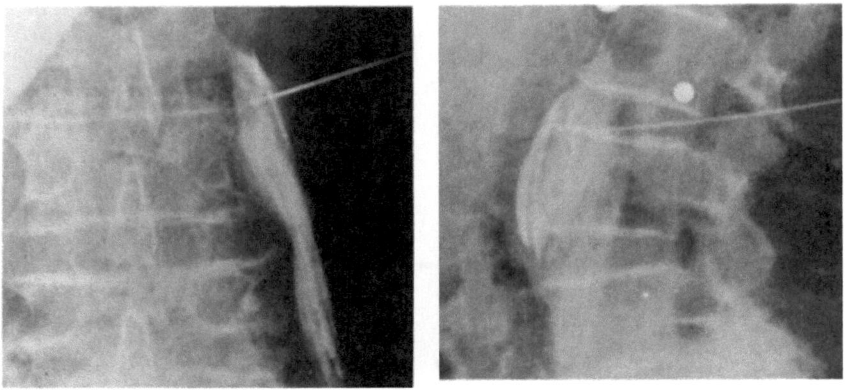

**Figure 6.9.** Lumbar sympathetic block confirmation of needle placement prior to injection of local anesthetic or neurolytic solution. Anterior and lateral views.

## Oral Therapies

In contrast to sympathetic blockade, oral agents have not proven themselves particularly efficacious in the treatment of RSD and, therefore, we strongly believe oral narcotic analgesics have no place in RSD treatment. We do routinely employ aspirin, acetaminophen, and nonsteroidal anti-inflammatory oral agents.

Several groups have reported reasonable results with systemic corticosteroids.[45-47] Unfortunately, many of these studies were performed on small groups of patients without adequate control and are, therefore, hard to interpret. In a controlled prospective study, Christensen and co-workers had 75% of their patients show good-to-excellent improvement in symptoms. Unlike our typical patient, their patients had symptoms consistent with sympathetic hypofunction for which corticosteroids may be useful.[47]

There are multiple reports of various oral antisympathetic drugs, beta blockers, alpha blockers, and calcium channel blockers being used in RSD treatment.[48-50] These case reports are isolated, however, and no systematic investigation of the efficacy of these agents has been made.

One new oral drug of particular interest is ketanserin. Ketanserin is a type I seratonin receptor antagonist that interacts with a specific receptor to cause vasodilation. There have been case reports from Europe of its efficacy in treating refractory RSD.[51] Currently, the drug is administered orally, but it may have potential use in IV regional techniques followed by oral administration.

## Physical Therapy

In our practice, physical therapy is the mainstay of RSD treatment. Patients with acute and chronic pain are involved in an appropriate physical therapy program. When symptoms interfere with adequate physical therapy, one of the interventions discussed above is used to aid the patient in continuing his or her program. The orthopedic literature advocates early postinjury physical therapy to avoid RSD development and physical therapy for treating RSD if it occurs. We believe in this approach and convey this attitude to all our patients.

## Behavior Modification

We believe our patients with chronic pain should be involved with behavior therapy administered by a professional. We assure all our patients from the start that we believe in the validity of their pain and explain to them the pathophysiology of their disease and treatment modalities and also explain the effect chronic pain has on life-styles, and how life-styles can affect their pain. Many of our patients have had pain despite multiple therapeutic interactions. Our goal is to have them function despite their pain.

Psychological factors play an important role in the way anyone perceives pain.[2] We inform our patients that behavioral therapy can help them manage their pain with such techniques as biofeedback, relaxation, and coping strategies. These can easily be taught to patients, allowing them to effectively manage situations that previously exacerbated their pain.

The diagnosis of RSD (see above) includes specific pathophysiologic findings. Treatment of RSD can and should occur even in psychiatric patients, who should be treated on an outpatient basis unless they require inpatient services for other reasons.

In summary, we feel that all our chronic patients need behavioral therapy. Without it, our other services provide them little benefit. The presence of a psychologist who acknowledges the patient's pain and keeps a positive attitude is easily accepted by our patients in their treatment and greatly benefits them.

### References

1. Rowlingson, J.C. (1985). Management of the patient with intractable pain. *American Society of Anesthesiologists. Refresher Course Lectures No. 256*:1–7.
2. Bonica, J.J. (1980). Pain research therapy: Past and current states and future needs. In L.K.Y. Ng and J.J. Bonica (Eds.), *Pain, Discomfort and Humanitarian Care.* New York: Elsevier/North Holland, pp. 1–46.
3. Black, R. (1980). The clinical syndrome of chronic pain. In L.K.Y. Ng and J.J. Bonica (Eds.), *Pain, Discomfort and Humanitarian Care.* New York: Elsevier/North Holland, pp. 207–220.
4. Arnoff, G. (1982). The use of non-narcotic drugs and other alternatives for analgesia as part of a comprehensive pain management program. *Journal of Medicine* 13:191–202.

5. Winnie, A.P. (1987). Regional anesthesia as a diagnostic maneuver. *Cook County Graduate School Review Course.* Evanston, IL: Northwestern University Medical School.
6. McCollum, D., Stephen C.R. (1964). Use of graduated spinal anesthesia in the differential diagnosis of pain of the back and lower extremities. *South Medical Journal* 57:410.
7. Winnie, A., Collins, V. (1968). The pain clinic I: Differential neural blockade in pain syndromes of questionable etiology. *Medical Clinics in America* 52:123–129.
8. Halpern, L. (1982). Substitution-detoxification and its role in the management of chronic benign pain. *Journal of Clinical Psychiatry* 43:10–14.
9. Williams, N. (1981). Current views on the pharmacological management of pain. In M. Swerdlow (Ed.), *The Therapy of Pain, Vol. 6*, Philadelphia: Lippincott Co., p. 87.
10. Evans, J.A. (1947). Reflex sympathetic dystrophy. Report in 57 cases. *Annals of Internal Medicine*, 26:417.
11. Rowlingson, J.C. (1983). The sympathetic dystrophies. *International Anesthesiology Clinics* 21(4):117–128.
12. Fergason, J.L. (1964). Liquid crystals. *Scientific American* 211:76–82.
13. Uematsu, S., Hendeler, N., Hungerford, D. (1981). Thermography and electromyography in the differential diagnosis of chronic pain syndrome and reflex sympathetic dystrophy. *Electromyographic Clinical Neurophysiology* 21:165–182.
14. Boas, R.A. (1978). Sympathetic blocks in the clinical practice. *International Anesthesiology Clinics* 16(4):149.
15. Carlson, D.H., Simon, H., Wegner, W. (1977). Bone scanning and diagnosis of RSD secondary to herniated lumbar discs. *Neurology* 27:791–793.
16. Mersky, H. et al. (1979). Pain terms: A list with definitions and notes on usage. *Pain* 6:249–252.
17. Sunderland, S. (1976). Pain mechanisms in causalgia. *Journal of Neurology, Neurosurgery, and Psychiatry* 39:471–481.
18. Thomas, A., Davis, F., Davis, R. (1987). Reflex sympathetic dystrophy syndrome association questionnaire statistics. Information not published.
19. Visitsunthorn, U., Prete, P. (1981). Reflex sympathetic dystrophy of the lower extremity—A complication of herpes zoster with dramatic response to propranol. *The Western Journal of Medicine* 135:62–66.
20. Ott, A., Ott, H. (1983). Three brothers with algodystrophy of the hip. *Annals of Rheumatoid Disease* 42:421–424.
21. Grosslight, K.R., Rowlinson, J.D., Broaden, R.W. (1986). Herpes zoster and reflex sympathetic dystrophy. *Anesthesia and Analgesia* 65:309–311.
22. Zimmerman, M. (1979). Peripheral and central nervous mechanisms of noeiception, pain and pain therapy: Fact and hypotheses. In J.J. Bonica, J.C. Liebeskind, D.G. Albe-Fressard. (Eds.), *Advances in Pain Research and Therapy, Vol. 3*. New York: Raven Press, pp. 3–32.
23. Abram, S.E. (1983). Common pain syndromes and their therapy. In S.G. Hershey (Ed.), *Refresher Courses in Anesthesiology, Vol. 11*, American Society of Anesthesiologists, Massachusetts, pp. 1–12.
24. Doupe, J., Cullen, C.H., Chance, G.Q. (1944). Posttraumatic pain and causalgia syndrome. *Journal of Neurology, Neurosurgery and Psychiatry* 7:33–44.
25. Melzack, R., Wall, P. (1968). Gate control theory of pain. In A. Soulaire, J. Cahn, and J. Charpentier. (Eds.), *Pain*. London: Academic Press.

26. Melzack, R., Wall, P. (1965). Pain mechanisms: A new theory. *Science* 150:971–979.
27. Bonica, J.J. (1979). Causalgia and other reflex sympathetic dystrophies. In *Advances in Pain Research and Therapy, Vol. 3*. New York: Raven Press, pp. 141–166.
28. Eriksen, S. (1981). Duration of sympathetic blockade. Stellate ganglion block versus intravenous regional guanethidine block. *Anaesthesia* 36:768–771.
29. Patman, R.D., Thompson, J.E., Persson, A.V. (1973). Management of post-traumatic pain syndrome: Report 113 cases. *Annals of Surgery* 117:780–787.
30. Thompson, J.E., Patman, R.D., Persson, A.V. (1975). Management of post-traumatic pain syndromes (Causalgia). *American Surgeon* 41:599–602.
31. Pak, T.J., Martin, G.M., Magness, J.L., Kavanaugh, G.J. (1970). Reflex sympathetic dystrophy: Review of 140 cases. *Minnesota Medicine* 53:507–512.
32. Moore, D.C. (1981). *Regional Block. A Handbook for Use in the Clinical Practice of Medicine and Surgery*, 4th ed. Springfield, IL: Charles C Thomas.
33. Hannington-Kiff, J.G. (1974). Intravenous regional sympathetic block with guanethidine. *Lancet* 1:1019–1020.
34. Hannington-Kiff, J.G. (1977). Relief of Sudek's atrophy by regional intravenous guanethidine. *Lancet* 1:1132–1133.
35. Hannington-Kiff, J.G. (1979). Relief of causalgia in limbs by regional intravenous guanethidine. *British Medical Journal* 2:367–368.
36. Glynn, C.J., Basedow, R.W., Walsh, J.A. (1981). Pain relief following postganglionic sympathetic blockade with IV guanethidine. *British Journal of Anesthesiology* 53:1297–1302.
37. Bonelli, S., Conoscente, F., Movilia, P.G., Restelli, L., Francucci, B., Grossi, E. (1983). Regional intravenous guanethidine vs. stellate ganglion block in reflex sympathetic dystrophies: A randomized trial. *Pain* 16:297–307.
38. Hannington-Kiff, J.G. (1984). Antisympathetic drugs in limbs. In P.D. Wall and R. Melzack (Eds.), *Textbook of Pain*. New York: Churchill Livingstone, pp. 566–573.
39. Driessen, J.L., Vander Werken, C., Nicolai, J.P., Crul, J.F. (1983). Clinical effects of regional intravenous guanethidine in reflex sympathetic dystrophy. *Acta Anaesthesiologica Scandinavica* 27:505–509.
40. Loh, L., Nathan, P.W., Schott, G.D., Wilson, P.G. (1980). Effects of regional guanethidine infusion in certain pain states. *Journal of Neurology, Neurosurgery, and Psychiatry* 43:446.
41. Burnstock, G., Costa, M. (1975). *Adrenergic Neurons*. London: Chapman and Hall.
42. Leipzig, T.J., Mullan S.F. (1984). Causalgic pain relieved by prolonged procaine amide sympathetic blockade. *Journal of Neurosurgery* 60:1095–1096.
43. Visitsunthorn, U., Prete, P. (1981). Reflex sympathetic dystrophy of the lower extremity. A coplication of herpes zoster with dramatic response to propranolol. *Western Journal of Medicine* 135:62–66.
44. Lewis, R., Racz, G. (1985). Therapeutic approaches to reflex sympathetic dystrophy of the upper extremity. *Clinical Issues in Regional Anesthesia* No. 2, 1:1–6.
45. Kozin, F., Ryan, L.M., Carerra, G.F., Soin, J.S., Wortmann, R.L. (1981). The reflex sympathetic dystrophy syndrome (RSDS). *American Journal of Medicine* 70:23
46. Mowat, A.G. (1974). Treatment of the shoulder–hand syndrome with corticosteroids. *Annals of Rheumatic Diseases* 33:120–123.
47. Christensen, K., Jensen, E.M., Noer, I. (1982). The reflex dystrophy syndrome response to treatment with systemic corticosteroids. *Acta Chirurgica Scandinavica* 148:653–655.

48. Thompson, J.E. (1979). The diagnosis and management of post-traumatic pain syndromes (causalgia). *Australia New Zealand Journal of Surgery* 49:299–304.
49. Prough, D.S., McLeskey, C.H., Poehling, G.G., Koman, L.A., Weeks, D.B., Whitworth, T., Semble, E.L. (1985). Efficacy of oral nifedipine in the treatment of reflex sympathetic dystrophy. *Anesthesiology* 62:796–799.
50. Ghostine, S.Y., Comair, Y.G., Turner, D.M., Kassell, N.F., Azar, C.G., (1984). Phenoxybenzamine in the treatment of causalgia. Report of 40 cases. *Journal of Neurosurgery* 60:1263–1268.
51. Davies, J.A.H., Beswick, T., Dickson, G. (1987). Ketanserin and guanethidine in the treatment of causalgia. *Anesthesia and Analgesia* 66:575–576.

# 7

# Pharmacologic Treatment of Chronic Pain

*Richard G. Fessler*

The pharmacologic treatment of chronic pain can be achieved through a multifaceted approach that enables selection of specific pharmaceutical preparations within a specific drug family, as well as selection between several independent families of drugs. In addition, combinations of drugs chosen from different families can be utilized to maximize pain relief while minimizing undesirable side effects. Several principles should be kept in mind when prescribing medications for the treatment of chronic pain. First, pharmacotherapy is only one part of a comprehensive approach to chronic pain. Pain relief can be augmented by combining physical therapy, psychological assessment, behavior modification, TENS, etc., with appropriate medication. Second, pain medication only reduces symptoms—it does not definitively treat the underlying problem(s). Third, minimize the number and frequency of medications whenever possible. This reduces potential side effects, and confusion regarding dosing schedules. Fourth, use drug combinations that do not have additive side effects. For example, aspirin and ibuprofen both have predominantly gastrointestinal side effects. Using them in combination can put the patient at increased risk of developing gastric or duodenal ulcers. Acetaminophen, however, has lower incidence of ulcerogenesis and, therefore, is a better agent for combining with ibuprofen and/or similar medications. Fifth, side effects may increase over time. Finally, narcotics should be avoided in treatment of chronic pain syndromes, with the possible exception of short-term treatment of acute pain exacerbations.

The most commonly prescribed medications for treatment of chronic pain disorders fall into one of several categories: (1) salicylates, (2) aniline derivatives, (3) nonsteroidal anti-inflammatory agents, (4) muscle relaxants/anxiolytics, (5) anti-depressants, and (6) mild narcotics. This chapter

acetylsalicylic acid

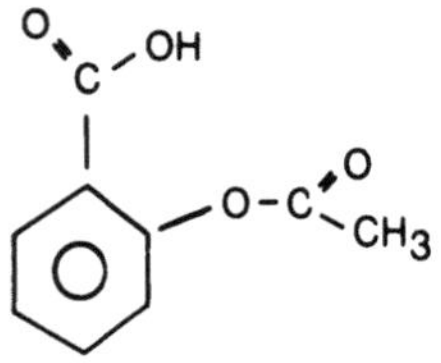


**Figure 7.1.** Structural formula of acetylsalicylic acid.

will review the history, basic pharmacology, therapeutic uses, and side effects/toxicities of these compounds. Tables in each section will list representative examples from each group, and detail recommended doses and dosing schedules. Side effects are discussed and are listed in tables when appropriate. Finally, Figures 7.1 to 7.7 demonstrate the structural formulas for representative examples from each of these drug families.

## Non-Narcotic Analgesics

### Salicylates

#### *History*

Aspirin (acetylsalicylic acid, Fig. 7.1) is the most widely prescribed analgesic-antipyretic and anti-inflammatory agent in the United States. Estimates place the quantity used as high as 30 million pounds annually. The analgesic affect of the salicylates has been known for centuries in the form of willow tree bark (salix). In 1763, Edmund Stone reported the effect of white willow in reducing fever. The active ingredient of the willow bark was then isolated in 1829 by Leroux, as Selicin. Salicylic acid was also prepared from oil of wintergreen in extracts of other plants such as spiraea. Finally the synthetic form of salicylic acid was prepared in 1860 by Kolbe and Lautemann. After this drug was demonstrated to be anti-inflammatory as well as antipyretic it was introduced by Dreser into common medical usage in 1899 under the name of aspirin.

#### *Pharmacokinetics*

*Absorption.* Oral salicylates are rapidly absorbed from both the stomach and upper gastrointestinal system, with significant plasma concentrations reached in less than 30 minutes, and peak concentrations in approximately 2 hours. Salicylate absorption occurs primarily from passive diffusion of the nonassociated lipid soluble molecule across GI membranes.

Rates of absorption, therefore, are influenced by multiple factors including gastric pH, gastric emptying time, the presence or absence of food, and the rates of dissolution of the tablets administered. Rate of absorption is increased by increasing pH and the solubility of salicylate; however, increasing pH also increases ionization of salicylate and thus tends to decrease absorption. Functionally, changes in absorption have minimal clinical significance, since the rate-limiting step in the effect of salicylate is the accumulation of this compound at its site of action. Applying salicylate dermally to the skin through ointments is an effective means of obtaining rapid therapeutic levels. Absorption by a rectal administration, however, results in unreliable absorption and is not a preferred route of administration.

Following absorption and transfer of the nonionized form of salicylate acid into the mucosal cell, ionization occurs and significant intracellular accumulation of salicylate can occur. This accumulation of intracellular salicylate may be responsible for mucosal damage.

*Distribution.* Following absorption, salicylate is rapidly distributed throughout most body tissues, with an average volume of distribution of 160 ml/kg of body weight. Although ingested aspirin is absorbed in the acetylated form, it is rapidly hydrolyzed to salicylic acid, thus aspirin levels in plasma are generally lower than 20 μg per ml at therapeutic doses. Eighty to 90% of salicylate is bound to plasma protein, particularly albumin, thus hypoalbuminemia predisposes to increased concentrations of free salicylate in the plasma and hence salicylate toxicity. In binding with human plasma albumin in vivo, salicylate competes with thyroxine, triiodothyronine, penicillin, thiopental, Dilantin, sulfinpyrazone, bilirubin, peptides, steroids, and nonsteroidal anti-inflammatory agents.

*Metabolism and Excretion.* Salicylate is metabolized predominantly in hepatic endoplasmic reticulum. The major metabolic by-products are the glycine conjugate salicylurate and the phenol- and acylglucuronides.

Excretion then occurs mainly by the kidney as salicyluric acid (75%), salicylic acid (10%), phenolic salicylate, and glucuronides (10%), acyl glucuronides (5%), and gentisic acid (1%). Salicylurate excretion is significantly affected by urinary pH, however. Alkalinization of the urine is associated with an increase in excretion of free-salicylurate of up to 85% of total excretion. Acidification, on the other hand, can decrease the concentration of free-salicylurate in urine to as low as 5%.

The urinary excretion of salicylurate is dose dependent and limited by the ability of the hepatic microsomal system to form salicyluric acid and phenolic glucuronides. Thus, whereas the plasma half-life of aspirin is approximately 15 minutes and that for salicylurate 2 to 3 hours, at low therapeutic doses, at high therapeutic or toxic doses the plasma half-life of salicylurate may be as long as 15 to 30 hours.

*Toxicity*

Salicylates are more frequently involved in poisonings than any other compound. Signs and symptoms of toxicity are poorly correlated with serum salicylate concentration or total daily dose, but rarely occur below concentrations of 15 mg/100 ml or doses of 3 g/day and usually are present at concentrations above 35 mg/100 ml and doses of 10 g/day. Serious poisoning is rare below concentrations of 50 mg/100 ml, but common at concentrations between 50 and 100 mg/100 ml. Fatalities have been reported with ingestions of 10 to 30 g of sodium salicylate in adults, although quantities up to 130 g of aspirin have been ingested without fatal outcome. Over 10,000 cases of salicylate intoxication are reported yearly, some of them fatal, and many occurring in children.

Symptoms of salicylate intoxication include headache, dizziness, tinnitus, difficulty hearing, dimness of vision, confusion, lethargy and drowsiness, hyperventilation, hyperhidrosis, nausea and vomiting, and diarrhea. Severe intoxication is characterized by marked central nervous system alterations, (including seizure, coma, and EEG abnormalities), alternations in systemic acid-base balance (including fever, dehydration, and acidosis), petechial hemorrhages, pulmonary edema, acneform eruption, GI symptoms, and cardiovascular decompensation. These signs and symptoms are summarized in Tables 7.2 and 7.3.

*Therapeutic Effects*

Aspirin is an effective analgesic for the relief of certain types of pain such as headache, arthritis, dysmenorrhea, neuralgia, and myalgia. Tolerance does not develop and dependence is rather unusual, even with chronic use. To be effective, plasma concentrations of 150 to 300 mg/ml are desired. These can generally be achieved using doses ranging from 325 to 650 mg orally every 4 hours for adults and 65 mg/kg/day divided in 4 to 6 doses for children.

At these doses aspirin is also an effective antipyretic without affecting normal body temperatures. Moreover, salicylates are still regarded as the standard to which other drugs are compared for the treatment of inflammatory diseases such as rheumatoid arthritis. In addition to analgesia, salicylates also produce inflammation in joint tissues and surrounding structures, thereby decreasing or delaying the development of joint crippling. Table 7.1 lists some of the aspirin products currently available, as well as added active ingredients and usual adult daily doses. Added ingredients generally potentiate analgesia (e.g., caffeine), produce analgesia independently of aspirin (e.g., codeine, hydrocodone, acetaminophen) stimulate (e.g., caffeine, pseudoephedrine), sedate (e.g., butalbital, meprobamate) or buffer (e.g., aluminum hydroxide, $NaHCO_3$[2]). In addition, aspirin cold formulas usually contain antihistamines. The following

**Table 7.1.** Adult Oral Aspirin Preparations

| Product | Quantity (mg) | Additional Ingredient (mg) | Recommended Dosage |
|---|---|---|---|
| Alka Seltzer | 324 | $NaHCO_3^{-2}$ 1916<br>Citric acid 1000 | 2 tablets every 4 hours |
| A.S. Extra Strength | 500 | $NaHCO_3^{-2}$ 1985<br>Citric acid 1000 | 2 tablets every 4 hours |
| A.S. Plus Cold Medicine | 324 | $NaHCO_3^{-2}$<br>Citric acid<br>Phenylpropanolamine 24.08<br>Chlorpheniramine 2 | 2 tablets every 4 hours, max. = 8/24 hours |
| A.S. Plus Nighttime Medicine | 324 | $NaHCO_3^{-2}$<br>Citric acid<br>Phenylpropanolamine 24.08<br>Diphenhydramine 38.33 | 2 tablets at bedtime |
| Anacin | 400 | Caffeine 32 | 2 tablets every 4 hours, max. = 10/24 hours |
| Anacin Maximum Strength | 500 | Caffeine 32 | 2 tablets every 6–8 hours, max. = 8/24 hours |
| Arthritis Pain Formula | 500 | Aluminum hydroxide 33<br>Magnesium hydroxide 100 | 2 tablets every 6–8 hours, max. = 8/24 hours |
| Axotol | 650 | Butalbital 50* | 1 tablet every 4 hours, max. = 6/24 hours |
| B-A-C tablets | 650 | Caffeine 40<br>Butalbital 50* | 1 tablet every 4 hours, max. = 6/24 hours |
| Bayer tablets | 325 | | 1–2 tablets every 4 hours, max. = 12/24 hours |
| Bayer Maximum Strength | 500 | | 1–2 tablets every 4 hours, max. = 8/24 hours |
| Bufferin Analgesic Tablets | 324 | Aluminum glycinate<br>Magnesium carbonate | 2 tablets every 4 hours, max. = 12/24 hours |
| Bufferin Arthritis Strength | 486 | Aluminum glycinate<br>Magnesium carbonate | 2 tablets every 4 hours, max. = 8/24 hours |

**Table 7.1.** (*Continued*)

| Product | Quantity (mg) | Additional Ingredient (mg) | Recommended Dosage |
|---|---|---|---|
| Bufferin Extra Strength | 500 | Aluminum glycinate<br>Magnesium carbonate | 2 tablets every 4 hours, max. = 8/24 hours |
| Damason-P | 224 | Hydrocodone5*<br>Caffeine 32 | 1 tablet every 4–6 hours |
| Easprin (enteric coated) | 975 | | 1 tablet every 6–8 hours |
| Ecotrin (enteric coated) | 325 | | 2 tablets every 4 hours |
| Ecotrin Maximum Strength | 500 | | 2 tables every 6 hours |
| Empirin | 325 | | 1–2 tablets every 4 hours |
| Empirin with codeine | 325 | Codeine #2 15* | 1–2 tablets every 4 hours |
| | | Codeine #3 30* | 1–2 tablets every 4 hours |
| | | Codeine #4 60* | 1 tablet every 4 hours |
| Equagesic | 325 | Meprobamate 200* | 1–2 tablets every 6 hours |
| Exedrin Extra Strength | 250 | Acetaminophen 250<br>Caffeine 65 | 2 tablets every 4 hours, max. = 8/24 hours |
| 4-Way Cold Tablets | 324 | Phenylpropanolamine 12.5<br>Chlorpheniramine | 2 tablets every 4 hours, max. = 8/24 hours |
| Fiogesic | 325 | Pseudoephedrine 30 | 2 tablets every 4 hours, max. = 8/24 hours |
| Fiorinal | 325 | Butalbital 50*<br>Caffeine 40 | 1–2 tablets every 4 hours, max. = 6/24 hours |
| Fiorinal with Codeine | 325 | Butalbital 50*<br>Caffeine 40 | 1–2 tablets every 8 hours, max. = 6/24 hours |
| | | Codeine #1 7.<br>#2 15.0<br>#3 30.0 | |
| Midol | 454 | Cinnamedrine 14.9<br>Caffeine 32.4 | 2 tablets every 4 hours, max. = 8/24 hours |

**Table 7.1.** (*Continued*)

| Product | Quantity (mg) | Additional Ingredient (mg) | Recommended Dosage |
|---|---|---|---|
| Midol Maximum | 500 | Cinnamedrine 14.9<br>Caffeine 32.4 | 2 tablets every 4 hours, max. = 8/24 hours |
| Norgesic | 385 | Orphenadrine 25<br>Caffeine 30 | 1–2 tablets every 6–8 hours |
| Norgesic Forte | 770 | Orphenadrine 50<br>Caffeine 60 | ½–1 tablet every 6–8 hours |
| Supac | 230 | Acetaminophen 160<br>Caffeine 33<br>Calcium gluconate 60 | 1–2 tablets every 4 hours, max. = 16/24 hours |
| Synalgas-DC | 356.4 | Dihydrocodeine*<br>Caffeine 30 | 2 capsules every 4 hours |
| Talwin | 325 | Pentazocine* 125 | 2 caplets every 6–8 hours |
| Vanquish | 227 | Acetaminophen 194<br>Caffeine 33<br>Aluminum hydroxide 25<br>Magnesium hydroxide 50 | 2 caplets every 4 hours, max. = 12/24 hours |

*Prolonged use of these compounds may be habit forming.

discussion pertains to only the acetylsalicylic acid component of these analgesics and refers only to their analgesic indications for adults.

### *Side Effects*

*Respiration.* Salicylates increase respiration both directly and indirectly. Indirectly salicylates increase oxygen consumption and $CO_2$ production by uncoupling oxidative phosphorylation primarily in skeletal muscle. Increased $CO_2$ production stimulates respiration while plasma $CO_2$ concentration is held constant through increased alveolar ventilation. If the respiratory response to $CO_2$ has been depressed by opiates or barbiturates, a marked increase in plasma $pCO_2$ occurs causing respiratory acidosis.

Respiration is stimulated directly by salicylates through stimulation of the medullary respiratory center. This causes hyperventilation, characterized by both increased depth and rate of respiration, and respiratory alkalosis ensues. At toxic doses of salicylates a depressant effect occurs on the medulla causing central respiratory paralysis and respiratory acidosis.

**Table 7.2.** Reported Side Effects of Salicylic Acid in Therapeutic Doses

| | |
|---|---|
| *Respiratory* | |
| | Increased $O_2$ consumption |
| | Increased $CO_2$ production |
| | Increased alveolar ventilation |
| | Dose-dependent stimulation or depression of medullary respiratory center |
| *Acid-base balance* | |
| | Primary effect = intra and extracellular respiratory alkalosis |
| | Compensation = increased renal excretion of $HCO_3$, $Na^+$, $K^+$ |
| *Cardiovascular* | |
| | Rare in therapeutic doses |
| | Peripheral vasodilation in large doses |
| | Increased plasma volume in large doses |
| | Increased cardiac output in large doses |
| *Gastrointestinal* | |
| | Nausea |
| | Vomiting |
| | Anorexia |
| | Erosive gastritis |
| | Gastric and duodenal ulcers |
| | Gastric hemorrhage |
| *Hematologic* | |
| | Anemia |
| | Increased bleeding time |
| | Decreased platelet function |
| | Decreased formation of thromboxane $A_2$ |
| *Hepatic* | |
| | Increased plasma SGOT and SGPT |
| | Hepatomegaly |
| | Jaundice |
| *Renal* | |
| | Decreased glomerular filtration rate |
| | Decreased renal blood flow |
| | Nephropathy |

**Table 7.3.** Signs and Symptoms of Aspirin Toxicity

| |
|---|
| *Early or Mild Toxicity* |
| Vertigo |
| Tinnitis |
| Decreased hearing |
| *Moderate Toxicity* |
| Nausea |
| Vomiting |
| Sweating |
| Diarrhea |
| Fever |
| Drowsiness |
| Headache |
| Dimming of vision |
| Confusion |
| Excitement |
| Restlessness |
| Talkativeness |
| *Severe Toxicity* |
| Pulmonary edema |
| Cardiovascular decompensation |
| Petechial hemorrhages |
| Seizure |
| Hallucination |
| Coma |

*Acid Base Balance*

At therapeutic doses of salicylates extracellular and intracellular respiratory alkalosis is the primary event, which is rapidly compensated by increased renal excretion of bicarbonate, sodium, and potassium. Toxic ingestions of salicylates, however, result in a combination of respiratory and metabolic acidosis. Uncompensated respiratory acidosis is produced by enhanced production and decreased renal excretion of $CO_2$ in the setting of a low plasma bicarbonate concentration (secondary to increased renal bicarbonate excretion). Metabolic acidosis is the result of accumulation of acids resulting from (1) dissociated salicylate acid derivatives, (2) accumulating sulfuric and phosphoric acids secondary to decreased renal excretion, (3) accumulation of pyruvic, lactic, and aceto-acetic acids secondary to impaired carbohydrate metabolism. In addition to these acid-base disturbances, it should be noted that hyperventilation and hyperhydrosis increase the amount of free water loss, thereby superimposing dehydration and hypernatremia upon these acid base disturbances.

*Cardiovascular Effects*

Therapeutic doses of salicylates have little or no effect upon cardiovascular function. Toxic doses of aspirin, however, have been reported to cause peripheral vasodilation secondary to a direct effect on vascular smooth muscle, and increased plasma volume and cardiac output.

*Gastrointestinal Effects*

The most frequently reported symptom arising from salicylate ingestion is gastrointestinal distress associated with nausea and sometimes vomiting. Aspirin ingestion in therapeutic doses may also cause erosive gastritis, gastric and duodenal ulceration, and gastric hemorrhage. Salicylate-induced gastric hemorrhage is generally painless and can lead to iron deficiency anemia secondary to prolonged blood loss, although average fecal blood loss is usually less than 3 to 8 ml/day. The gastrointestinal effects of aspirin appear as cell damage resulting from penetration of the lipid membrane of the gastric mucosal cell by salicylate and inhibition of gastric mucous secretion as well as reduced synthesis of prostaglandin. Damage to the gastric mucosal cell allows back diffusion of hydrochloric acid resulting in enhanced cellular and capillary injury. Gastric acid secretion, moreover, is enhanced since prostaglandin normally inhibits secretion.

*Hematologic Effects*

A single dose of 650 mg of aspirin approximately doubles the mean bleeding time for normal individuals for a period of 4 to 7 days. This is probably due to acetylation of platelets' cyclooxygenase and, subsequently, reduced formation of thromboxane A2.

*Hepatic and Renal Effects*

Hepatotoxicity has been reported in normal individuals although more commonly it is seen in patients with connective tissue disorders.[1] Elevated levels of SGOT and SGPT in the plasma are the primary indicators of hepatic damage, and patients are generally symptom-free. Approximately 5% of patients do experience hepatomegally, anorexia, jaundice, and nausea.

Therapeutic doses of aspirin have been reported to decrease both renal blood flow and glomerular filtration rate.[2] These effects are generally insignificant in normal individuals, but may become important in patients with underlying renal dysfunction. In large doses, or when given in combination with other analgesics, "analgesic" nephropathy may result.

## Mechanism of Action of Aspirin and Aspirin-Like Drugs

The analgesic effect of aspirin is attributed to the inhibition of prostaglandin biosynthesis. In vivo, dietary essential fatty acids are esterified to form arachidonic acid (5, 8, 11, 14-Eicosatetraenoic acid). Arachidonic acid is then oxygenated and cyclized by fatty acid cyclooxygenase to form the cyclic endoperoxide prostaglandin G ($PGG_2$). This chemically unstable compound, $PGG_2$, is then rapidly isomerized into several products including PGE, PGF, and PGD (Fig. 7.2).

Aspirin-like drugs inhibit the conversion of arachidonic acid to the unstable endoperoxide intermediate $PGG_2$. Although various pharmacologic agents have different mechanisms of inhibition of these cyclooxygenase enzymes, aspirin acetylates serine at the active site of the cyclooxygenase enzyme.[3] Aspirin and most aspirin-like drugs irreversibly inhibit cyclooxygenase. Since prostaglandins are associated especially with the development of pain that accompanies injury or inflammation, inhibition of its synthesis is an effective means of analgesia. For example, $PGE_2$ and $PGF_2$ cause intense local pain and headache when injected intramuscularly or subcutaneously. $PGE_1$, injected intradermally, produces a long lasting hyperalgesia that is believed to result from a lowering of the threshold of the polymodal nociceptive C fibers.[4]

### Paraaminophenol Derivatives

#### *History*

The parent member of this family of compounds, acetanilid, was introduced into medicine in 1886 as "antifebrin," an antipyretic compound. Its excessive toxicity was rapidly noted, however, and alternative compounds were sought. The first effective paraamino phenol derivative with reasonably acceptable toxicity was introduced in 1887 as Phenacetin (Fig. 7.3). Although it is still available in analgesic preparations, its popularity has been overshadowed by the less toxic compound, acetaminophen. Acetaminophen was first used in medicine by Von Mering in 1893; however, it gained popularity and become available as an over-the-counter drug in the United States only since 1949, after it was recognized as the major active metabolite of both acetanilid and Phenacetin.

#### *Therapeutic Effect*

Acetaminophen is an effective analgesic and anti-pyretic agent, but it is only weakly anti-inflammatory. It functions as a suitable substitute for aspirin for the relief of pain or fever, especially in patients for whom aspirin is contraindicated (i.e., those with a bleeding diathysis). Because it

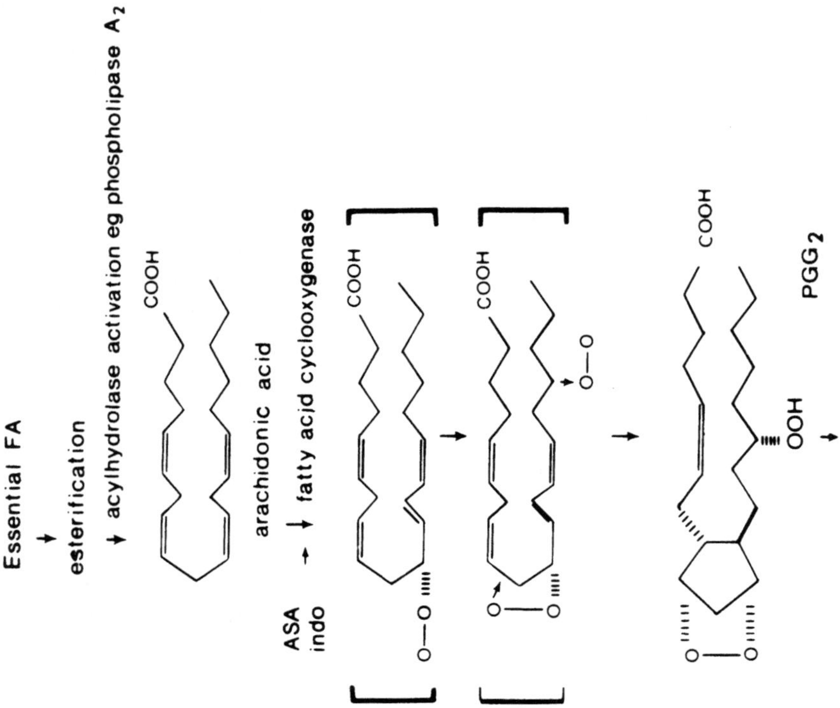
Essential FA
esterification
acylhydrolase activation eg phospholipase A2
COOH
arachidonic acid
ASA
indo
fatty acid cyclooxygenase
COOH
O—O
COOH
O—O
O—O
COOH
OOH
O—O
PGG2

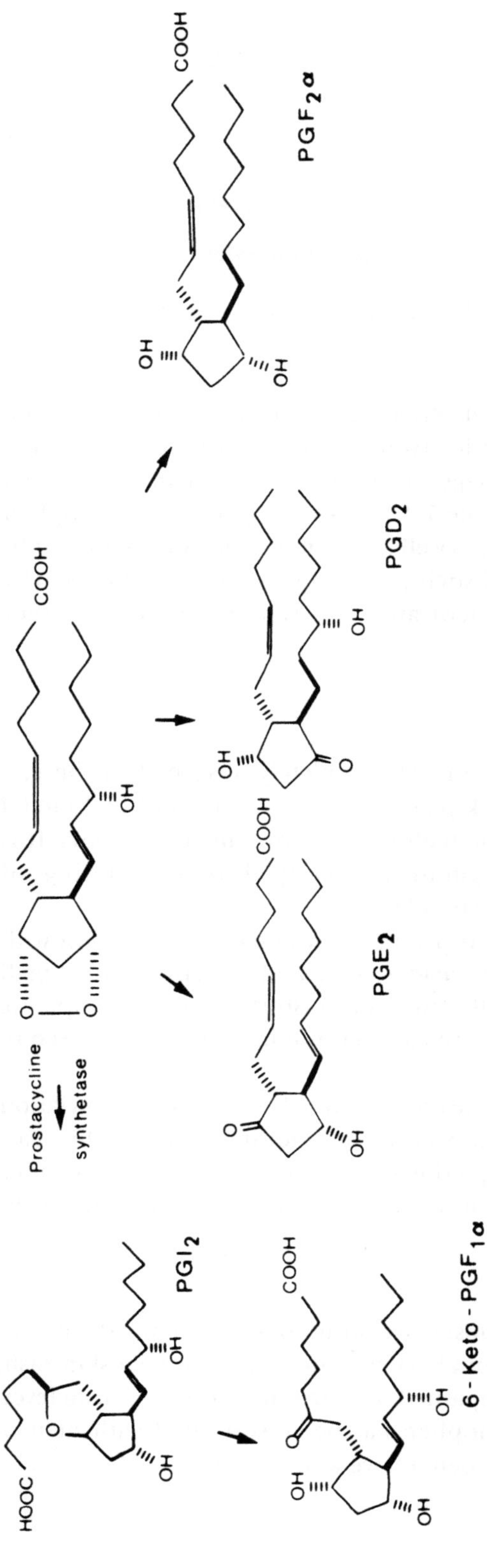


**Figure 7.2.** Metabolic pathway of arachadonic acid to several prostaglandin derivatives. Point of interruption of sequence by ASA (aspirin) and indo (indomethacin) inhibition of fatty acid cyclooxygenase is indicated. See text for further discussion.

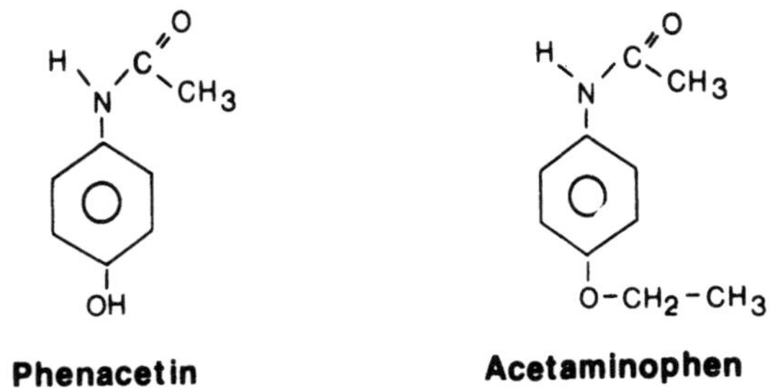


**Figure 7.3.** Structural formula of para-aminophenol compounds.

lacks many of the undesirable side effects of aspirin, it is rapidly becoming the preferred oral analgesic. However, its association with fatal hepatotoxicity in acute overdosage must always be kept in mind when prescribing this medication. Table 7.4 lists some of the acetaminophen preparations and combinations, as well as recommended doses for adults. Because there are well over 100 such preparations this list is necessarily limited. Consult appropriate medication references for various other alternatives.

*Pharmacokinetics*

Acetaminophen is rapidly and almost completely absorbed in the gastrointestinal tract, reaching peak plasma concentrations within 30 to 60 minutes, and achieving a plasma half-life of approximately 2 hours. It is uniformly distributed throughout the body. Protein binding of acetaminophen varies between 20 to 50%.

Acetaminophen is metabolized primarily by hepatic conjugation with glucuronic acid (60%), sulfuric acid (35%), and cysteine (3%). Small amounts are hydroxylated. Following administration of a therapeutic dose, 90 to 100% of the administered acetaminophen can be recovered in these forms from urine.

Toxic doses of acetaminophen are also metabolized via N-hydroxylation to form the reactive intermediate N-acetyl-benzoquinoneimine. This reactive intermediate results in a depletion of hepatic glutathione and various hepatic proteins. Depletion of these proteins results in hepatic necrosis.

*Side Effects*

In recommended therapeutic doses, acetaminophen has few side effects. Those reported include occasional erythematous or urticarial skin rash, which may sometimes be accompanied by mucosal lesions and drug fever. A few cases in which acetaminophen has been associated with neutropenia, pancytopenia, and leukopenia have also been reported.

**Table 7.4.** Adult Oral Acetaminophen Preparations

| Product | Quantity (mg) | Additional Ingredients (mg) | Recommended Dosage |
|---|---|---|---|
| Anacin-3 | 325 | | 2–3 tablets every 4 hours, max. = 12/24 hours |
| Anacin-3 Maximum Strength | 500 | | 2 tablets every 6–8 hours, max. = 8/24 hours |
| Cogesic | 500 | Hydrocodone 5* | 1 tablet every 6 hours |
| Comtrex | 500 | Pseudoephedrine 30<br>Chlorpheniramine 2 | 2 tablets every 6 hours, max = 8/24 hours |
| Datril | 500 | | 2 tablets every 4 hours, max. = 8/24 hours |
| Dristan Advanced Formula | 325 | Phenylephrine 5<br>Chlorpheniramine 2 | 2 tablets every 4 hours, max. = 12/24 hours |
| Empracet with Codeine | 300 | #3 Codeine 30* | 1–2 tablets every 4 hours |
| | | #4 Codeine 60* | 1 tablet every 4 hours |
| Esgic | 325 | Butalbital 50*<br>Caffeine 40 | 1–2 tablets every 4 hours, max. = 6/24 hours |
| Esgic with Codeine | 325 | Butalbital 50*<br>Caffeine 40<br>Codeine 30* | 1–2 capsules every 4–6 hours, max. = 6/24 hours |
| Extra-strength Sine-aid | 500 | Pseudoephedrine 30 | 2 tablets every 6 hours, max. = 8/24 hours |
| Fioricet | 325 | Butalbital 50*<br>Caffeine 40 | 1–2 tablets every 4 hours, max. = 6/24 hours |
| Hydrocet | 500 | Hydrocodone 5* | 1–2 capsules every 4–6 hours, max. = 8/24 hours |
| Hyphen | 500 | Hydrocodone 5* | 1–2 capsules every 4–6 hours, max. = 8/24 hours |
| Isocom | 325 | Isometheptene 65<br>Dichloralphenazone 100 | 1–2 tablets every 4 hours, max. = 8/24 hours† |

**Table 7.4.** (*Continued*)

| Product | Quantity (mg) | Additional Ingredients (mg) | Recommended Dosage |
|---|---|---|---|
| Migralam | 325 | Isometheptene 65<br>Dichloralphenozone 100 | 1–2 tablets every 4 hours, max. = 8/24 hours |
| Percoset | 325 | Oxycodone 5* | 1 tablet every 6 hours |
| Percogesic | 325 | Phenyltoloxamine 30 | 1–2 tablets every 4 hours, max. = 8/24 hours |
| Phenaphen with Codeine | 325 | #2 codeine 15*<br>#3 codeine 30* | 1–2 tablets every 4 hours |
| | | #4 codeine 60* | 1 tablet every 4 hours |
| Phrenilin | 325 | Butalbital 50* | 1–2 tablets every 4 hours, max. = 6/24 hours |
| Phrenilin Forte | 650 | Butalbital 50* | 1 tablet every 4–6 hours, max. = 3/24 hours |
| Roxicet | 325 | Oxycodone 5* | 1 tablet every 6 hours |
| Talacen | 650 | Pentazocine 25* | 1 tablet every 4 hours, max. = 6/24 hours |
| Tylenol | 325 | | 1–2 tablets every 4 hours, max. = 12/24 hours |
| Tylenol Extra Strength | 500 | | 2 tablets every 6–8 hours, max. = 8/24 hours |
| Tylenol with Codeine | 300 | #1 codeine 7.5* | 1–2 tablets every 4 hours |
| | | #2 codeine 15* | 1–2 tablets every 4 hours |
| | | #3 codeine 30* | 1–2 tablets every 4 hours |
| | | #4 codeine 60* | 1 tablet every 4 hours |
| Tylox | 500 | Oxycodone 5* | 1 tablet every 6 hours |
| Vicodin | 500 | Hydrocodone 5* | 1 tablet every 6 hours |

**Table 7.4.** (*Continued*)

| Product | Quantity (mg) | Additional Ingredients (mg) | Recommended Dosage |
|---|---|---|---|
| Wygesic | 500 | Propoxyphene 65 | 1 tablet every 4 hours, max. = 390 mg propoxy/24 hours |
| Zydone | 500 | Hydrocodone 5 | 1 capsule every 4–6 hours, max. = 8/24 hours |

*May be habit forming.
† Particularly useful for chronic vascular headaches.

*Toxicity*

The most significant adverse effect of acute overdose of acetaminophen is the potentially fatal hepatic necrosis. In adults, hepatotoxicity has been reported following ingestion of a single dose of 10 to 15 grams of acetaminophen. Ingestion of 25 gm or more is potentially fatal. Early symptoms of acute toxicity include nausea, vomiting, anorexia, and abdominal pain followed in 24 to 48 hours later by clinical indications of hepatic damage including elevation of plasma transaminases, and bilirubin, and an increase in prothrombin time. Symptoms of hepatotoxicity may progress to encephalopathy, coma, and death. Other findings reported in the setting of severe hepatotoxicity include transient hypoglycemia, glycosuria, metabolic acidosis or alkalosis, cerebral edema, and myocardial depression.[5] It is estimated that 10% of patients experiencing acetaminophen poisoning go on to develop severe liver damage, and of these 10 to 20% eventually die in hepatic failure.

The mechanism of acetaminophen-induced hepatotoxicity is believed to be production of toxic metabolites in excess of the available glutathione for inactivation. The resulting necrosis is centrilobular with periportal sparing. If nonfatal, hepatic regeneration occurs over a period of weeks to months.[6]

Chronic use of high doses of acetaminophen (or more commonly Phenacetin) in combination with other analgesics has also been associated with renal disease (i.e., "analgesic nephropathy"). Histologically, the lesions appear as papillary necrosis, interstitial nephritis, and capillary sclerosis, all resulting from microangiopathy-induced compromise of vascular supply. Clinically these become apparent as decreased concentrating ability and eventually can progress to renal insufficiency. The exact nephrotoxic factor in the mixtures has not yet been identified, although phenacetin, aspirin, and caffeine have all been implicated.[7] A recent study

**Table 7.5.** Side Effects and Toxic Effects of Acetominophen

| |
|---|
| *Side Effects* |
| Skin rash, urticarial or erythematous |
| Mucosal lesions |
| Drug fever |
| Neutropenia |
| Pancytopenia |
| Leukopenia |
| *Toxic Effects* |
| *Early* |
| Nausea |
| Vomiting |
| Anorexia |
| Abdominal pain |
| *Delayed* |
| Elevated serum transaminases |
| Elevated serum bilirubin |
| Elevated prothrombin time |
| Transient azotemia |
| Hypoglycemia |
| Glycosuria |
| Metabolic acidosis or alkalosis |
| Myocardial arrythmia |
| Cerebral edema |
| Encephalopathy |
| Coma |
| Death |

by Emkey[8] failed to demonstrate impaired renal function in a group of patients taking aspirin (alone) for greater than 10 years. This would suggest that aspirin, taken alone, would not cause renal disease, but does not prove that it is free of nephrotoxic effects when taken in combination with other analgesics.

## Nonsteroidal Anti-inflammatory Agents

### *History*

Nonsteroidal anti-inflammatory agents are frequently used in place of, or as an adjunct to, the analgesics already discussed.

Indomethacin was first utilized as an anti-inflammatory and analgesic agent in the treatment of rheumatoid arthritis in 1963, following its laboratory synthesis in a search for drugs with such properties. Since then numerous drugs have been synthesized in several families (Table 7.6 and

**Table 7.6.** Nonsteroidal Anti-inflammatory Drugs

| Generic Name | Product Name | Chemical Family | Recommended Dosage | Plasma Half-life (hours) |
|---|---|---|---|---|
| Diflunisal | Dolobid | Salicylic acid | 500 mg every 8–12 hours | 8–12 |
| Fenoprofen | Nalfon | Phenyl-propionic acid | 200 mg every 4–6 hours | 3 |
| Ibuprofen | Advil | Phenyl-propionic acid | 200 mg every 4–6 hours | 3–4 |
| | Medipren<br>Midol<br>Motrin<br>Nuprin<br>Rufen | | | |
| Indomethacin | Indocin | Indole-acetic acid | 25–50 mg every 8–12 hours, max. = 150–200 mg/24 hours | 2 |
| Ketoprofen | Orudis | Propionic acid | starting dose 75 mg every 8 hours, max. = 300 mg/24 hour | 2–4 |
| Meclofenamate | Meclomen | Anthranilic acid | starting 50 mg every 6–8 hours, max. = 400 mg/24 hours | 2–3 |
| Meclofenamic acid | Ponstel | Anthranilic acid | 250 mg every 6 hours, max. = use for 1 week | 2 |
| Naproxen | Naprosyn<br>Anaprox | Propionic acid | 250 mg every 6–8 hours, max. = 1250 mg/24 hours | 13 |
| Piroxicam | Feldene | Oxicam | 20 mg once daily | 50 |
| Sulindac | Clinoril | Indene | 150 mg every 12 hours, max. = 400 mg/24 hours | 7.8 |

**Table 7.6.** (*Continued*)

| Generic Name | Product Name | Chemical Family | Recommended Dosage | Plasma Half-life (hours) |
|---|---|---|---|---|
| Suprofen | Suprol | Arylacetic acid | 200 mg every 6–8 hours, max. = 800 mg/24 hours | 2–4 |
| Tolmetin | Tolectin | Arylacetic acid | 400 mg every 6–8 hours, max. = 2000 mg/24 hours | biphasic early 2 delayed 5 |

Fig. 7.4). Diflunisal (Dolobid) is a difluorophenyl derivative of salicylate acid. Doses of 500 mg give analgesia equivalent to 650 mg of aspirin and 650 mg of acetaminophen with 100 mg propoxyphene, 1000 mg of diflunisal has yielded analgesia equivalent to 600 mg acetaminophen with 60 mg codeine. Its relatively long half-life of 8 to 12 hours gives the advantage of less frequent dosing.

Fenoprofen, ibuprofen, ketoprofen, naproxen, suprofen, and tolmetin are all propionic or acetic acid derivatives. At the recommended doses each provides analgesic potency approximately equivalent to 650 mg of salicylic acid or 600 mg of acetaminophen. Other nonsteroidal anti-inflammatory agents available include meclofenamate and meclofenomic acid (anthranilic acid derivatives), piroxicam (oxicam derivative), and sulindac (indene derivative).

The pharmacologic profile of all these compounds is similar in that: (1) all provide analgesia roughly equivalent to aspirin and acetaminophen, (2) all are believed to function via inhibition of prostaglandin synthesis, (3) all are rapidly and extensively absorbed from the gastrointestinal tract following oral administration, (4) most are extensively protein bound in plasma (90 to 99%), and (5) elimination is predominantly via renal excretion of glucuronidated or hydroxylated metabolites. Notable exceptions, however, are: (1) ibuprofen is eliminated as free derivatives of proprionic acid, (2) sulindac is eliminated as the sulfone or sulfide derivative, and (3) meclofenamate, meclofenamic acid, piroxicam, and sulindac are each eliminated via both renal (66%) and fecal (33%) routes.

Table 7.7 reviews the reported side effects common to the entire group of nonsteroidal anti-inflammatory drugs. The most common side effects reported are gastrointestinal symptoms, followed by mild neurologic symptoms (e.g., lightheadedness). These symptoms have resulted in dis-

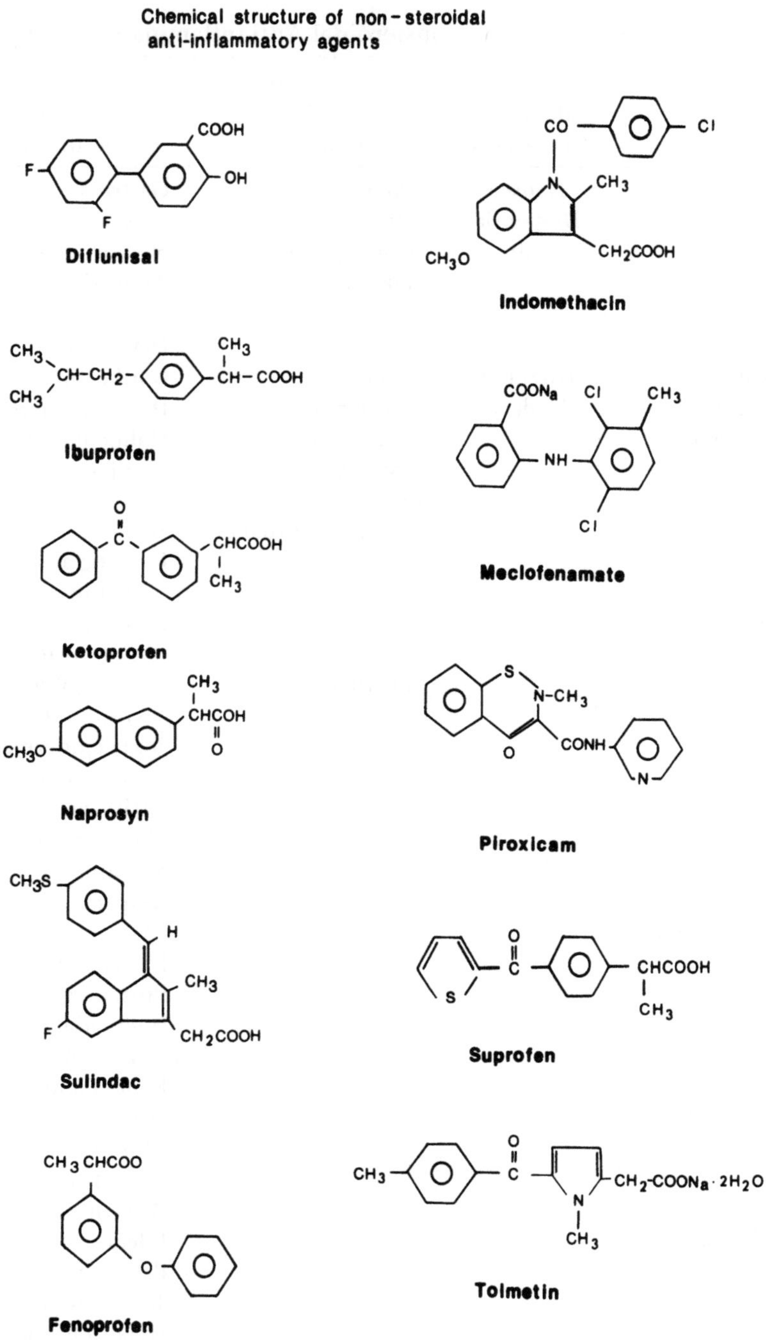


**Figure 7.4.** Structural formula of several parent nonsteroidal anti-inflammatory compounds.

**Table 7.7.** Adverse Effects of Nonsteroidal Anti-inflammatory Drugs

| | Greater than 3% Occurrence | Between 1 and 3% Occurrence | Less than 1% Occurrence |
|---|---|---|---|
| Gastrointestinal | Nausea | Vomiting | Gastritis |
| | Dyspepsia | Diarrhea | Ulceration |
| | Pain | Constipation | Hemorrhage |
| | | Flatulence | Anorexia |
| | | | Stomatitis |
| | | | Dry mouth |
| Neurologic | Dizziness | Somnolence | Confusion |
| Psychiatric | Headache | Insomnia | Disorientation |
| Special sensory | | Nervousness | Hallucination |
| | | Fatigue | Vertigo |
| | | Tinnitis | Depression |
| | | Visual disturbance | Seizure |
| | | | Hearing and taste alteration |
| Dermatologic | | Rash | Erythema multiforme |
| | | Pruritis | Stevens-Johnson syndrome |
| | | | Toxic epidermal necrolysis |
| | | | Urticaria |
| | | | Photosensitivity |
| | | | Sweating |
| | | | Alopecia |
| Genito-urinary | | | Dysuria |
| | | | Hematuria |
| | | | Proteinuria |
| | | | Interstitial nephritis |
| | | | Renal failure |
| Respiratory | | | Dyspnea |
| | | | Rhinitis |
| | | | Hemoptysis |
| | | | Bronchospasm |
| Cardiovascular | | | Edema |
| | | | Palpitations |
| | | | Tachycardia |
| | | | Hypertension |
| | | | Pulmonary edema |
| | | | Atrial fibrillation |
| | | | Congestive heart failure |

**Table 7.7.** *(Continued)*

| | Greater than 3% Occurrence | Between 1 and 3% Occurrence | Less than 1% Occurrence |
|---|---|---|---|
| | | | Chest pain |
| Musculoskeletal | | | Myalgia |
| Hepatic/ pancreatic | | | Jaundice |
| | | | Hepatitis |
| | | | Cholestasis |
| | | | Pancreatitis |
| Hematologic | | | Thrombocytopenia |
| | | | Agranulocytosis |
| | | | Neutopenia |
| | | | Aplastic anemia |
| | | | Eosinophilia |
| Hypersensitivity | | | Acute anaphylaxis |

continuing the medications in 3 to 20% of patients in trial studies. When given in recommended doses, serious side effects of these drugs are rare. Because indomethacin is the most well known of this group, its pharmacologic profile is discussed in more detail below. Representative details are also given for each of the other major families of these drugs.

*Pharmacokinetics*

Indomethacin has been the most extensively studied of the nonsteroidal anti-inflammatory agents. It is rapidly and completely absorbed from the gastrointestinal tract following oral ingestion, obtaining a peak plasma concentration within 2 hours. Ninety percent of Indomethacin is bound to plasma protein. Metabolism of Indomethacin results in its conversion to inactive metabolites, 50% by O-demethylation, 10% by glucuronic acid conjugation, and also by N-deacylation. These metabolites are then eliminated in the urine, bowel, and feces. Ten to 20% of the drug is excreted unchanged.

Following oral administration of Sulindac, about 90% of the drug is absorbed from the G.I. tract obtaining peak plasma concentrations within 1 hour. Sulindac then undergoes 2 transformations, first being oxidized to sulfone and then reversibly reduced to the active metabolite sulfide. The plasma half-life of the active sulfide is as long as 18 hours. Sulindac is excreted in both urine and feces, mostly as the sulfone and its conjugates.

Naproxen and Fenoprofen are rapidly absorbed following oral administration. Naproxen is fully absorbed, whereas Fenoprofen is incompletely absorbed. Peak concentrations in plasma appear within 2 to 4 hours. The half life of Naproxen is 14 hours, whereas that of Fenoprofen is 3 hours.

They are both extensively bound to plasma proteins, and extensively metabolized and conjugated. Both are excreted almost entirely in the urine.

Piroxicam is completely absorbed following oral administration, reaching a peak concentration in 2 to 4 hours. The major advantage of Piroxicam appears to be that its plasma half-life ranges up to 45 hours. It is extensively bound to plasma proteins, and extensively metabolized and conjugated. It is excreted both in the urine and the feces.

*Therapeutic and Side Effects*

All the agents listed above are effective analgesic, antipyretic, and anti-inflammatory agents used in the treatment of rheumatoid arthritis, osteoarthritis, acute musculoskeletal disorders, and ankylosing spondylitis, and several are very effective in the treatment of acute gout. Their major advantage in the treatment of chronic pain syndromes is their lack of addictiveness. Their major limiting factor is their side effects. The most significant side effects have been reported for Indomethacin. These will be described below. In general, the side effects for Sulindac, Ibuprofen, Fenoprofen, and Piroxicam are significantly less than those Indomethacin.

Approximately 35 to 50% of the patients receiving therapeutic doses of Indomethacin experience unacceptable side effects. About 20% eventually must discontinue its use. The most frequent complaints are gastrointestinal including anorexia, nausea, abdominal pain, ulceration, anemia secondary to occult blood loss, and diarrhea. Severe headache occurs in 25 to 50% of patients. Other central nervous system symptoms include dizziness, vertigo, lightheadedness, confusion, depression, psychosis, hallucinations, and suicide. Hematologic side effects have included neutropenia, thrombocytopenia, and aplastic anemia. Dermatologic reactions have included rashes and itching. Hypersensitivity has also been demonstrated as acute asthmatic attacks.

Indomethacin is contraindicated for use in pregnant women, nursing mothers, persons operating heavy machinery, psychiatric patients, patients with epilepsy or Parkinsonism, and patients with renal or ulcerative disease. Although the remaining nonsteroidal anti-inflammatory agents are generally much better tolerated than Indomethacin, several other side effects have been reported with them. Ibuprofen has been associated with several cases of blurred vision, toxic amblyopia, fluid retention, and edema. Jaundice, impaired renal function, ototoxicity, and angioneurotic edema have been reported with Naproxen.

Indomethacin is generally prescribed beginning with 25 mg b.i.d. or t.i.d., and increasing by 25 mg increments at weekly intervals until a maximum total daily dose of 100 to 200 mg is achieved. Sulindac is generally prescribed as 150 to 200 mg b.i.d. for adults. Ibuprofen is prescribed as

**Figure 7.5.** Structural formula of propoxyphene, a mild narcotic with relatively low-addictive potential which can be used in chronic pain syndromes.

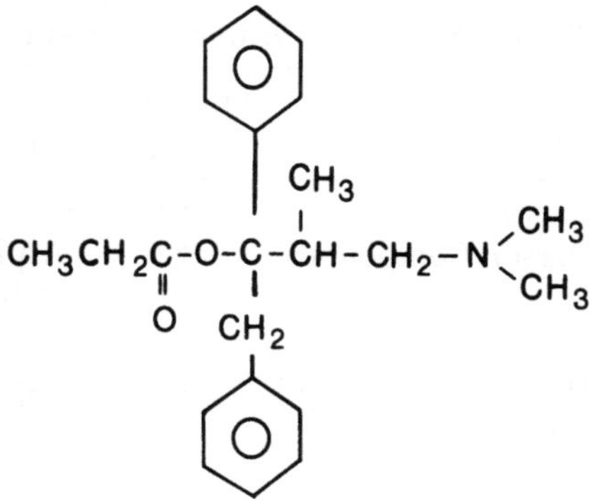

400 mg every 4 to 6 hours as needed for mild to moderate pain. The usual total daily dose is 1200 to 1600 mg. Naproxen is administered in 250 to 375 mg b.i.d. to t.i.d. as needed. Therapeutic doses of Fenoprofen are achieved with 300 to 600 mg t.i.d. to q.i.d., as needed with a maximum of 3.2 grams per day. Piroxicam is administered 10 mg to 20 mg given once daily.

## Narcotic Analgesics

In general, narcotic analgesics are not indicated in the treatment of chronic pain syndromes. However, for the short-term treatment of acute exacerbations of musculoskeletal pain, several mild narcotic analgesics are available. Specifically, Darvon and its various combinations with aspirin, acetaminophen, and codeine in combination with aspirin and acetaminophen are effective analgesics with relatively low addictive potential. Combinations of these compounds are listed in Tables 7.1 and 7.4. It must be kept in mind, however, that use of these medications in chronic pain patients should be limited to short-term use during acute exacerbations of pain.

### Propoxyphene

Propoxyphene is a mild, centrally acting, narcotic analgesic, structurally similar to methadone (Fig. 7.5). Its analgesic potency is between two-thirds and fully as effective as codeine. When given in combination with salicylic acid or acetaminophen, it produces greater analgesia than any given individually.

*Pharmacokinetics*

Propoxyphene (Darvon) is rapidly absorbed following oral administration and reaches peak plasma concentrations in 1 to 2 hours. Plasma half-

**Table 7.8.** Propoxyphene Preparations

| Product | Quantity (mg) | Additional Ingredients (mg) | Recommended Dosage |
|---|---|---|---|
| Darvon | 65 | | 65 mg every 4 hours |
| Darvon Compound | 32 | Aspirin 325<br>Caffeine 32.4 | 1 tablet every 4 hours, max. = 390 mg/24 hours |
| Darvon Compound 65 | 65 | Aspirin 325<br>Caffeine 32.4 | 1 tablet every 4 hours, max. = 390 mg/24 hours |
| Darvon w/aspirin | 65 | Aspirin 325 | 1 tablet every 4 hours, max. = 390 mg/24 hours |
| Wygesic | 65 | Acetaminophen 650 | 1 tablet every 4 hours, max. = 390 mg/24 hours |
| Darvocet-N 50 | 50 | Acetaminophen 325 | 1 tablet every 4 hours, max. = 600 mg/24 hours |
| Darvocet-N 100 | 100 | Acetaminophen 650 | 1 tablet every 4 hours, max. = 600 mg/24 hours |
| Darvon N with aspirin | 100 | Aspirin 325 mg | 1 tablet every 4 hours, max. = 600 mg/24 hours |

life has been estimated between 3.5 to 15 hours. Bioavailability is limited by first pass metabolism ranging between 30 to 70% in humans. Metabolism to nor-propoxyphene is via n-demethylation.

*Therapeutic and Side Effects*

Propoxyphene binds to opiate receptors producing analgesia as well as other CNS effects. It has no significant antipyretic or anti-inflammatory actions.

Propoxyphene is a respiratory depressant with approximately one-third the potency of codeine. As with other narcotic analgesics, in addition to respiratory depression propoxyphene has been reported to cause nausea, vomiting, somnolence, confusion, hallucinations, and delusions. In addition, seizures, pulmonary edema, and cardiovascular toxicity including ventricular bigeminy and tachycardia have been reported with propoxyphene. Naloxone effectively antagonizes the respiratory depression, seizure, and some of the cardiotoxic effects of propoxyphene.

Although propoxyphene is generally regarded as a relatively safe and effective analgesic, discontinuation of chronic propoxyphene use has resulted in withdrawal symptoms. Physical dependence has been pro-

**Table 7.9.** Tricyclic Antidepressants Potentially Useful as Adjuncts to Other Pain Medications

| Generic Name | Product Name | Initial Recommended Daily Dose (mg) | Usual Maintenance Daily Dose (mg) |
|---|---|---|---|
| Imipramine | Tofranil<br>Presamine | 25–100 | 75–300 |
| Desipramine | Norpramine<br>Pertofrane | 50–150 | 75–300 |
| Amitryptilene | Elavil<br>Endep<br>Etrafon<br>Limbitral<br>Triavil | 25–100 | 75–300 |
| Nortryptilene | Pamelor<br>Aventyl | 25–50 | 50–100 |
| Protriptylene | Vivactyl | 10–30 | 15–60 |
| Doxepin | Sinequan<br>Adepin | 50–100 | 75–150 |

duced with as little as 500 to 800 mg per day of propoxyphene hydrochloride or 800 to 1200 mg per day of the napsylate salt.

Propoxyphene is generally prescribed as 65 mg to be administered orally every 4 hours as needed. Combination forms of propoxyphene containing 32.5 or 65 mg of propoxyphene are available.

## Tricyclic Antidepressants

### *History*

Although the basic structure of the iminodibenzyl molecule was synthesized in the late 19th Century, its pharmacological properties were not investigated until the 1940s. At that time Haflinger and Chinlur synthesized a series of derivatives, including imipramine, to test as potential antihistamines, sedatives, analgesics, and anti-Parkinsonian drugs (Fig. 7.6). In 1958 Kuhn discovered that although these compounds were not effective anti-psychotics, they were very effective in the treatment of certain depressed patients. Since the early 1960s, numerous reports have demonstrated effective pain relief with tricyclic antidepressants as well as adjunctive pain relief with these compounds when used in combination with other known analgesics.[2,9–11]

### *Therapeutic Effects*

In addition to their use in the treatment of depression, tricyclic antidepressants have also been used in the treatment of enuresis in children, severe obsessive-compulsive neurosis, and recently as adjunctive therapy

**TRICYCLIC ANTIDEPRESSANTS**

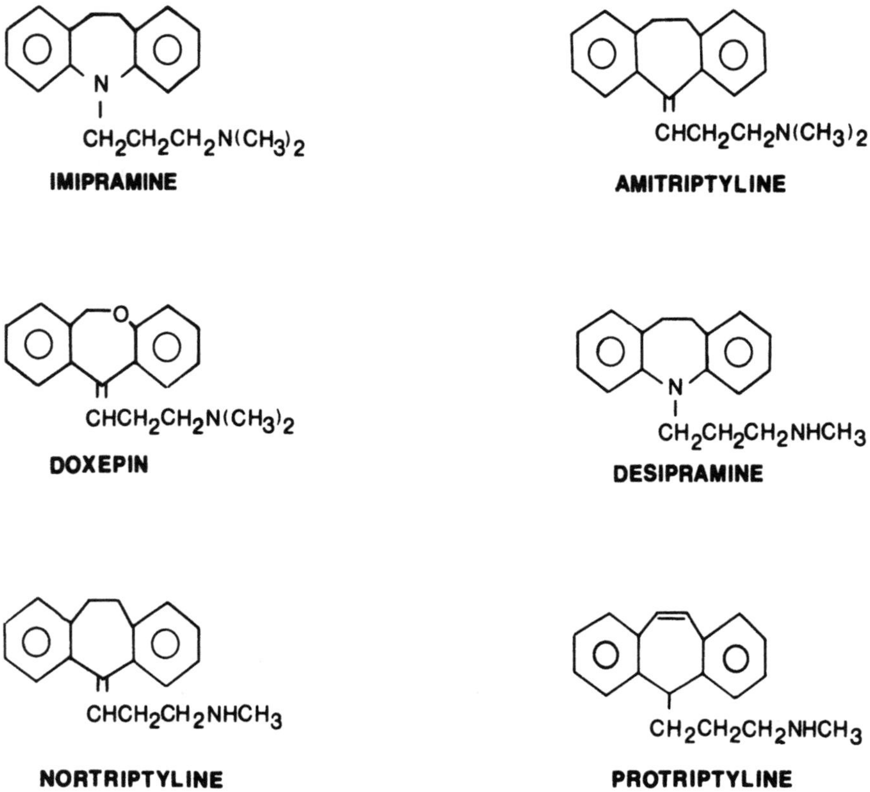


**Figure 7.6.** Structural formula of several tricyclic antidepressant agents useful in treatment of pain, as well as depressive symptoms common to chronic pain syndromes.

in the treatment of chronic pain. Amitryptilene,[10] imipramine,[11,12] and doxepin[13] have each been reported to induce or augment analgesia.

The mechanism of action of tricyclic antidepressants is related to blockade of re-uptake of serotinin and norepinephrine into the presynaptic nerve terminal. Re-uptake blockade physiologically antagonizes the major route of inactivation of these neurotransmitters. Desipramine is the most potent tricyclic antidepressant in blocking the re-uptake of norepinephrine but is 100 to 1000 times less potent in blocking the re-uptake of serotonin. In contrast, amitryptilene inhibits the re-uptake of serotonin and norepinephrine approximately equally well. Based on the anatomy of descending serotonergic influences as spinal cord afferent pain fibers, presumably blockade of serotonin re-uptake is the key factor in producing tricyclic induced analgesia.

*Pharmacokinetics*

Tricyclic antidepressants are moderately well absorbed following oral administration. Peak-plasma concentrations are reached within 2 to 8 hours. Following absorption, they are rapidly distributed throughout the body and are extensively bound to plasma proteins. Metabolism of the tricyclic antidepressants is via oxidation by the hepatic microsomal enzyme system followed by conjugation with glucuronic acid. Amitrytilene (Elavil) and Doxepin (Adapin), antidepressants frequently used for pain relief, are both converted to active metabolites by demethylation. The ratio of methylated to demethylated products following administration is quite variable, and it is presumably the result of genetic differences in metabolism of the drugs. The half-life of amitryptilene in plasma is approximately 16 hours with the majority of metabolites being excreted in the urine.

*Side Effects*

The predominant early effect of tricyclic antidepressants is sedation. Therefore, imitation of tricyclic antidepressant treatment is generally begun at a low dose, such as 25 to 50 mg orally at bedtime, and advanced slowly over a period of weeks to doses in the range of 75 to 150 mg orally, at bedtime or undivided doses.

Significant toxic effects of tricyclic antidepressants are relatively common. Antimuscarinic effects of these compounds includes dry mouth, metallic taste, epigastric distress, constipation, dizziness, tachycardia, cardiac arrhythmias, blurry vision, and urinary retention. Central nervous system effects include weakness, fatigue, sedation, hypomania, and tremor. Cardiovascular side effects include postural hypotension, cardiac arrhythmias secondary to prolonged repolarization, prolongation of the PR interval, widening of the QRS complex, bundle branch block, complete heart block, supraventricular or ventricular arrhythmias, as well as bradycardia.[14] Finally, acute intoxication with tricyclic antidepressants can induce mental status changes from confusion to coma, as well as hyperpyrexia, hyperactivity, athetoid and choreiform movements, muscular rigidity, and increased intestinal activity.

## Muscle Relaxants

Drugs that produce muscle relaxation or prevent flexor and extensor muscle spasms have been shown to effectively decrease musculoskeletal pain. Figure 7.7 demonstrates that there are several families of compounds that are used for this purpose. Among the various alternatives, the three most frequently prescribed medications are the benzodiazepines, baclofen, and dantrolene. It is generally preferable to avoid benzodiazepine for prolonged treatments secondary to their predominance of central ner-

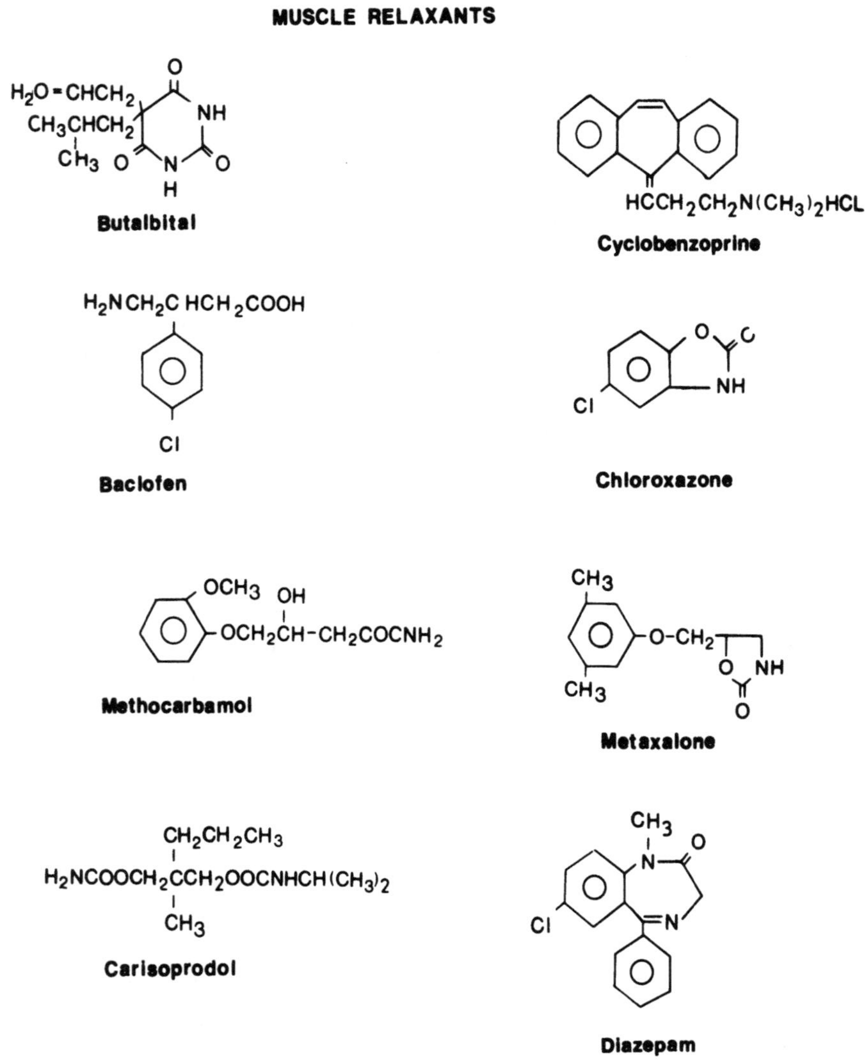


**Figure 7.7.** Structural formula of several muscle relaxants useful as adjunctive therapy in chronic pain disorders.

vous system side effects. Dantrolene, although the drug of choice for muscle spasm secondary to upper motor neuron disorders, is less frequently used for spasm resulting from musculoskeletal disorders.

Baclofen, a derivative of gamma-aminobutyric acid (GABA), effectively reduces the frequency and severity of flexor and extensor spasms and reduces increased flexor tone. The mechanism of action is believed to be depression of monosynaptic and polysynaptic neural transmission at the level of the spinal cord, by decreasing excitatory post-synaptic potentials in motor neurons of the anterior horn.

**Table 7.10.** Muscle Relaxants Potentially Useful as Adjuncts to Other Pain Medications

| Generic Name | Product Name | Quantity | Additional Ingredients (mg) | Recommended Dosage (mg) |
|---|---|---|---|---|
| Butalbital | B-A-C | 50 | Aspirin 650<br>Caffeine 40 | 1 tablet every 4 hours, max. = 6/24 hours |
| Cyclobenzaprine | Flexoril | 10 | | 1 tablet every 6–8 hours, max. = 60 mg/24 hours |
| Baclofen | Lioresal | 10, 20 | | 10–20 mg every 6–8 hours, max. = 80 mg/24 hours |
| Chloroxazone | Paraflex | 250 | | 1 tablet every 6–8 hours |
| Chloroxazone | Parafon Forte | 500 | | 1 tablet every 6–8 hours |
| Methocarbamol | Robaxin | 500, 750 | | 2 tablets every 6 hours, max. = 4–8 gms/24 hours |
| Methocarbamol | Robaxisal | 400 | Aspirin 325 | 2 tablets every 6 hours |
| Metaxalone | Skelaxin | 400 | | |
| Carisoprodol | Soma | 350 | | 1 tablet every 6 hours |
| Carisoprodol | Soma Compound | 200 | Aspirin 325 | 1–2 tablets every 6 hours |
| Diazepam* | Valium | 2, 5, 10 | 2–10 mg every 6–12 hours | |

*Benzodiazepines may not provide muscle relation beyond placebo or aspirin (Med. letter, 1973).

*Pharmacokinetics**

Baclofen, and each of the compounds listed in Table 7.10, is rapidly absorbed following oral administration, achieving a peak concentration within 1 to 2 hours. Half-lives vary among the groups from 3 to 4 for

*Portions of the pharmacokinetic, therapeutic, and side-effect data, and toxicity of several compounds were summarized from references 15 and 16. For further details, these references should be consulted.

baclofen, 1 to 3 days for flexoril, and 2 to 8 days for valium. Most of these compounds have significant inter-subject variation in plasma half-life, and dose-dependent rates of metabolism. All are excreted in the urine following conjugation, with the exception of baclofen, which is excreted unchanged.

### *Side Effects*

Most frequently noted side effects of these compounds include drowsiness, insomnia, dizziness, weakness, ataxia, and confusion. Overdose can result in coma, respiratory depression, and seizures. It is significant that the threshold for initiation of seizures may be lowered in epileptic patients. Sudden withdrawal of these compounds following chronic administration can cause anxiety, tachycardia, and hallucinations.

## References


1. Benson, A. (1983). Antipyretic analgesic therapy. Current worldwide status. *American Journal of Medicine* 75 (No. 5A):1–140.
2. Mathes, R.S., & Bennett, W.M. (1980). Effects of aspirin on glomerular filtration rate in normal humans. *Annals of Internal Medicine* 92:386–387.
3. Roth, G.R., & Siok, C.J. (1978). Acetylation of the $NH_2$ terminal serine of prostaglandin synthetase by aspirin. *Journal of Biological Chemistry* 253:3782–3784.
4. Perl, E.R. (1976). Sensitization of nociceptors and its relation to sensation. *Advances in Pain Research and Therapy*. Vol. I. In (Eds.) J.J. Bonica, and D. Albe-Fessard, New York: Raven Press.
5. Proudfoot, A.T., & Wright, N. (1970). Acute paracetamol poisoning. *British Medical Journal* 3:557–558.
6. Prescott, L.F., Wright N., Roscoe P., & Brown, S.S. (1971). Plasma paracetamol half-life and hepatic necrosis in patients with paracetamol overdosage. *Lancet* 1:519–522.
7. Prescott, L.F. (1965). Effects of acetylsalicylic acid, phenacetin, paracetamol, and caffeine on renal tubular epithelium. *Lancet* 2:91–96.
8. Emkey, R.D., & Mills, J.A. (1982). Aspirin and analgesic nephropathy. *Journal of the American Medical Association* 247:55–57.
9. Regalado, R.G. (1976). Anafranil in the management of long-term pain: A preliminary report. *Journal of Internal Medicine Research* 3:54–55.
10. Montgomery, B.J. (1978). Psychotropic agents finding analgesic use. *Journal of the American Medical Association* 240:1225.
11. Gringas, M. (1976). A clinical trial of tofranil in rheumatic pain in general practice. *Journal of Internal Medicine Research* 4:41–49.
12. Scott, W.A.M. (1969). The relief of pain with antidepressants in arthritis. *Practitioner* 202:802–807.
13. Chapman, C.R., Butler, S.H. (1978). Effects of doxepin on perception of laboratory induced pain in man. *Pain* 5:253–262.

14. Kantor, S.J., Bigger, T., & Glassman, A.H. (1975). Imipramine induced heart block. A longitudinal case study. *Journal of the American Medical Association* 231:1364–1366.
15. *Physicians Desk Reference.* Oradell, N.J. Medical Economics Company, Inc.
16. Goodman, L.S., & Gilman, A. (1985). *The Pharmacological Basis of Therapeutics.* Seventh Edition. New York: Macmillan.

# 8

# Psychiatric Examination and Treatment Determination

*Ruth M. Benca*

Psychological influences are almost always involved in shaping an individual's response to pain. Even for pain syndromes with readily identifiable organic etiologies, it is clear that psychological factors are inextricably linked to the subjective experience of pain. However, the psychological component of pain is usually not addressed until the physician is unable to determine the cause of or successfully treat the pain, at which time the nonresponding patient is all too often told by a frustrated physician that "There's nothing wrong with you," "The pain is all in your head," and "I can't do anything more for you." The patient may then be referred to a psychiatrist for evaluation of his or her psychological problems. Unfortunately, at this point, the patient is probably the least likely to accept the referral because of anger and frustration based on feelings that the pain complaint is not "believed" and that the patient has been abandoned by the physician. Furthermore, by failing to perform a psychiatric assessment early in the course of the patient evaluation, psychiatric illness, which may be etiologically related or secondary to the pain complaint, may go unrecognized and untreated. This chapter will discuss the major psychiatric etiologies and complications of chronic pain and how to assess the need for psychiatric intervention by the nonpsychiatric health professional.

Pain syndromes are often classified on the basis of duration (acute vs. chronic) and etiology. Psychogenic factors seem to be most significant in patients with chronic "benign" pain (i.e., pain not attributable to progressive or terminal illness); in this chapter, the term chronic pain refers to individuals with chronic "benign" pain syndromes. Pain may either be a presenting complaint of an underlying, primary psychiatric illness, or may be complicated by the development of secondary psychiatric symptoms such as anxiety, depression, or substance abuse. In many patients—perhaps the majority—a definitive psychiatric or other medical diagnosis cannot be made; these patients have received a variety of labels, including Engel's classification of the "pain-prone patient."[1] An understanding of the psychiatric conditions associated with chronic pain is necessary to provide an adequate evaluation of the pain complaint.

## Psychiatric Disorders Associated with Chronic Pain

Psychological factors are usually assumed to be significant etiologic factors for pain when an individual's pain complaints seem out of proportion to or without underlying pathology. The process by which psychological factors are transformed into physical symptoms of pain is somatization; it is a ubiquitous phenomenon, in which physical complaints (most often pain) express emotional distress and/or obtain relief from responsibility.[2] Somatization may occur with or without underlying physical illness, and the process itself becomes pathologic when the somatizing individual becomes dysfunctional at work or home, and/or seeks medical attention. Somatizing patients disproportionately account for both use of medical resources and loss of work days.[3]

It has been postulated that individuals may somatize because of an inability to understand and describe their internal, emotional states. Such individuals have been described as alexithymic—without words for feelings.[4] The alexithymic patient is unable to experience normal emotions such as anger, sadness, or joy, and tends to express negative internal states as pain. Both alexithymia and somatization are descriptive terms for cognitive and behavioral abnormalities that may be involved in the generation of pain complaints; they are not specific diagnoses themselves, but are processes involved in many of the psychiatric disorders that present as chronic pain syndromes.

The following descriptions of some of the psychiatric disorders associated with chronic pain syndromes are based on the *Diagnostic and Statistical Manual of Mental Disorders*, Third Edition-Revised (DSM-III-R).[5] The diagnostic categories of DSM-III-R are widely accepted as standard terminology for the medical profession in general and the mental health field specifically. For further discussion of the clinical syndromes and diagnostic criteria, the reader is referred to DSM-III-R.

### Depression

Depression is, by far, the psychiatric disorder most commonly associated with chronic pain. Investigations of chronic pain populations show that a proportion of pain patients meet diagnostic criteria for major depression, with most estimates ranging from approximately 10 to 80%,[6,7] depending on the populations sampled. Conversely, when groups of patients with major depression are studied, a significant number of individuals are found to be suffering from chronic pain.[8] Some authors have suggested that chronic pain may be a form of major depression, and have proposed the descriptive terms "masked depression,"[9] "depression-spectrum disease,"[10] and "pain-prone disorder"[1]; others believe that depression occurs secondarily, as a response to the experience of chronic pain.[11] Evidence in support of an etiologic connection between depression and pain includes the presence of similar biological markers, such as failure to inhibit cortisol secretion during the dexamethasone suppression test and decreased REM sleep latency.[12] Family histories show an increased incidence of affective illness and alcohol abuse.[7] Finally, it has also been suggested that antidepressant medication is useful in the treatment of chronic pain. Some studies find that pain patients respond to tricyclic antidepressants vs. placebo with significant pain relief independent of co-existing depressive symptoms, while other studies indicate that patients who have symptoms of both depression and pain tend to have more subjective pain improvement than do nondepressed patients.[13,14] The purported mechanism for the efficacy of tricyclics in chronic pain is through increase in central nervous system serotonin levels, since serotonin seems to be involved in CNS pathways involved in pain perception.

The evaluation of depression in chronic pain patients is often difficult because of the overlap of symptoms. Diagnosis of depression requires the presence of depressed mood, or loss of interest or pleasure, and at least four more complaints from a group that includes "vegetative" signs and symptoms: appetite disturbance, sleep disturbance, and fatigue or energy loss. However, diagnostic criteria require that the symptoms not be due to a physical condition. Chronic pain, like many medical illnesses, characteristically can interfere with sleep, appetite, energy, and the ability to enjoy normal activities, which makes definitive diagnosis of major depression unclear in the context of chronic pain; for example, is a patient unable to sleep at night because he or she is in pain or depressed? Diagnosis is easier in patients who express feelings of guilt, worthlessness, suicidal ideation, or other of the nonvegetative symptoms of depression.

Recognition of depression in individuals with chronic pain has important implications for treatment, whether one views pain as being distinct from or a variant of depression. Treatment of depression is most often successful, and the reduction of depressive symptoms and cognitions in chronic pain patients may affect significantly their perception of the pain experience. Certainly, "quality of life" is often improved if a reduction of depression can be achieved. The idea that pain may be a form of depression argues more strongly in favor of consideration of depression treatment for all chronic pain patients, particularly for those in whom the risks of antidepressant therapy are minimal.

## Anxiety Disorders

Like depression, symptoms of anxiety are quite common accompaniments to chronic pain syndromes.[15] The symptom of anxiety is known to exacerbate the subjective experience of pain, and uncontrolled pain can increase an individual's level of anxiety. However, some pain patients have specific anxiety disorders that can complicate or present as chronic pain disorders. Generalized anxiety disorder, characterized by excessive and unrealistic worrying, may include physical symptoms of muscle soreness (from motor tension) or abdominal pain (from autonomic hyperactivity). Individuals with panic disorder may have significant chest pain during their panic attacks, and may go to emergency rooms, where they are usually evaluated for a possible heart attack. After repeated episodes (with normal electrocardiograms), they may be referred for psychological evaluation of their pain.

## Somatoform Disorders

It is often assumed that an individual who somatizes has a somatoform disorder. As described earlier, somatization is a process that can occur with a variety of psychiatric conditions, and the most likely diagnoses for somatizing pain patients are probably depression or anxiety disorders. However, some patients with pain complaints will have evidence of somatoform disorders after diagnoses of depression and anxiety disorders have been ruled out. In general, the somatoform disorders are more common in women than men, generally begin in early to mid-adulthood, and tend to be chronic. The production of symptoms is involuntary; that is, patients are not consciously aware of what they are doing. Individuals with somatoform disorders tend to have little insight into their psychological problems, even independently of their physical complaints, and are, therefore, extremely difficult to engage in psychological treatment. The somatization disorders that most commonly present as chronic pain are somatization, somatoform pain, and hypochondriasis.

### *Somatization Disorder*

Formerly referred to as Briquet's Syndrome, somatization disorder involves the production of at least thirteen of a list of specific symptoms (some of which include pain) without underlying pathology and with a significant response to the symptoms by the patient (i.e., seeking medical attention, missing school or work, etc.). Symptoms most commonly associated with somatization disorder include vomiting, pain in the extremities, shortness of breath, amnesia, difficulty swallowing, burning sensation in sexual organs, and dysmenorrhea. Patients with the disorder tend to undergo multiple surgeries with vague indications other than chronic pain, and usually report no lasting improvement (or often worsening) of their conditions after surgery.

*Somatoform Pain Disorder*

This diagnosis was included in DSM-III-R to replace the former category of psychogenic pain disorder. Both diagnoses specify that the pain complaint be long standing (six months or longer) and be either without or in excess of physical findings. Diagnosis of psychogenic pain required that psychological factors be identified as etiologic; that is, that they were temporally related to the appearance of symptoms or reinforced the pain behavior through secondary gain. Although psychological precipitants or secondary gain may also occur in somatoform pain, definitive identification of them is not required to make a diagnosis, which makes the category potentially applicable to a broader group of individuals. Somatoform pain is the diagnosis that probably best accounts for most of the various psychological descriptions of chronic pain patients who were psychiatrically "undiagnosable" in the past. Patients with somatoform pain disorder may have a variety of presentations based on the underlying psychodynamic forces responsible for the pain symptoms. At one end of the spectrum are the alexithymic individuals who appear obsessional, ruminative, and seem constricted in their expression of emotion; at the other extreme are the highly emotional, dramatic individuals who use the defense mechanisms of repression and dissociation to deal with conflictual situations.

*Hypochondriasis*

There is still a great deal of controversy as to whether hypochondriasis is a separate diagnostic entity rather than a symptom of a variety of other disorders.[16] It involves an unrealistic interpretation of physical signs and symptoms as indications of illness; patients are overly focused on physical sensations and may, therefore, complain of pain, although in contrast to the previous disorders, the patient may be more concerned with the potential significance of the pain rather than its intensity.

In general, the somatoform disorders are often accompanied by a variety of associated features. Chronic pain patients with somatoform disorders tend to "doctor-shop," become dependent on narcotics and/or minor tranquilizers, and undergo multiple unsuccessful surgeries. They often have coexisting personality disorders, and may have a history of physical or sexual abuse in childhood.

Their treatment is best achieved through an empathic and long-term relationship with a primary-care physician, with the goal of treatment to "protect" the patient from unnecessary diagnostic tests, procedures, and medications. Behavioral and supportive therapies are useful for motivated patients; psychotherapy is rarely successful because of the general lack of psychological insight found in this population, combined with their intense insistence that the problems are of a physical nature.

*Associated Disorders*

Other disorders that also involve production of physical symptoms (often pain) for psychological reasons include factitious disorders and malingering. Unlike the somatoform illnesses, these disorders are characterized by voluntary or self-induced production of symptoms.

*Factitious Disorder.* Individuals sometimes create signs or symptoms of physical illness for the primary purpose of maintaining a "sick" role; in contrast to malingering (described below), obvious secondary gain is usually not present. The term Munchausen's syndrome has been used for those in whom the maintenance of a factitious illness becomes a way of life. These individuals tend to have a characteristic presentation, including vague and fantastic histories, often having wandered from place to place in search of medical care, a history of multiple surgeries, and possible drug dependence. Patients with factitious disorders may also engage in self-destructive behavior in their attempts to simulate illness, including self-inflicted trauma, injection or ingestion of toxic substances, and self-bleeding. Factitious disorders are often difficult to diagnose because of the conscious determination of the patient not to be "discovered." Interestingly, a significant number of individuals with factitious disorders have a history of working in health-care fields; their sophisticated knowledge makes their illness more convincing than in some cases of somatoform disorders.

*Malingering.* Malingerers also fabricate signs and symptoms of illness, but do so for more obvious reasons; secondary gains usually involve release from responsibilities and/or increased attention from others. Malingering itself is not a mental illness, and may be a more or less pathological adaptive response to environmental stressors. Malingerers can be confused with those experiencing conversion (i.e., an alteration or loss of physical function which is an expression of an underlying psychological conflict), and it is often difficult to distinguish the "conscious" or "unconscious" nature of the symptoms. (A conversion disorder cannot be limited to pain, however.)

## Psychological Factors Affecting Physical Condition

In contrast to the somatoform and related disorders described above, in which underlying pathophysiology is not primarily responsible for the symptoms, this category requires that an individual have a true, "organic" illness. For some individuals with chronic illnesses, it seems clear that flare-ups are highly correlated with psychosocial stressors.

Some authors have suggested that "compensation neurosis" falls under this heading.[17] In this situation, patients who are eligible for disability or workmen's compensation payments, or who may be beneficiaries in a lawsuit related to an accident, may have a prolonged experience of pain following an illness or injury, out of proportion to underlying pathology. Unlike malingerers, these patients do not consciously feign symptoms; and as in somatoform disorders, the pain is an unconscious mechanism for dealing with psychosocial conflicts.

## Evaluation of Patients with Chronic Pain

Because of the high prevalence of psychiatric disorders in chronic pain patients,[18] the physician must maintain a high index of suspicion toward psychiatric illness when evaluating these patients. Some nonpsychiatric physicians who treat chronic pain require psychiatric evaluation of all patients; this usually is possible in multidisciplinary clinics specializing in the treatment of chronic pain. However, it is not feasible for every chronic pain patient to be evaluated thoroughly by a psychiatrist, particularly in primary care settings. It is therefore useful for physicians working with this patient population to be aware of particular aspects of the history that may help in deciding which patients would most benefit from psychiatric referral. Although some physicians suggest focusing on a few, specific items that tend to indicate "psychogenic" pain, there is, in fact, data potentially relevant to underlying psychiatric illness in all parts of a standard medical history. With an understanding of which aspects of the history may be most useful, and how best to elicit the information, a fairly effective psychological screening evaluation can be performed.

There are several reasons for addressing potential major psychological contributions to pain in the context of the medical examination. First, attempting to perform a medical history and physical without attention to psychological factors is both incomplete and reinforces the idea that pain is either physical or psychological; it may delay accurate diagnosis and appropriate treatment. Second, by spending the extra time to get an understanding of psychosocial contributions to pain, the physician can begin to develop an empathic relationship with the patient, which is a crucial step toward the establishment of the therapeutic alliance, itself vital for the successful treatment of chronic pain.

The most important factor in eliciting a history that will be useful in evaluating whether psychological factors are etiologically significant in a chronic pain syndrome is spending adequate time with the patient. A hurried or "short-cut" approach makes it virtually impossible to have access to all the relevant data. Furthermore, time and patience are especially required in sorting through the histories of chronic pain patients because most of the cognitive work of determining possible psychological influences on the physical problem must be done by the examiner; as a group, chronic pain patients have little insight or understanding into their emotional states and, in fact, tend to deny associations between their pain and psychosocial factors.

In addition to spending enough time, there are several other general guidelines for obtaining the history. First, questioning in each area should always begin in an open-ended way (as recommended for all good medical history-taking); it is particularly necessary for this group of patients. Second, the history should be organized in a chronological fashion, partly with the aid of the patient. It is sometimes helpful for the examiner to elicit and organize medical and psychosocial histories separately and then look for possible associations, rather than expect the patient to be able to do so. Without a clear sense of the temporal sequence of events in all spheres of the patient's life, it is impossible to infer relationships between psychological and physical events.

Finally, the attitude of the examiner can play a significant role in affecting the nature of the information elicited. The examiner should display a genuine and professional interest in hearing the patient's story; he or she should be at neither extreme of displaying too much emotion or involvement (i.e., overly identifying with the patient or trying to "save" the patient), or being too distant and aloof. It is extremely important not to see the interview as a challenge to prove that the patient is "not really sick" or, in other words, that the examiner "wins" and the patient "loses" if it can be shown that the pain complaint has a psychological etiology. A more accurate way to view the situation is that the goal of the interview is to arrive at the correct diagnosis, whether it be psychiatric or other medical; in this way, the process can avoid becoming adversarial and both parties "win."

Several issues should be addressed in the initial interview by any medical professional who evaluates chronic pain patients. Listed below are some of the more important areas to cover, including suggestions for specific lines of questioning, and the kinds of answers that may indicate the need for further psychiatric assessment.

## Description of Pain Complaint

There is almost universal consensus that obtaining a careful history of the pain itself is vital for consideration of psychogenic factors. Begin by asking the patient to describe the pain, or "tell the story" of the pain. In addition to asking the usual questions about the pain (e.g., location, quality, intensity; see Chapter 4), be sure to ask about variability of the pain or what makes the pain better or worse, including medications, activities (sleeping, resting, eating, exercise, sex, work, etc.), locations (home, work, school, etc.), and time (day vs. night, morning vs. evening, weekdays vs. weekends, etc.). For individuals who report that the pain appears to worsen according to a specific parameter, it is important to consider the potential psychosocial factors that may be contributing to the symptoms, particularly in cases that don't seem to make sense physiologically—for example, a patient whose pain is incapacitating at work but doesn't interfere with an active social life.

In addition to asking about factors that influence the pain, the clinician must personally be watchful for potential influences that the patient will be unable to report. For example, the pain may worsen acutely in the presence of certain family members or medical staff, or in particular situations.

The possibility of psychiatric disorders should also be considered for individuals who state that their pain never changes or nothing helps. Similarly, further psychiatric evaluation should be considered for those whose complaints are vague and nonspecific, or when the pain seems to move from location to location.

For patients whose pain is subsequent to an accident or injury, find out whether the event occurred at work and whether litigation is pending or the patient is thinking of filing a suit. Is the individual on Workmen's Compensation? If the pain syndrome has appeared subsequent to a surgery or procedure, is the patient involved in malpractice proceedings? All of these may be powerful reinforcers for pain complaints, either at a conscious or unconscious level.

## History of Treatment

Ask the patient to describe everything that has been done to date for the pain, even if the patient brings in medical records of previous treatment. Watch for excessive use of narcotics or benzodiazepines, and be sure to inquire specifically about use of, and response to, street drugs and alcohol. Consider urine or blood drug screens if unsure about the veracity of the patient's report. Those with current substance abuse problems may require both detoxification and further evaluation of underlying affective or anxiety disorders.

Listen to the patient's description of previous care by medical personnel; patients who repeatedly express extreme hostility or patterns of idealization and subsequent devaluation toward previous caretakers may have underlying personality disorders. For example, a patient may say something like, "Dr. A. was supposed to be the best in his field, and I thought he was going to be able to help me, but he turned out to be no good, just like all the others." Some patients may even express degrees of paranoia about former doctors, occasionally reaching delusional proportions (e.g., "The doctor was performing secret experiments on me") and may have a psychotic illness.

Finally, compare the patient's version of treatment outcome with the medical record or the previous physician's report. Look for great discrepancies between reports of the patient and physician, and cases where everything works for a brief period or while the patient is in close contact with a physician or other medical therapist.

## Psychiatric Symptoms

All patients merit an inquiry into general psychiatric symptomatology. A possible introduction to the topic is to ask the patient how he is coping with his pain, in what ways the pain has affected his life or how his spirits have been. Some patients may readily report symptoms of depressed mood, hopelessness, or excessive anxiety while others may deny problems with their mood but still have underlying affective disorders. Such individuals may be alexithymic and use the process of somatization to express their emotional state. It is, therefore, important to question all patients, including those without an apparent mood disorder, about other symptoms of depression. Specifically, one should inquire about sleep and appetite disturbances (increased or decreased), energy, change of level of interest in activities, sexual relationships, and self-esteem. All patients must be questioned about possible thoughts of suicide.

Patients should also be questioned about symptoms of anxiety; do they worry excessively, feel tense physically, or have panic attacks? Often patients will admit to difficulties concentrating or remembering things, which can be seen with anxiety or may suggest an underlying organic brain disorder. Patients who report subjective problems with memory or concentration should be tested briefly on their short-term memory (remembering three objects or a name and address for five minutes) and ability to concentrate (e.g., serial sevens).

Screening for psychotic symptoms may be useful for patients who seem suspicious, paranoid, or disorganized. Ask if they have noticed difficulties with thinking, or unusual thought or experiences, such as hallucinations.

Finally, all patients should be asked about a history of psychiatric or emotional problems. This includes inquiry about family history of psychiatric problems, and alcohol or other substance abuse.

## Family and Social History

A detailed, chronological social history is invaluable for attempting to link psychosocial stressors with the pain syndrome. With the medical history in mind, look for temporal associations between life events and pain episodes. Ask about other family members, with whom the patient may be identifying, who have had chronic illnesses or pain syndromes. It is also important to inquire about the quality of the patient's relationships with significant family members—are there conflicts or responsibilities that the patient can escape from through his or her pain?

### Level of Insight

An extremely useful approach to assessing the patient's level of insight into his situation, which often yields valuable psychological information, is to ask the patient what his understanding is of what is wrong with him. This question is not necessarily equivalent to asking what the doctors have told the patient is wrong with him, although it is usually helpful to ask that question as well. Often the patient will respond with an answer like, "I have no idea" or "That's what I'm here to find out." The interviewer can acknowledge the patient's uncertainty and gently press him to answer by asking him to describe his worst fear of what is wrong. Occasionally, a patient may use the pain to identify with a relative or close friend who has been ill recently, for example, "My headaches feel just like the ones my aunt had before she died of a brain tumor last year." Other patients may reveal hypochondriacal preoccupations less clearly related to a specific event, suggesting a somatoform disorder or depression. Rarely, a patient may respond to such questioning with a frank delusion, indicating an underlying psychotic process.

## Referral for Psychiatric Evaluation

Psychiatric referral should be considered for any patient with chronic pain with symptoms suggestive of psychiatric illness, as described earlier. Specifically, the physician should be alert for signs of significant anxiety or depression, powerful psychosocial reinforcers of illness behavior, and pain that is unexplained by known pathophysiologic mechanisms. A careful initial examination will often provide enough information for the determination of whether or not psychiatric input may be needed.

It is often easier to identify chronic pain patients in need of psychiatric intervention than it is to make the actual referral to the psychiatrist, however. The success of the psychiatric evaluation probably is most dependent on getting the psychiatrist involved early in the evaluation process, and the manner in which the referral is made. As indicated in the beginning of the chapter, telling patients that their medical evaluation revealed no underlying problem and, therefore, they are being sent to a psychiatrist to find out what is wrong with them tends to make patients angry, defensive, and unlikely to follow through with the referral.

A potentially more successful way to get the patient involved in the psychological component of the assessment is to begin the process concurrently with the medical evaluation, and introduce the psychiatrist as a member of the treatment team. The reason for the psychiatric consultation can be stated in a number of ways, including (1) to understand the patient's unique situation as well as possible, (2) to help the patient cope with the pain, (3) to evaluate and treat the patient's concurrent depression or anxiety, (4) to make recommendations on how to help control the patient's pain, etc.; it is generally preferable not to tell a patient that a pain is "psychological" or "not physical" in suggesting referral to the psychiatrist.

When consulting a psychiatrist in the course of evaluation of a chronic pain patient, it is imperative that the primary physician remain involved. The potential outcomes of psychiatric evaluation range from having the patient enter a psychotherapeutic treatment (in which case the primary physician should maintain a role as the provider of medical services when indicated) to having the patient managed primarily by the primary-care physician. Most patients with chronic pain and psychiatric disorders (e.g., depression, anxiety, somatoform disorders) are, in fact, taken care of by nonpsychiatrists. In these cases, the psychiatrist serves as a consultant, to establish the psychiatric diagnosis and make recommendations to the primary physician regarding appropriate management.

The treatment of chronic pain presents a difficult challenge to both medical physicians and psychiatrists. Everyone involved in the treatment of patients with chronic pain needs to watch for signs of possible psychiatric disorders, which may be the primary source of the pain complaint or secondarily complicate a chronic pain syndrome. Timely referral to psychiatrists can lead to accurate diagnosis and appropriate treatment planning for this demanding group of patients.

## References


1. Engel, G. (1959). "Psychogenic" pain and the pain-prone patient. *American Journal of Medicine* 26:899–918.
2. Lipowski, Z.J. (1987). Somatization: medicine's unsolved problem. *Psychosomatics* 28:294–297.
3. Ford, C.V. (1986). The somatizing disorders. *Psychosomatics* 27:327–337.
4. Lesser, L.M., Ford, C.V., & Friedmann, C.T.H. (1979). Alexithymia in somatizing patients. *General Hospital Psychiatry* 1:256–261.
5. *Diagnostic and Statistical Manual of Mental Disorders.* (1987). Third Edition—Revised. Washington, D.C.: American Psychiatric Association.
6. Kramlinger, K.G., Swanson, D.W., & Maruta, T. (1983). Are patients with chronic pain depressed? *American Journal of Psychiatry* 140:747–749.
7. Magni, G. (1987). On the relationship between chronic pain and depression when there is no organic lesion. *Pain* 31:1–21.
8. Von Knorring, L., Perris, C., Eisemann, M., Eriksson, U., & Perris, H. (1983). Pain as a symptom in depressive disorders. I. Relationship to diagnostic subgroup and depressive symptomatology. *Pain* 15:19–26.
9. Lopez-Ibor, J.J. (1972). Masked depression. *British Journal of Psychiatry* 120:245–258.
10. Winokur, G., Behar, D., Van Valkenburg, M.D. et al. (1978). Is a familial definition of depression both feasible and valid? *Journal of Nervous and Mental Disorders* 166:764–768.

11. Hendler, N. (1984). Depression caused by chronic pain. *Journal of Clinical Psychiatry* 45:30–36.
12. Blumer, D., Zorick, F., Heilbronn, M., & Roth, T. (1982). Biological Markers for depression in chronic pain. *Journal of Nervous and Mental Disorders* 170:425–428.
13. Dworkin, R.H., Richlin, D.M., Handlin, D.S., & Brand, L. (1986). Predicting treatment response in depressed and non-depressed chronic pain patients. *Pain* 24:343–353.
14. Getto, C.J., Sorkness, C.A., & Howell, T. (1987). Antidepressants and chronic nonmalignant pain: A review. *Journal of Pain and Symptom Management* 2:9–18.
15. Fishbain, D.A., Goldberg, M., Meagher, B.R., Steele, R., & Rosomoff, H. (1986). Male and female chronic pain patients categorized by DSM-III psychiatric diagnostic criteria. *Pain* 26:181–197.
16. Kellner, R. (1986). Functional somatic symptoms and hypochondriasis. *Archives of General Psychiatry* 42:821–833.
17. Hackett, T.P., & Cassem, N.H. (Eds.) (1987). *Massachusetts General Hospital Handbook of General Hospital Psychiatry.* Second Edition. Littleton, Mass.: PSG Publishing Co., Inc.
18. Reich, J., Tupin J.P., & Abramowitz, S.I. (1983). Psychiatric diagnosis of chronic pain patients. *American Journal of Psychiatry* 140:1495–1498.

# 9

# The Conservative Medical Management of Pain

*Robert K. Erickson*

Few would argue with the premise that every attempt should be made to manage the painful condition conservatively before considering surgical procedures or other invasive maneuvers. Exceptions to this rule would include conditions caused by progressive mass effect, such as cauda equina and cord compression syndromes. Additionally, many feel that the causalgic syndromes should be treated as early as possible to prevent progression of the disease.

In the case of disc disease or other mechanical lesions of the spinal nerve roots, most conservative treatment regimens center about strict bedrest, mild analgesic medication, and avoidance of physical activities that exacerbate the pain. Secondary muscle spasm may be successfully treated with a short course of muscle relaxant medication. Many patients will also benefit from the use of a cervical collar or lumbar corset. Painful recurrences of root compression may be diminished by instructing the patient in exercises designed to strengthen the abdominal and paraspinal musculature. Persistent or chronic problems may respond to transcutaneous stimulation, epidural injection, or physiotherapeutic maneuvers. It is well known that the great majority of patients who suffer from radiculopathy secondary to disc disease will improve under conservative therapy. When symptoms are associated with spinal stenosis, conservative measures are less likely to be of lasting value. Chronic arachnoiditis and epidural fibrosis are particularly difficult problems that are generally poorly responsive to conservative therapy.

The diagnosis of a myofascial pain syndrome will lead to the institution of a treatment regimen that is entirely conservative. These problems will often respond to local treatment directed at the involved muscles or trigger points. The administration of topical or intramuscular anesthesia in conjunction with muscle relaxation techniques such as massage, progressive stretching, or biofeedback may be quite beneficial. In some instances, limited manipulation may prove effective. Although most myofascial problems will improve with systematic physical measures, there are several conditions such as the chronic flexion-extension injury ("whiplash") that may frustrate any intervention.

There exists no effective conservative treatment for deafferentation pain. Carbamazepine (Tegretol) may occasionally reduce some of the spontaneous sharp pain associated with the thalamic syndrome; dysesthesia and hyperpathia are generally not reduced, however. Neuroleptic and psychotropic medications have not been shown to be of benefit, although the tricyclic antidepressants may diminish the insomnia that frequently accompanies the pain.[22] Peripheral blocks with alcohol or anesthetics often will result in temporary relief of pain, which in the long run is quite disappointing. Some patients may benefit from psychotherapeutic support.

The present chapter will review the available non-invasive methods of pain treatment. The pharmacology of pain, specific injection techniques, and cognitive-behavioral approaches will be reviewed elsewhere in the text.

## Bedrest and Immobilization

Rest and immobilization remain the mainstay of conservative treatment in cases of degenerative disc disease. The treatment is most likely to be efficacious in acute cases of disc herniation, however. The rationale behind the treatment is clear, based on the pathological progression from nuclear degeneration and nuclear displacement to eventual fibrosis of the disc material.[2] Bedrest and immobilization serve to protect the abnormal disc from strain and to encourage healing by fibrosis and desiccation of the disc material[26,27] It is thought that even completely herniated fragments will eventually respond to rest. Early surgery is not indicated unless there is evidence for a persistent or progressive neurologic deficit.

Those with severe symptoms are maintained on strict bedrest with the knees slightly elevated. Analgesics are generally prescribed during the acute stage. The addition of a muscle relaxant may be beneficial. When the symptoms have subsided somewhat, the patient is allowed to resume careful general activity that avoids lifting, bending, and twisting. Many patients will benefit from the use of a well-fitted lumbosacral corset. Pelvic traction may be useful only in keeping a noncompliant patient in bed or if enough weight is applied to equal at least half the body weight. There is no evidence that traction for lumbar disc disease hastens resolution of symptoms. Extreme pelvic manipulation may potentially be harmful.[18] Once the symptoms have subsided, the patient is instructed in back exercises designed to develop the abdominal and erector spinae muscles; the maintenance of good abdominal muscle tone again serves to reduce strain at the disc level.[16,19] Correct posture and lifting techniques are emphasized. Disc disease in the cervical area is treated in a similar fashion. The use of a cervical collar or other external immobilization will reduce the amount of repetitive flexion and extension. In contrast to pelvic traction, cervical traction is quite commonly used, although not everyone finds this treatment effective.[17] The compliant patient may be instructed in the use of intermittent halter traction at home; this treatment, although convenient, depends upon the experience of the instructor and the cooperation of the patient. Generally, if cervical traction is to be effective, there will be a positive response within the first week of treatment. While rest, immobilization, and restricted activity are well established as treatment for acute disc disease or other conditions arising from mechanical instability, it is difficult to rationalize similar treatment for patients with nonradiating back pain or exacerbations of chronic back pain. Often these patients benefit no more from extended periods of inactivity than they do from a few days of rest.[4] These patients with primarily myofascial syndromes should be encouraged to be as active as possible. Inappropriately long periods of inactivity may serve to reduce the effective muscle mass and may actually render the patient more vulnerable to subsequent injuries. Of course, extended periods of inactivity may also interfere with motivation and add to reactive depression. The patient with chronic back pain should be reassured that discomfort is unlikely to be harmful, and that meaningful activity should be pursued.

## Myofascial Pain Syndromes

Chronic pain associated with myofascial disease may be temporarily relieved by periods of rest or immobilization only to recur as soon as normal activity is resumed. In general, extended periods of bedrest for myofascial disease are not effective; in fact, prolonged immobility may leave the muscle in a fully shortened position which may increase the probability of recurrence. The diagnosis of a primary myofascial syndrome is made based on the presence of palpable trigger points and the verification of a typical pain referral pattern. The diagnosis is confirmed during therapeutic maneuvers directed at the chronic trigger points.

The techniques of trigger-point treatment have been thoroughly reviewed by Travell and Simons.[29] Treatment involves progressive stretching of the involved musculature as the patient moves the muscle actively through its full range of motion. The normal reflex shortening of the painful muscle is avoided either by topical vapocoolant (chlorofluoromethane or ethyl chloride), or by precise trigger-point injection with a suitable local anesthetic. Often, local heat is applied to the area during stretching maneuvers, again to reduce the post-injection soreness. It has been reported that dry needling or simple saline injection of trigger points without local anesthesia are also effective modes of treatment.[10] Deep massive, ischemic compression of the muscle, and the application of ultrasound are other techniques that have been used in various combinations to relieve myofascial pain.

Although the above maneuvers may be definitively therapeutic, it is generally most important that any perpetuating factors in the problem be corrected. The most common perpetuating factors include poor posture, obesity, or prolonged immobility. A sedentary lifestyle punctuated by infrequent heavy work or exercise is all too common; the institution of a regular exercise program specifically designed to strengthen the involved muscles is required. Structural inadequacy may lead to mechanical stresses that overload certain muscles. Scoliosis, pelvic asymmetry, and limb-length discrepancy all are conditions capable of imposing intolerable muscular stress.[28]

## Transcutaneous Electrical Nerve Stimulation

Although the classic gate control theory of Melzack and Wall is a simplification of events that occur in the dorsal horn of the spinal cord,[21] one of its major assertions has been confirmed. The theory predicted that activity in the large myelinated primary afferent fibers (the A fibers) would inhibit the transmission of activity in the small unmyelinated primary afferent fibers (the C fibers) via inhibitory circuits in the dorsal horn of the spinal cord.

The gate control theory was first tested clinically by Wall and Sweet in 1967 at which time they reported on the prolonged stimulation of peripheral nerves with percutaneous electrodes in normal volunteers. The percutaneous stimulation clearly modified the reaction to acute noxious stimuli without any untoward discomfort.[30] Following this report, there has been an explosion in the use of transcutaneous electrical nerve stimulation (TENS) with the advent of modern solid state technology. TENS is a convenient and relatively inexpensive pain treatment. The location of the surface electrodes may be easily changed, and the amount of current varied, in order to achieve low-threshold stimulation which typically produces nonpainful paresthesia in the region of the body where the pain is located. Unless the patient feels adequate paresthesia at the sight of the pain, it is unlikely that the pain will be reduced to a satisfactory degree.

Often it is not possible to predict the most effective site for the stimulating electrodes; the patient should be trained in the use of the stimulator by an experienced practitioner with time set aside for several adjustments.

In our clinic, the initial trial period is generally thirty to sixty days. Most patients will prefer frequencies between 40 and 70 Hz with pulse-widths of 0.1 to 0.5 ms. It is possible to use high-intensity stimulation if the trains of high frequency bursts are repeated at a fairly low frequency.[5]

Analgesia following TENS may be produced immediately, or a beneficial effect may not be noted for several hours or days following continuous stimulation. The average time to a positive response is approximately 20 minutes. Because of the great variability in the onset of benefit, a brief trial with a negative result is almost meaningless. Some patients find that TENS produces analgesia only during stimulation, while others are relieved for a significant periods following stimulation.

Both acute pain states and chronic pain conditions are responsive to TENS. Postoperative pain is particularly amenable to TENS. Sterilized electrodes are placed adjacent to the incision by the surgeon at the end of the operation. The use of TENS postoperatively decreases narcotic requirements and provides continuous relief. TENS has also been used to treat the pain of childbirth and acute oral pain associated with dental procedures. Acute pain can be significantly diminished by the use of TENS in many patients.

Because of the non-invasive nature of TENS, it has been applied to virtually every chronic pain condition. TENS is commonly used as the first form of treatment in the pain clinic. It is particularly suited to the treatment of neurogenic pains, such as peripheral nerve injury, causalgia, intercostal neuritis, and post-herpetic neuralgia.[21] TENS is also indicated in cases of backpain, radiculopathy, and in central pain states such as brachial plexus avulsion.[5,32] Even the pain of spinal cord injury can be successfully treated if sufficient paresthesia can be generated.[25]

TENS is contraindicated in patients with pacemakers or other implanted electrical devices that could be affected by the stimulator. TENS also works poorly in chronic states that affect multiple somatic areas or are poorly localized. Similarly, visceral and nonorganic pain do not respond to TENS. There is often a negative response to TENS in the presence of significant hyperesthesia.

There are hundreds of reported studies that document successful treatment of widely different pain conditions with TENS. Most of these studies center on the efficacy of stimulation, and certainly a trial of TENS is warranted in almost any pain condition because of its safety. Although the response of chronic pain states to TENS is significantly better than that of placebo stimulation, on the average only approximately 30% of chronic pain patients will respond significantly. In addition, the efficacy of the treatment tends to diminish with time. Wolff[31] has summarized the experience of several authors, noting that in the early stages TENS generally produces a 60 to 80% positive response rate, which on the average falls off over the first year of treatment until a stable long-term success rate of

20 to 30% is achieved. Of course, part of the response is due to placebo effect; the placebo effect, however, seems to fall off very rapidly, and contributes very little to the long-term benefit.[11,31]

## Acupuncture and Hyperstimulation Analgesia

The control of pain by intense stimulation which in itself may be quite painful is not a new method. Various techniques of "counter-irritation" have been practiced for centuries in many different cultures including our own. Examples of these techniques include trephination of the skull for headache, scarification of the skin, cauterization, and the application of strong astringent solutions that blister the skin.

Acupuncture has also been in continuous practice in China for thousands of years, and is currently the subject of revitalized interest. Briefly, acupuncture involves insertion of fine needles at specific locations following which the needles are twirled slowly. The needles may be left in place for varying periods of time, or may be used to administer electrical stimulation ("electro-acupuncture"). The stimulation points are based on complex charts consisting of 361 points that lie on 14 meridians, most of which are thought to correspond to specific internal organs.[8]

Recent systematic studies of acupuncture have shown that its effect is neither miraculous or mysterious. Most acupuncture points when displayed according to the treated syndrome lie at or near the site of pain.[15] Although in China it is sometimes used as surgical anesthesia, it is only carried out on very select patients who have been thoroughly exposed to the method of acupuncture before the procedure.[3] Acupuncture has not provided sufficient anesthesia for surgical procedures in Western countries. It has been shown that stimulation of nerves by the needles rather than a specific location on meridians is necessary for effective pain relief.[7] The analgesic effect of acupuncture may be blocked by procaine infiltration of the respective acupuncture points, and subsequent neuropharmacological studies have shown specific alterations in neurotransmitter levels in cerebrospinal fluid. Generally, experimental evidence shows that acupuncture produces significantly greater analgesia than comparable placebo treatment, and that stimulation close to the sight of pain is more effective than distant stimulation.[1,24] Finally, the pain response of experimental animals is also favorably altered by acupuncture-like stimulation. These experimental effects may be produced by various kinds of intense stimulation, including the application of heat.[9,23] Thus acupuncture seems to be an effective method of producing a fairly intense sensory input that results in analgesia.

The term "hyperstimulation analgesia"[13] includes all of the methods based on counter-irritation, such as acupuncture. It is likely that many of our physiotherapeutic methods such as icepacking, ice massage, deep heat, and ischemic compression also fall into this category. Dry needling and saline injection may be best categorized as forms as hyperstimulation analgesia.

The effects of brief intense transcutaneous electrical stimulation at trigger points or acupuncture points on pain have been examined by Melzack.[14] Most investigators feel that intense TENS utilized as "electro-acupuncture" is at least as effective as acupuncture itself, and has the further advantage of chronic, non-invasive application.[24]

The exact physiologic explanation for pain relief after intense stimulation has not been ascertained.[15] It is felt that both brain stem and spinal mechanisms must be operative in the effect, as it has been observed that naloxone reverses needle-acupuncture analgesia,[12] while it has also been found that spontaneous activity in dorsal horn cells can be inhibited by intense stimulation of the contralateral leg in experimental animals. Again, analgesia, resulting from hyperstimulation may be obtained at distant body sites, and the pain relief will typically outlast the period of stimulation.

## Physical Therapy

Physical therapy may be therapeutic, as in the relief of muscle spasm in myofascial syndromes, or may be purely palliative as in cases of causalgia or central pain. No attempt will be made here to review the wide scope of physical therapy which involves the use of multiple modalities in combination. Obviously, the success of the treatment will depend on the experience of the practitioner and the degree of communication maintained between physician and therapist.

When indicated, the rather simple application of heat or cold may be quite palliative. Heat may be applied in the form of ultrasound or shortwave radiation. Vapocoolant sprays are convenient methods of applying cold stimulation, and ice massage is a well-established physical therapeutic technique. The therapist may employ whirlpool treatments, deep massage, manipulation, and traction or splinting of the extremities as indicated.

The most crucial aspects of a physical therapy program are those directed at rehabilitation. Many patients will benefit from movement education and the institution of specific exercise programs directed at the particular complaint. Again this is particularly applicable to myofascial pain syndromes. Pain may recede as a person's functional capacity increases. A program designed to increase function ("work-hardening") may demonstrate that the patient can carry on normal daily and vocational function despite the presence of pain. Indeed, many practitioners feel that meaningful activity may well interfere with the abnormal, memory-like nature of the pain experience.[13]

## References

1. Anderson, A., & Holmgren, E. (1975). On acupuncture analgesia and the mechanism of pain. *American Journal of Chinese Medicine* 3:311–334.
2. Armstrong, J.R. (1965). *Lumbar Disc Lesions.* Third Edition. Baltimore: Williams and Wilkins.
3. Bonica, J.J. (1974). Anesthesiology in the People's Republic of China. *Anesthesiology* 40:175–186.
4. Deyo, R.A., Diehl, A.K., & Rosenthal, M. (1986). How many days of bed rest for acute low back pain? *New England Journal of Medicine* 315:1064–1070.
5. Eriksson, M.B.E., Sjolund, B.H., & Nielzen, S. (1979). Long-term results of peripheral conditioning stimulation as an analgesia measure in chronic pain. *Pain* 6:335–347.
6. Fitzgerald, M. (1982). The contralateral input to the dorsal horn of the spinal cord in the decerebrate spinal rat. *Brain Research* 236:275–287.
7. Han, J.S., & Terenius, L. (1982). Neurochemical basis of acupuncture analgesia. *Annual Review of Pharmacology and Toxicology* 22:193–220.
8. Kao, F.F. (1973). *Acupuncture Therapeutics.* New Haven, Conn.: Eastern Press.
9. LeBars, D., Dickerson, A.H., & Besson, J.M. (1979). Diffuse noxious inhibitory controls (DNIC). *Pain* 6:305–327.
10. Lewit, K. (1979). The needle effect in the relief of myofascial pain. *Pain* 6:83–90.
11. Long, D.M., Campbell, J.N., & Gurer, G. (1979). Transcutaneous electrical stimulation for relief of chronic pain. In: *Advances in Pain Research and Therapy.* Bonica, J.J. et al. (Eds.). Vol. 3. New York: Raven Press.
12. Mayer, D.J., Price, O.D., & Rafii, A. (1977). Antagonism of acupuncture analgesia in man by the narcotic antagonist naloxone. *Brain Research* 121:368–372.
13. Melzack, R. (1973). *The Puzzle of Pain.* New York: Basic Books.
14. Melzack, R. (1975). Prolonged relief of pain by brief, intense trancutaneous somatic stimulation. *Pain* 1:357–373.
15. Melzack, R. (1984). Acupuncture and related forms of folk medicine. In: *Textbook of Pain.* Wall, P.D. and Melzack, R. (Eds.). New York: Churchill Livingstone.
16. Morris, J.M., Lucas, D.B., & Bresler, B. (1961). Role of the trunk in stability of the spine. *Journal of Bone Joint Surgery* 43-A:327–351.
17. Murphey, F., Simmons, J.C.H., & Brunson, B. (1973). Ruptured cervical discs. *Clinical Neurosurgery* 20:9–17.
18. Nachemson, A.L., & Elfstrom, G. (1970). Intravital dynamic pressure measurements in lumbar discs. A study of common movements, maneuvers and exercises. *Scandinavian Journal of Rehabilitation Medicine, Supplement.* 1:1–40.
19. Nachemson, A.L. (1976). The lumbar spine. An orthopedic challenge. *Spine* 1:59–71.
20. Nathan, P.W. (1976). The gate control theory of pain. A critical review. *Brain* 99:123–158.
21. Nathan, P.W., & Wall, P.D. (1974). Treatment of post-herpetic neuralgia by prolonged electrical stimulation. *British Medical Journal* 3:645–647.
22. Pagni, C.A. (1984). Central pain due to spinal cord and brain stem damage. In: *Textbook of Pain.* Wall, P.D. and Melzack, R. (Eds.). New York: Churchill Livingstone.

23. Pomeranz, B., Cheng, R., & Law, P. (1977). Acupuncture reduces electrophysiological and behavioral responses to noxious stimuli: pituitary is implicated. *Experimental Neurology* 54:172–178.
24. Reichmanis, M., & Becker, R.O. (1977). Relief of experimentally induced stimulation at acupuncture loci. *Comparative Medicine East and West* 5:281–288.
25. Richardson, R.R., Meyer, P.R., & Cerullo, L. (1980). Neurostimulation in the modulation of intractable paraplegic and traumatic neuroma pains. *Pain* 8:75–84.
26. Semmes, R.E. (1964). *Ruptures of the Lumbar Intervertebral Disc*. Springfield, Ill.: Charles C. Thomas.
27. Shenkin, H.A., & Hash, C.J. (1976). A new approach to the surgical treatment of lumbar spondylosis. *Journal of Neurosurgery* 44:148–155.
28. Simon, D.G. (1984). Myofascial pain syndromes. In: *Textbook of Pain*. Wall, P.D. and Melzack, R. (Eds.). New York: Churchill Livingstone.
29. Travell, J.G., & Simons, D.G. (1983). Myofascial pain and dysfunction. *The Trigger Point Manual*. Baltimore: Williams and Wilkins.
30. Wall, P.D., & Sweet, W.H. (1967). Temporary abolition of pain in man. *Science* 155:108–109.
31. Wolff, C.J. (1984). Transcutaneous and implanted nerve stimulation. In: *Textbook of Pain*. Wall, P.D. and Melzack, R. (Eds.). New York: Churchill Livingstone.
32. Wynn-Parry, C.B. (1980). Pain in avulsion lesions of the brachial plexus. *Pain* 9:41–53.

# 10

# Neurosurgical Approaches to Chronic Pain

*Frederick D. Brown*

The past two decades have witnessed dramatic changes in the neurosurgical management of chronic pain. Previously, the neurosurgeon's approach was limited to one of destruction of a portion of the central or peripheral nervous system serving nociception. Currently, ablative procedures have been largely replaced by the implantation of electrical stimulation devices in the spine or brain and by implanted infusion devices that allow the delivery of analgesics intraspinally.

## Ablative Procedures for Control of Pain

Discoveries in the functional neuroanatomy of nociception laid the groundwork for the control of pain by neurosurgical ablation. It seemed logical to pioneering neurosurgeons that if one could define the nociceptive pathways that subserved a painful body part, one could relieve the pain by simply destroying one or more pathways. This line of reasoning led Wilder Penfield to once say "all pain can be relieved, if it is really required, by cutting the proper sensory nerves or nerve tract in the proper place at the proper time."[1] There are several factors that limit the applicability of destructive procedures. For one, the destructive procedure may produce an unacceptable loss of function; for example, if two or more dorsal roots that supply one of the extremities are cut, the patient is liable to experience significant loss of proprioception. Without proprioception, an extremity is rendered virtually useless. Thus, the procedure of dorsal rhizotomies is limited in the treatment of upper or lower extremity pain.

Another reason for failure of destructive procedures is that nociceptive fibers serving a certain area of the body may not be confined to specific roots or tracts. It has been discovered, for example, that a significant number of nociceptive fibers at a given spinal cord segment may enter through the ventral root rather than the dorsal root.[2] A lesion of the lateral spinothalamic tract may work only temporarily because of the potential of nociceptive fibers to travel in the anterior spinothalamic tract.

Another serious problem with the ablative approach is that ablative procedures to relieve pain may produce severe iatrogenic pain. Lesions of nociceptive peripheral fibers or central nervous system tracts may produce a deafferentation pain. In this case, the sensation of pain is referred to the appropriate denervated segment of the body. Deafferentation pain is typically described as continuous and burning, and it is especially refractory to medical or surgical interventions.[3] It may be seen following surgical or nonsurgical trauma, or following a nontraumatic event such as brain stem infarction. When a surgeon contemplates a destructive procedure for the relief of pain, he or she must always consider this complication, which may produce more severe pain than that associated with the patient's original problem.

Many ablative operations failed for the lack of proper patient selection. In reviewing the literature of early approved procedures, White and Sweet concluded that patients with pain of malignant origin faired much better than other patients.[4] On the surface, it would appear that good results in cancer patients are due to the fact that they have fairly short life expectancies so that pain relief occurs for an adequate period of time; whereas patients with longer life expectancies survive beyond the benefit from their ablative procedures. An alternative explanation is that patients with pain of the malignant origin have nociceptive (or non-deafferentation) pain. Many other patients presenting for pain relief have benign pain stemming from deafferentation lesions. It has not proven fruitful to treat deafferentation pain with an operation, which is actually a second deafferentation injury. For example, many patients have benefited from a lateral spinothalamic cordotomy for many pains of malignant origin, but this procedure is not generally effective when applied to patients whose malignancy has produced a deafferentation injury of the brachial plexus.[5]

Another significant problem in the selection of patients for ablative procedures has been the lack of a preoperative psychological assessment in many cases. Too often neurosurgeons have found retrospectively that their operative failures were because of significant psychological factors, which either generated or amplified the patient's complaint. After a procedure has failed, it is tempting for the surgeon to blame the failure on the "craziness of the patient" rather than on a deficient preoperative selection process.

For a thorough listing of the status of neuroablative procedures (circa 1982), the reader is referred to Wall and Melzack's *Textbook of Pain*.[6] It is evident that destructive procedures for pain have included many different levels throughout the central and peripheral nervous system, including dorsal nerve roots, the spinal cord, brain stem, and even psychosurgery. In the last 15 years, we have witnessed dramatic changes in the frequency of ablative procedures. In the 1970s, we saw a marked reduction in the number of ablative procedures performed for benign pain concurrent with the development of neuroaugmentative procedures, that is, electrical stimulation of the spinal cord and deep brain structures. Ablative procedures were applied mostly to patients with pain of malignant origin, however even in this latter group we have seen in the 1980s a dramatic reduction in ablative procedures because of the advent of implanted infusion systems that chronically deliver intraspinal analgesics.[7] The result has been that cerebral and brain stem therapeutic lesions are done only rarely at present, and there has been a dramatic reduction in the frequency of spinal cord and peripheral lesions. With the rapid change of events, the "lesion" chapters in Wall and Melzack accurately reflect the neurosurgical role in the management of pain in 1982,[6] but do not reflect the more limited role of destructive procedures by the end of that decade.

In this chapter, my comments will be restricted to two destructive procedures that would still appear to have a useful role in current neurosurgical practice, namely, the percutaneous anterolateral cordotomy (cordotomy)[8,9] and the dorsal root entry zone lesion (DREZ).[10]

The cordotomy involves a lesion of the lateral spinothalamic tract that produces a contralateral loss of pain and temperature sensation below the level of the lesion. Although this procedure was first described in 1912,[11] the percutaneous technique was not discovered until a full half century later.[8] Following the introduction of the percutaneous technique and its modifications, there occurred a widespread interest in its application. For example, in our institution more than a thousand procedures were done in the 1960s and early 1970s. The technique caught on quickly because of its appeal as a simple technique that could be done safely even in debilitated patients with far advanced malignancies.

At first, the cordotomy was applied somewhat indiscriminately to patients with either benign or malignant pain syndromes. As experience grew, it became clear that the analgesia obtained typically did not last more than two years. Therefore, it was not a satisfactory procedure for young or middle-aged patients, with benign disease. Also, a significant number of patients develop the dreaded complication of post-cordotomy dysesthesia,[4,12,13] a deafferentation pain syndrome that is frequently worse than the patient's original pain. The procedure did not prove applicable to bilateral pain syndromes since bilateral lesions in the spinal cord produced a host of complications including ventilatory insufficiency.[14] Given the incidence of complications and return to pain after a period of time, the procedure was eventually limited to only patients with malignant disease.

Another limitation is that the procedure is not effective for pain higher than the 4th or 5th cervical dermatomes. This limitation is due to the fact that after spinothalamic fibers enter the spinal cord, they ascend as they cross to the contralateral side. Therefore, a lesion at C1-2 would not be expected to produce analgesia higher than C4 or C5 on the opposite side. The ideal candidates for cordotomy were eventually defined as those patients with pain of malignant origin confined to one side of the body, no higher than C4 or C5, and who have less than two years of life expectancy and were willing to accept the potential risks of post-cordotomy dysesthesia. Given these potential risks and the limited application of the procedure, it is little wonder that now the majority of the patients with pain of the malignant origin, who are referred for surgery, prefer the alternative of intraspinal morphine infusion.[7] There still are some patients, however, in whom percutaneous cordotomy does remain a reasonable choice. One consideration is life expectancy. Patients who receive morphine infusions infrequently develop tolerance within three to six months. Therefore, patients with a life expectancy of greater than six months may not be good candidates. Patients who have developed tolerance to morphine that cannot be reversed may be candidates for cordotomy. Other issues include the fact that the cordotomy is relatively inexpensive as compared to the cost of an implanted infusion system. Also, the bulk of the latter may be a problem when placed subcutaneously in a cachectic patient. Thus, at least for now, the cordotomy would appear to have a role in the future of neurosurgical pain management.

The DREZ lesion is a relatively recent addition to the field of neurosurgical ablative procedures for pain. The lesion involves coagulation of the substantia gelatinosa of the dorsal horn of the grey matter of the spinal cord.[10] It has been applied for the treatment of various pain disorders that may be due to abnormal impulses arising in this area of the spinal cord. Whereas the cordotomy has been used primarily for patients with pain of malignant origin, the DREZ lesion has been applied mostly to patients with benign deafferentation pain syndromes. Whereas a cordotomy is usually done percutaneously in awake patients, the DREZ procedure requires an open laminectomy, usually under general anesthesia. The disorders treated include pain after injuries of the brachial plexus, transitional pain of paraplegics, and postherpetic neuralgia.

Experience has helped refine the indications for this procedure. For example, the procedure helps the majority of patients with phantom limb pain but is not effective in post-amputation stump pain or combined stump and phantom limb pain.[15] Fair to good results are achieved in approximately 85% of patients with avulsion injuries of the brachial plexus[16,17] and conus medullaris.[18] About two-thirds of patients with post-herpetic neuralgia[19] and about one-half of spinal cord injury patients will benefit.[20]

With any denervation procedure, the early results of surgery are frequently superior to those found in long-term follow-ups. In one series of eleven patients with brachial plexus avulsions, all reported substantial pain relief at early follow-up, but five had recurrence of the original pain after a mean follow-up of seventeen months.[21] The complications of the procedure relate to damage of the surrounding spinal cord, producing motor or sensory loss in the ipsilateral lower extremity. Only a small minority have persisting, mild deficits.[20] In summary, the DREZ lesion appears to have a significant role in well selected patients with deafferentation pain syndromes with the notable exception of stump pain.

## Stimulation of the Central Nervous System

After the introduction by Shealy of implantable spinal cord stimulation devices in 1967,[22] peripheral nerve stimulation (PNS), spinal cord stimulation (SCS), and deep brain stimulation (DBS) became widely available in neurosurgical practice by the early 1970s. Initial enthusiasm for these techniques soon waned as it became clear that many, if not the majority of patients, failed to enjoy long-term benefit from these techniques. Typical of many early workers, in the field, Long demonstrated that when SCS was employed for the treatment of severe intractable pain as the only criterion, that a very small percentage of the patients enjoyed long-term benefit. However, when stringent patient selection criteria were utilized, approximately 70% of the patients experienced lasting benefit. Long emphasized the following selection criteria: (1) an organic cause consistent with the magnitude of pain; (2) the lack of significant psychiatric or psychological factors in the pain complaints; (3) appropriate treatment of depression, anxiety, and insomnia; and (4) percutaneous stimulation of the spinal cord resulting in satisfactory pain relief for several days of temporary stimulation.[23]

There are several reasons why preoperative assessment is especially critical and difficult for patients under consideration for stimulation procedures. The vast majority of patients are those with benign causes of pain, and it is not always apparent that a particular clinical condition will result in severe incapacitating pain. Listed below are the selection criteria that are used in the University of Chicago Pain Clinic and their rationale.

### A Clear Etiology of the Pain

Burton noted that the most important element of initial screening is to verify the previous medical diagnosis, which is incorrect in over one-half of the patients referred to his practice.[24] For example, in a neurosurgical or orthopedic practice, as well in a chronic pain center, we frequently see patients who have failed to respond to low back surgery. Of 200,000 low back operations done per year, 40,000 to 60,000 of these patients do not improve. Clearly, one of the major causes of failed back procedures is that many of these operations were done without proper indications.[25] For example, a patient may have low back pain with pain referred to a portion of the lower extremity and have a coincidental bulging disc seen on a radiological study. When "lesions" are excised that are coincidental to and not the cause of pain, it is not surprising if the pain complaint remains the same or is even increased following the added operative insult. Thus, patients are frequently referred to as "low back surgery failures" or as having pain secondary to "post-operative scarring" when the original diagnosis was actually wrong, and the patient underwent an unnecessary operation. Another example is a patient who has undergone multiple abdominal operations without a confirmed diagnosis and had subsequent operations in which only "adhesions" were found. In both examples, important psychological factors may have been overlooked, as well as a failure to consider other diagnoses prior to subjecting the patient to an operation. Furthermore, a clear etiology is important because certain organic diagnoses are consistent with severe pain; whereas others are not frequently associated with severe debilitating pain. Finally, when the diagnosis is clear, the surgeon can provide the patient with a reasonable assessment of potential benefit since references can be made to comparable patients who have undergone the procedure in question.

### Absence of Secondary Gain

A great many patients seen in a pain clinic derive benefits from their pain. For example, some patients who receive workmen's compensation benefits may dislike their present employment and would like to avoid returning to work. Obviously, such a patient would likely persevere with a complaint of pain, and maintain pain-related behavior. Other patients may benefit from the attention provided by a caring, doting spouse who protects the patient from avoiding stressful situations. Another good example is a patient who pursues litigation in which he or she stands to receive substantial financial compensation for pain following a personal injury. We do not exclude all patients who have workmen's compensation or personal injury claims, but we are especially cautious and operate only when all members of the pain team, including the psychologist, feel that secondary gain plays a minor role in the patient's overall pain experience.

### Other Psychological Factors

It has been generally recognized that the patients referred to a chronic pain center will frequently manifest significant depression. It is important to assess whether or not the depression is excessive, and may be a significant factor that amplifies the patient's complaint of pain. When there is no clear etiology for complaint of pain, it is very important to rule out the possibility of hysteria or malingering. Clearly, a patient should not undergo an operation who has psychologically generated pain or pain that is greatly amplified by psychological factors. Our current recommendation is that all patients with benign pain syndromes should undergo a psychological interview and testing prior to an operation. Even if we find that psychological factors play a minor role, we will be prepared to continue psychological or behavioral treatment in the postoperative period, to give the patient potential to enjoy maximal pain relief and increased functioning.

### Cognitive Factors

Patients should not be subjected to stimulation procedures if they do not understand the risks/benefits. The patient needs to be able to communicate sensory data: almost all of the electrical implants are done under local anesthesia, and the patient must be able to tell the surgeon in what part of the body electrically generated paresthesias are perceived. Also, the patient must be intelligent enough to control the amplitude, frequency, and on-off switch, which are external to the body in many of the implant devices.

### Failure of Appropriate and Thorough Medical Management of the Underlying Disease

In most cases, it is preferable to treat the underlying disease rather than a symptom. If the original diagnosis is wrong, it may be appropriate to refer the patient to a specialist outside of the pain clinic or back to the original referring doctor, as indicated. One obvious pitfall to avoid, for example, would be treating angina pectoris in a pain clinic if the underlying cause of the cardiac ischemia could be safely treated. Another example would be the patient referred for an SCS procedure following a failed lumbar disc surgery if radiological studies indicated that the patient had an operation performed at the wrong disc level, or that a large extruded fragment had been missed during the original operation. On the other hand, in some cases treating the symptom may be safer than treating the underlying cause, particularly in an elderly or otherwise medically fragile patient.

### Failure of Conservative Pain Management Treatment

Frequently, patients are referred for an operation to relieve pain without any consideration of less invasive techniques of pain management. Prior to considering the patient for a SCS or DBS procedure, we always assess the patient's previous conservative management. Good conservative management generally includes such approaches as physical therapy, transcutaneous electrical nerve stimulation, acupuncture, injections of local anesthetics, steroids, or alcohol by a qualified anesthesiologist, and behavioral medicine approaches, including stress reduction techniques, such as biofeedback.

### Established Chronicity and Severity

As a general rule we do not consider patients for SCS or DBS procedures unless their pain has been well established for at least six months. We feel that if the pain has been present for at least that time, it is liable to become a permanent problem. Waiting at least six months gives the patient a chance to improve through the natural history of the disease or, as is often said, "the tincture of time." Also, the pain should be severe and nearly continuous. It is very difficult to evaluate, over a short period, the effect of any intervention on an episodic pain. Furthermore, we believe that if the pain is not severe enough to produce disability or to interfere significantly with one's recreational activities, we are not justified in performing invasive procedures.

### The Lack of Dependence on Narcotics

All too frequently patients who have benign pain receive excessive narcotic analgesics. We have found in some cases that simply tapering the patient off narcotics may reduce the perception of pain to the point that the patient no longer needs to be considered for an operative procedure. It would appear that prolonged usage of endogenous opiates leads to an elevation in the pain threshold, or a decrease in the ability to cope psychologically with pain, or perhaps interfere with the ability of endogenous opiates to relieve pain: There is evidence to suggest the presence of cross tolerance between endogenous opiates and stimulation-produced analgesia.[26] This cross tolerance is probably associated with the role of endorphins and enkephalins as neurotransmitters in inhibitory pain pathways.

## Spinal Cord Stimulation

Although implants for pain include PNS, SCS, and DBS, PNS has not endured as an efficacious approach. Therefore, the following discussion of electrical implants will be limited to SCS and DBS procedures. The clinical introduction of SCS quickly followed the dissemination of Melzack and Wall's Gate Control Theory of Pain.[27] Shealy was the first to describe implantation of electrodes over the dorsal column in patients for the control of pain.[22] Following this introduction, the early 1970s were characterized by a flurry of activity in this field by a number of neurosurgeons.[28] As has already been emphasized, many of these early investigators did not achieve long-term success in their patients because of nonstringent or vague selection criteria.[23] The current success achieved by many centers in the SCS procedure is due not only to thorough preoperative assessment, but also the refinement of surgical techniques. Originally, electrodes were placed over the spinal cord via a laminectomy. Failures of this procedure were often caused by problems with the technique itself. Since a laminectomy was required, the patients were typically operated under a general anesthetic, which did not allow physiological confirmation of electrode location. It has been generally accepted that a necessary requirement for success in this procedure is the production of induced paresthesias into the painful area of the body. Therefore, patients who experience stimulation that did not cover the painful area did not benefit. The later development of percutaneous techniques obviated the need for laminectomy and allowed the surgeon to place an electrode in the spinal epidural space under a local anesthetic.[29] After percutaneous placement, a patient can be tested intraoperatively to determine the optimal location of the electrode(s) that produces electrically induced paresthesias over the entire painful area of the patient's body. After anchoring the electrode to the fascia, a percutaneous extension is applied and brought out through an opening in the skin. This percutaneous extension allows postoperative testing with the patient ambulatory in the hospital ward. This situation will allow the patient and the doctor to determine whether the device will relieve pain brought on by activity, as well as pain at rest. Following a few days of testing, the patient undergoes a second procedure under a local or general anesthetic in which the internal or permanent portion of the electrode(s) is connected to a subcutaneous radiofrequency receiver or a pulse generator. The former requires the application of stimulation via an external transmitter-antenna system, which allows the patient to control the amplitude and frequency of stimulation. The latter is similar to a heart pacemaker and is programmed non-invasively via telemetry. The early percutaneous systems were mono- or bipolar, but most of the present SCS systems are quadripolar. With the "floating" electrode in the epidural space, there is sometimes a problem with adequate contact of the tip of the electrode. For example, the patient may lose paresthesias during a change of body position. If this problem persists, we have the option of placing an electrode via a laminectomy for a better contact. Unless this last procedure is done under local anesthetic, we again face the possibility of a less than optimal placement in the epidural space.

One of the most appealing aspects of the SCS procedure is that the patient is subjected to an extremely low risk of any neurological complications; whereas patients undergoing ablative procedures, by definition, experience an iatrogenic (ideally therapeutic) injury to the central or peripheral nervous system. Should a failure occur, we can console our patients and ourselves by the fact that we have done no harm. Unfortunately, many patients who have had ablative procedures have been made more disabled or more miserable than they were prior to an attempted therapy. SCS does have some significant drawbacks, however. We are still faced with the complication of infection, which can happen with any implanted device. Also, electrode migration or breakage remain problems. Thus, patients should be prepared for the fact that a strong possibility exists that although success is achieved with the procedure, there is a high chance that they will need revisional operations.[29] The description of the ideal patient for SCS would be someone with benign non-deafferentation pain of the torso or lower extremities. Malignant pain seems to be so potent that it overrides the benefit that may result from electrically induced paresthesias. With deafferentation pain the appropriate target fibers for stimulation may have degenerated, such as is seen with cervical root evulsion. The majority of successfully treated patients in most series are those who have had failed low back procedures and are left with low back or lower extremity pain. Many of these patients are typically classified as having persistent pain on the basis of "epidural fibrosis" or "arachnoiditis." As previously stated, with usage of stringent preoperative selection criteria and in experienced hands, significant pain relief can be achieved in 70 to 80% of the patients.[23]

## Deep Brain Stimulation

Although therapeutic electrical stimulation of the brain was apparently used as early as the mid-1950s,[30] interest in totally implanted stimulation units was not popularized until the early 1970s. The usage of DBS to control chronic pain in humans followed closely the discovery by Reynolds of stimulation-produced analgesia in the rat.[31] Subsequent studies revealed that electrical stimulation of the periaqueductal grey matter of the midbrain activated descending inhibitory systems,[32,33] which relied on beta-endorphin and serotonin as key transmitters. These basic science discoveries led several surgeons to pioneer the use of electrical stimulation in a periaqueductal grey and periventricular grey matter regions in humans for the treatment of chronic pain.[34,35] A variety of other surgeons discovered that stimulation of the sensory thalamus could be effective in pain patients as well.[36-38] Further work led most surgeons to agree that periaqueductal grey or periventricular grey stimulation was most effective in patients with nociceptive pain occurring in the presence of an intact central nervous system.[39] The deafferentation pain syndromes therefore typically did not respond to stimulation of this target but were thought to be responsive to stimulation of the sensory thalamus.[40] Thus, given the flexibility of different target sites in the brain, it would appear that DBS has the potential to treat pain at any site in the body and in any of the major categories of malignant pain, benign nociceptive pain, or benign deafferentation pain.

Patients are selected according to the same criteria that preceded the discussion of spinal cord stimulation. Patients who have failed to respond to SCS are among the candidates for DBS.

The procedure is done under a local anesthetic and by a stereotactic technique. Unless one uses stereotaxis guided by computerized tomography, the surgeon must rely on intraoperative ventriculography. The procedure then is generally done by placing a burr hole in the skull, generally contralateral to the side of the patient's pain. In the case of thalamic electrical stimulation, the electrode is always placed contralateral to the side of the pain. Prior to electrode placement, a radio-opaque contrast agent is injected into the ventricular system to localize the target. An electrode with four uninsulated stimulating sites is passed to the desired target. The stimulation is then applied to the electrode via a transmitter to determine whether the patient feels relief with stimulation. Generally with PVG or PAG stimulation, the patient feels a warm pleasant sensation and possibly paresthesias in the painful area. With thalamic stimulation, the patient must receive paresthesias in the painful area in order to have a success.

Depending on the nature of the patient's pain, one or two electrodes may be placed: sometimes bilaterally or sometimes on the same side with one electrode in the thalamus and one in the PAG or PVG. Following the operation, the patient returns to the hospital room for several days of testing in which one determines whether the patient is able to achieve adequate pain relief to warrant internalization of the system; it is also determined which bipolar combination of electrode stimulation sites provides maximum pain relief. If pain relief is not obtained, the electrodes are removed in the second procedure. If pain relief is achieved, the patients undergo a second procedure in which the electrode(s) is tunneled subcutaneously and eventually connected to either a radiofrequency receiver or a pulse generator located in a subcutaneous pocket inferior to the clavicle.

The complications that one sees with an SCS system also pertain here. Infection and even erosion through the skin are possible. Also, breakage of a part of the system is a possibility. Neurological damage is a major concern with DBS as opposed to SCS. In the course of passing the electrode through the brain, there is always the possibility of a hemorrhage.[40] This complication could either be fatal or produce significant morbidity such as aphasia and hemiplegia. However, this risk is rare unless the patient has a coagulopathy. The study by Young illustrates the kind of long-term results that can be achieved with stringent preoperative selection criteria and good technique. In his study, 90% of patients felt significant pain relief and underwent a permanent implantation. In long-term follow-up (2 to 60 months) 73% of the original group of patients reported lasting significant pain relief. Thirty-three percent considered their pain had been completely relieved by stimulation, and 40% felt that at least 50% of their pain had been relieved.[41]

## Summary

Technological zealotry has often led to the hasty application of a procedure prior to understanding the indications for a given operation.[28] Certainly, this statement describes many of the neurosurgical procedures for intractable pain. It is now evident that the preoperative assessment is just as crucial as the technical aspects of a procedure. Those patients with severe, intractable pain of clear etiology, without major psychological maladjustments, would appear to be reasonable candidates for surgical interventions.

### References


1. Penfield, W. Foreword in White, J.C., & Sweet, W.H. (1969). *Pain and the Neurosurgeon. A Forty Year Experience*. Springfield, Ill.: Charles C. Thomas, pps. vii–ix.
2. Applebaum, M.L., Clifton, G.L., Coggeshall, R.E., Coulter, J.D., Vance, W.H., & Willis, W.D. (1976). Unmyelinated fibers in the sacral-3 and caudal-1 ventral roots of the cat. *Journal of Physiology* 256:557–572.
3. Tasker, R.R., Organ, L.W., & Haurylyshyn, P. (1980). Deafferentation and causalgia. In: *Pain*. Bonica, J.J. (Ed.). New York: Raven Press, pp. 305–329.
4. White, J.C., & Sweet, W.H. (1969). *Pain and the Neurosurgeon. A Forty Year Experience*. Springfield, Ill.: Charles C. Thomas.
5. Tasker, R.R. (1982). Percutaneous cordotomy—the lateral high cervical technique. In: *Operative Neurosurgical Techniques. Indication, Methods, and Results*. Volume 2. Schmidek, H.H., and Sweet, W.H. (Eds.). New York: Grune and Stratton, pp. 1137–1153.
6. Wall, P.D., & Melzack, R. (1984). *Textbook of Pain*. New York: Churchill Livingstone.
7. Onofrio, B.M., Yarksh, T.L., & Arnold, P.G. (1981). Continuous low-dose intrathecal morphine administration in the treatment of chronic pain of malignant origin. *Mayo Clinic Proceedings* 56:516–520.
8. Mullan, S., Harper, P.V., & Hekmatpanah, J. (1963). Percutaneous interruption of spinal pain tracts by means of a strontium 90 needle. *Journal of Neurosurgery* 20:931–939.
9. Rosomoff, H.L., Carrol, F., & Brown, J. (1965). Percutaneous radiofrequency cervical cordotomy. *Journal of Neurosurgery* 23:639–644.
10. Nashold, B., & Ostdahl, R.H. (1979). Dorsal root entry zone lesions for pain relief. *Journal of Neurosurgery* 57:59–69.
11. Spiller, W.G., & Martin, E. (1912). The treatment of persistent pain of organic origin in the lower part of the body by division of the anterolateral column of the spinal cord. *Journal of the American Medical Association* 58:1489–1490.

12. White, J.C. (1963). Anterolateral chordotomy—its effectiveness of relieving pain of non-malignant disease. *Neurochirurgia* 6:83–102.
13. Pagni, C.A,. & Nraspes, P.E. (1973). A critical appraisal of pain surgery and suggestions for improvement of treatment. In: *Recent Advances on Pain-Pathophysiology and Clinics.* Bonica, J.J., Procacci, P., and Pagni, C.A. (Eds.). Springfield, Ill.: Charles C. Thomas.
14. Mullan, S., & Hosobuchi, Y. (1968). Respiratory hazards of high cervical percutaneous cordotomy. *Journal of Neurosurgery* 28:291–297.
15. Saris, S.C., Iacono, R.P., & Nashold, B.S. (1985). Dorsal root entry zone lesions for post-amputation pain. *Journal of Neurosurgery* 62:72–76.
16. Thomas, D.G., & Jones, S.J. (1984). Dorsal root entry zone lesions (Nashold's procedure) in brachial plexus avulsion. *Neurosurgery* 15:966–968.
17. Thomas, D.G., & Sheehy, J.P. (1983). Dorsal root entry zone lesions (Nashold's procedure) for pain relief. *Journal of Neurology, Neurosurgery and Psychiatry* 46:924–928.
18. Moosy, J.J., Nashold, B.S., Osborne, D., & Friedman, A.H. (1987). Conus medullaris nerve root avulsions. *Journal of Neurosurgery* 66:835–841.
19. Friedman, A.H., & Nashold, B.S. (1984). Dorsal root entry zone lesions for the treatment of postherpetic neuralgia. *Neurosurgery* 15:969–970.
20. Friedman, A.H., & Nashold, B.S. (1986). DREZ lesions for relief of pain related to spinal cord injury. *Journal of Neurosurgery* 65:465–469.
21. Garcia-March, G., Sanchez-Ledesma, M.J., Diaz, P., Yagrie, L., Anaya, J., Goncalves, J., & Broseta, J. (1987). Dorsal root entry zone lesions versus spinal cord stimulation in the management of pain from brachial plexus avulsion. *Acta Neurochisurgia* [Suppl.] (Wien) 39:155–158.
22. Shealyl, C.N., Mortimer, J.T., & Resurik, J. (1967). Electrical inhibition of pain by stimulation of the dorsal column: Preliminary clinical reports. *Anesthesia and Analgesia* 46:489–491.
23. Long, D.M., Erickson, D., Campbell, J., & North, R. (1981). Electrical stimulation of the spinal cord and peripheral nerves for pain control. A ten year experience. *Applied Neurophysiology* 44:207–217.
24. Burton, C.V. (1977). Safety and clinical efficacy. *Neurosurgery* 1:214–215.
25. Long, D.M., Filtzer, D.L., Ben Debra, M., & Hendler, N.H. (1988). *Journal of Neurosurgery* 69:61–71.
26. Mayer, D.J., & Hayes, R.L. (1975). Stimulation-produced analgesia: Development of tolerance and cross-tolerance to morphine. *Science* 188:941–943.
27. Melzack, R., & Wall, P.D. (1965). Pain mechanisms: A new theory. *Science* 150:971–979.
28. Taub, A. (1975). Electrical stimulation for the relief of pain. Two lessons in technological zealotry. *Perspectives in Biology and Medicine* 19:125–135.
29. North, R.B., Fischell, T.A., & Long, D.M. (1977). Chronic stimulation via percutaneously inserted epidural electrodes. *Neurosurgery* 1:215–218.
30. Pool, J.L. (1956). Psychosurgery in elderly people. *Journal of the American Geriatric Society* 2:456–465.
31. Reynolds, D.V. (1969). Surgery in the rat during electrical analgesia induced by focal brain stimulation. *Science* 164:444–445.
32. Basbaum, A.I., & Fields, H.L. (1978). Endogenous pain control mechanisms: Review and hypothesis. *Annals of Neurology* 4:451–462.

33. Mayer, D.J., Wolfe, T.L., & Akil, H. (1971). Analgesia from electrical stimulation in the brainstem of the rat. *Science* 174:1351–1354.
34. Richardson, D.E., & Akil, H. (1977). Pain reduction by electrical brain stimulation in man. Part 2: Chronic self-administration in the periventricular grey matter. *Journal of Neurosurgery* 47:184–194.
35. Hosobuchi, Y., Adams, J.E., & Linchitz, R. (1977). Pain relief by electrical stimulation of the central gray matter in humans and its reversal by naloxone. *Science* 197:183–186.
36. Mazars, G. (1975). Intermittent stimulation of the nucleus ventralis posterolateralis for intractable pain. *Surgical Neurology* 4:93–95.
37. Tsubokawa, T., Yamamoto, T., Katayama, Y. (1982). Clinical results and physiological basis of thalamic relay nucleus stimulation for relief of intractable pain with morphine tolerance. *Applied Neurophysiology* 45:143–155.
38. Turnbull, I.M., Shulman, R., & Woodhurst, W.B. (1980). Thalamic stimulation for neuropathic pain. *Journal of Neurosurgery* 52:486–493.
39. Hosobuchi, Y., Rossier, J., Bloom, F.E., & Guillemin, R. (1979). Periaqueductal grey stimulation for pain suppression in humans. In: *Advances in Pain Research and Therapy.* Volume 3. Bonica J.J., Liebeskind, J.C., and Albe-Fessard, D.G. (Eds.). New York: Raven Press, pp. 515–523.
40. Turnbull, I.M. (1984). Brain stimulation. In: *Textbook of Pain.* Wall, P.D., and Melzack, R. (Eds.). New York: Churchill Livingstone, pp. 706–714.
41. Young, R.F., Kroenig, R., Fulton, W., Feldman, R.A., & Chambi, I. (1985). Electrical stimulation of the brain in treatment of chronic pain. *Journal of Neurosurgery* 62:389–396.

# 11

# Dental Pain: Diagnosis of Temporomandibular Joint Disorders

*LaDeane Fattore and Robert A. Strauss*

Pain and dysfunction of the temporomandibular joint apparatus afflict up to 20% of the population of Western countries.[1-3] The condition presents some of the most complex and frustrating diagnostic problems encountered by the dental and medical professions. In fact, the temporomandibular joint disorders have been termed "The Great Imposter" because they can mimic so many different conditions. For example, some patients may present with obvious and fundamental problems such as an inability to open or close the mouth; others may have pain suggesting migraine, sinusitis, temporal arteritis, trigeminal neuralgia, or neck and shoulder pain. Still others may suffer from vertigo, tinnitus, hearing loss, ear pain, nausea, or visual disturbances.[4]

It is not surprising, with such a wide array of sensory, motor, and autonomic possibilities, that misdiagnosis is not uncommon. As a result, it is also not surprising that many of these patients shop from doctor to doctor seeking relief from their symptoms without success. Many eventually begin to wonder whether their symptoms are not in fact psychosomatic—particularly if a frustrated practitioner infers that this must be the case. A number of these patients may have already been referred for psychiatric consultation, which tends to confirm their darkest suspicions—"The doctor thinks the pain is all in my mind; nobody can find anything wrong with me; maybe it *IS* all in my mind." The fact is, however, that in chronic pain disorders pain can often lead to psychological symptoms. Thus, an unfortunately all-too-common sequel is for the patient's mental state to progress from anxiety to depression, as the search for relief proves fruitless.[4]

Research in the area of temporomandibular joint (TMJ) disorders is particularly fascinating because it is not limited to any one discipline in either dentistry or medicine but rather encompasses disciplines of both professions.

Current approaches to the diagnosis and treatment of pain associated with temporomandibular joint disorders are multifactorial and multidisciplinary.

Twenty-five years ago TMJ was considered a mystery understood only by selected clinicians who could describe the anatomy and had some treatment experience. The prevailing concept was based on Costen's Syndrome,[5] espoused over forty years ago, recognizing that loss of posterior teeth with the resulting loss in vertical dimension could cause TMJ symptoms. Costen proposed that the overclosure caused distal displacement of the condyles of the mandible, which impinged on the auriculotemporal and chorda tympani nerves as well as obstructed the eustachian tube. Successful treatment was typically restoration of the bite. Costen's theory was a departure from the theories of other otolaryngologists who considered the problem nondental.[6]

However acute Costen's clinical observations were, his anatomical explanation did not hold up. In 1960, Harry Sicher[7] published the third edition of *Oral Anatomy*. Included was a chapter on TMJ attacking, as he did in his lectures, Costen's anatomical explanation. Sicher described the anatomy in a dynamic three-dimensional perspective with fascial planes and demonstrated that it was anatomically impossible for the well-protected chorda tympani to be pressured by overclosure since its entry through a small canal in the petrotympanic fissure is situated behind the articular capsule. He also discredited the anatomic concept of pressure against the tympanic bone or some influence on the eustachian tube and a disturbance of the function of the tensor palati muscle. He explained the pain as a result of pressure on the posterior part of the disc and on the loose connective tissue behind the disc. This highly vascular and innervated zone was a subject of much histologic investigation explaining the correlation of pain in the 1960s and, like arthrography, is discussed as a new concept today.[6]

Sicher further defined three causes of TMJ disorders: (1) overclosure, (2) occlusal disharmonies, (3) mental tension and, even more significantly, observed that the common denominator in all these cases is the mandibular musculature. Sicher pressed to precisely narrow the issues and characterized regions of pain with specific muscle involvement. For example: pain in the region of the temple is pain in the temporal muscles; pain in the throat is pain in the pterygoids; pain in the cheek is pain in the masseter; pain in the tongue is pain in the geniohyoid muscles. Although Sicher correctly refuted the anatomic basis for Costen's theory, almost every dentist can attest to the clinical acuity of Costen's observations. Both physicians, Costen and Sicher operated at the frontiers of medical knowledge and their contributions are significant and clinically applicable today.[6]

Discrepancies in occlusion (bite), in maxillomandibular relationships, or in both, formed the basis for most of the early theories of temporomandibular disorders.[8]

In 1959 Laslow Schwartz introduced stress and emotional components as more important causes of TMJ dysfunction than malocclusion.[8]

In 1969, Daniel Laskin introduced the term myofascial pain-dysfunction (MPD) syndrome to identify a subgroup of temporomandibular joint pain patients having spasm of the masticatory musculature, rather than intrinsic pathology of the temporomandibular joint itself. He felt this group comprised the bulk of patients having pain and dysfunction.[8]

In the 1970s, chiropractors, kinesiologists, myofunctional therapists, nutritionists and health personnel trained in biofeedback techniques appeared on the TMJ/MPD treatment scene. Many of the treatments were empirical and some were of limited effectiveness but focus was placed on multiple etiologies and multiple treatments of TMJ/MPD rather than one etiology, one treatment to which many theorists adhered.

In the 1980s two important milestones were reached. With the advent of new radiographic techniques, the temporomandibular joint, a difficult anatomical structure to visualize radiographically, became amenable to closer scrutiny. Tomograms have virtually eliminated the problem of overlap of bony structures and have made it possible to examine the articulating surfaces as well as the nearby surrounding bony structures of the temporomandibular joint.

Advances in fiberoptic technology have allowed the arthroscopic examination of the TMJ for accurate diagnosis of internal derangements and clinical research has now begun into the use of arthroscopy for therapeutic meniscoplasty, menisectomy, and articular surface surgery within the temporomandibular joint.

The meniscus can be viewed through the injection of radiopaque dye into the upper and lower joint spaces of the TMJ. The dye will outline the meniscus, which may then be examined statically using conventional tomography or dynamically using fluoroscopy. This technique is highly useful in detecting both meniscal derangements and perforation.

Utilizing advanced techniques, Computerized Tomography Scanning (CT) has made it possible to obtain diagnostic images of both hard and soft structures of the joint and Magnetic Resonance Imaging (MRI) is extremely effective in delineating soft tissue abnormalities of the joint.

The second milestone was reached in the 1980s with the development of the multidisciplinary team approach to the management of TMJ/MPD disorders. The disciplines of medicine, dentistry, psychology, and physical therapy have become equal partners in the management of a complicated craniomandibular disorder that, in chronicity, becomes an extremely debilitating one affecting the lifestyles of both the patient and family.

The multifactorial etiology of temporomandibular joint disorders and the multidisciplinary approach of the 1980s for the management of these disorders are rapidly replacing the single practitioner with his or her limited knowledge in only one narrow health discipline. The effectiveness of treatment and the prevention of the development of chronic pain

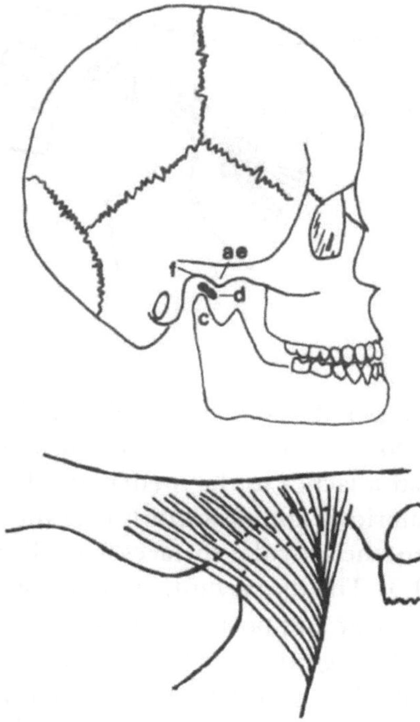


a

b

**Figure 11.1.** (A) Anatomy of temporomandibular joint: (f) glenoid fossa, (ae) articular eminence, (d) disc, (c) condyle. (B) Temporomandibular ligament.

promises to increase the number of such teams in the local community as well as in the large medical center.

## Applied Anatomy of the Temporomandibular Joint

It is essential for the practitioner evaluating patients with pain in the TMJ to first understand the basic anatomy of this complex joint. The TMJ is unique in that it acts as both a rotating hinge joint and a sliding joint, and has two separate articulating surfaces (one on each side of the face) that function as a single joint.[9] This unique anatomical configuration allows the complicated motions and forces necessary for mastication.

The joint itself is composed of four main elements: the glenoid fossa and articular eminence (which form the roof); the condylar process of the mandible; the intervening meniscus; and the surrounding fibrous connective tissue capsule (Fig. 11.1). Of great importance is that unlike most joints, the articular surfaces of the TMJ are not covered by hyaline cartilage, but rather by a layer of dense fibrous connective tissue (which may explain why this joint reacts to stresses differently than other joints).[10,11]

Under normal conditions the condylar head functions and slides against, and down, the posterior slope of the articular eminence rather than the roof of the fossa, as might be expected (Fig. 11.2). Intervening

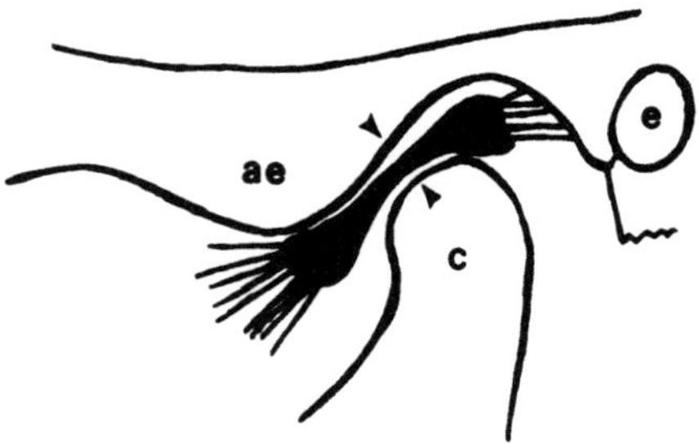


**Figure 11.2.** Function of condyle against posterior slope of articular eminence (ae). Arrows indicate point of maximum function, (e) ear canal, (c) condyle.

between the condyle and glenoid fossa is the articular disc, or meniscus (a historic but less accurate term), a pliable piece of dense connective tissue that attaches to the medial and lateral poles of the condyle and rotates anteriorly and posteriorly over the condylar head during function to prevent the articular surfaces from directly rubbing against one another (Fig. 11.3). The disc is quite thin and avascular centrally, and thickens to form anterior and posterior "bands."

During function, the disc translates down the eminence along with the condyle to maintain the central zone in juxtaposition with the head of the condyle.[12] Smooth, uninterrupted, and coordinated movement by both the condyle and meniscus is absolutely necessary for normal, painless function of the joint.

The disc divides the joint into inferior and superior compartment spaces. The superior space acts like a sliding joint and allows condylar and disc translation, while the inferior space primarily functions as a hinge joint and allows condylar rotation. The disc is attached posteriorly to the temporal bone by a thick pad of fibrous and elastic connective tissue known as the posterior attachment or bilaminar zone. This tissue is highly innervated and when impinged upon may account for much of the pain associated with internal derangements of the TMJ. Anteriorly, the disc and condyle are attached to the lateral pterygoid muscle which functions to traction the condyle anteriorly for opening and stabilize the disc during closing.[13]

The joint is surrounded by a fibrous connective tissue capsule that aids in limiting the condyle within the joint. This capsule is reinforced laterally, where it is called the temporomandibular ligament, and is quite thin and loose medially and anteriorly. This area of weakness in the capsule may in fact be the Achille's heel of the TMJ, allowing pathologic hypertranslation of the condyle or disc. It is also highly innervated and may induce pain if stretched (i.e., if the joint space is pathologically widened).

The muscles of mastication that manipulate the joint must also act in a coordinated fashion to appropriately move both condyles and discs, if function is to be smooth and without undue stresses on these components. These muscles are the medial and lateral pterygoids, the temporalis,

**Figure 11.3.** Disc moving simultaneously with condyle during anterior excursion to maintain central zone between the condyle and eminence. Small arrows indicate point of maximum function.

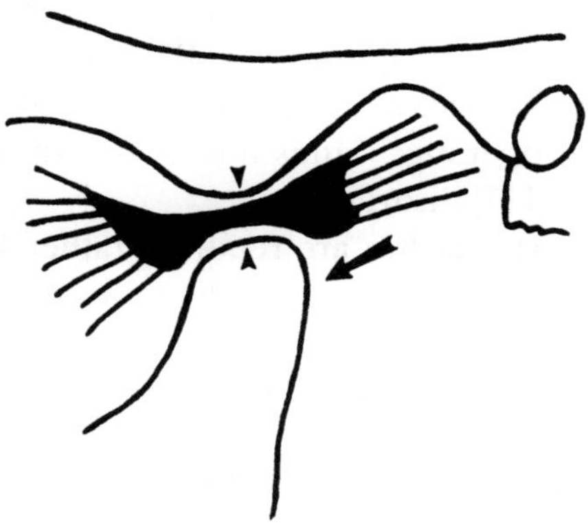

the masseter and, to a lesser extent, the anterior digastric and mylohyoid muscles. Discoordinate function of these muscles may lead to myospasm and pain, abnormal disc function, or both.[14] Palpation of these muscles for pain and myospasm should be routinely undertaken when examining patients with TMJ disorders.

Finally, one must keep in mind the proximity of the TMJ to the middle ear and ear canal. When one considers this anatomical relationship it is easy to see why diseases of each structure may present with symptoms of the other.[15]

## History Taking

A patient's history is divided into the general past history that includes the patient's medical, surgical, psychological, occupational, social, and family background and the history relating to the patient's chief complaint.[16]

Because of the nature of temporomandibular joint disorders, patients with this type of problem often have had consultations with otolaryngologists, neurologists, dentists, physical therapists, and even psychologists and psychiatrists when no treatment has been satisfactory. The present examiner should become familiar with past diagnoses and treatments because this information is quite useful in the differential diagnosis and in selection of the appropriate treatment.

### Pertinent Medical History

1. Systemic disease that may affect the TMJ must be considered in the differential diagnosis. Rheumatoid arthritis and osteoarthritis, for example, can affect the temporomandibular joints just as any other joint. If the patient suffers from such a disorder, this information would be pertinent to the present complaint.[17]

2. Infections in the ear such as otitis media and furuncle can have the same symptoms as TMJ disorders, i.e., tinnitus, a sensation of fullness in the ear, and, in more advanced infections, limitation of mandibular opening.[17] Sinus infections can also mimic some of the symptoms of TMJ disorders.
3. Headaches are reported rather frequently by patients with TMJ disorders. If a patient has a history of vascular headache, this condition must be ruled out or considered to be another condition that exists independently of the TMJ disorder. The treatments are quite different.[17]
4. Trauma to the condyles, the jaws, the dentition, and the neck must be considered as a possible etiologic factor in the patient's present complaint.[17]
5. Stress may be important as a causative factor in the development of TMJ disorders (MPD in particular). Emotional stress may take the form of parafunctional activity (nonphysiologic activity) such as clenching, bruxism (grinding of the teeth, gum chewing, nail biting, etc.) that cause fatigue and muscle spasm.[17]
6. Emotional states are important in evaluating how the patient may react to another clinician's attempts to treat the patient's TMJ disorder. A history of depression, suicide, anxiety, and the prescription of psychotropic medications are important information because these emotional states as well as the medications to treat them will all have an impact on the management of TMJ disorders.[17]

### Chief Complaint

Patients are first asked to state their reason for seeking another medical opinion. Pain and dysfunction are the two main symptoms of disorders of the masticatory system and are the two symptoms most frequently reported. The location of symptoms should be determined such as unilateral or bilateral pain and the area(s) of pain should be delineated. Masticatory pain is typically not well localized. Because of the diffuse, spreading characteristics of TMJ pain, it is important to ask the patient where the pain was first noticed and if any changes have occurred in location or character of the symptoms.[17]

### Referred Pain

The arthralgia of disorders of the TMJ and the myalgia of MPD are typical forms of deep pain that have certain characteristics. The location of pain is not always where the source lies. The pain is rather steady but variable and has a dull, aching quality. The pain of TMJ disorders spreads by central excitation so that, before long, the referred pain in otherwise normal structures and muscles constitutes the main complaint. It is important for the clinician examining the patient to not be duped by this referred pain because at times, such pain can be well localized and superficial, masking its source.[17]

### Onset of Symptoms

Gradual onset of dysfunction and pain is characteristic of intrinsic pathology of the temporomandibular joints (with the exception of trauma).[1]

Sudden onset of pain and dysfunction is usually caused by injury or muscle spasm and specific events.[17]

1. Dental treatment may induce a sudden onset of pain and muscle spasm if the patient had extensive procedures that require that the mouth be open for long periods of time. Fillings or cast restorations (bridge, crown, etc.) may cause a sudden onset of pain if the restorations are "high" and hit before the other teeth do. This can cause the masticatory muscles to avoid the prematurity by a shift of mandibular position that could result in muscle spasm and pain. "High" dental restorations can also predispose some patients to brux on the premature spot resulting in muscle spasm and pain.[17]
2. Stressful events can bring on the sudden onset of pain and dysfunction through parafunctional activity. If a patient reports pain in the early morning or upon waking, bruxing or clenching may be occurring while the patient sleeps. Daytime parafunctional activity may cause pain and muscle spasm in the early evening hours. Most patients will not be aware of these habits unless brought to their attention.[17]
3. Trauma, of course, will cause a sudden onset of pain and dysfunction, but the patient usually is immediately aware of the problem.[17]

### Chronologic Record of Symptom Behavior

A chronological progression of symptoms should be elicited from the patient because the location, character of pain, and degree of dysfunction may change with time. With MPD, if the patient currently has limitation of jaw movement, no clicking will be present but clicking will be in the history.[17]

### Pertinent Information That May Indicate the Presence of Myofascial Pain Dysfunction Syndrome

1. Parafunctional activity such as bruxing, clenching, lip, pencil, or pipestem biting, and wind instrument playing.
2. Employment in stressful occupations.
3. Previous dental treatment such as orthodontia and/or extensive restorations that may have changed the original occlusion (bite) of the patient.

4. Loss of posterior teeth with no replacement and occlusal anomalies that result in overclosure of the vertical dimension[17]

### Pertinent Information That May Indicate the Presence of Disc-Interference Disorders

Besides pain, the symptoms of disc-interference disorders include: (1) sensations of binding, rubbing, or catching that the patient can detect subjectively as well as the examiner can through use of a stethoscope; (2) joint noises such as clicking, popping, or crepitus (grating) that the patient can hear just as the clinician can with a stethoscope; and (3) altered translation (movement of mandible downward and forward to its maximum opening), such as rough or irregular movement, momentary locking, hard, discrete locking, or soft locking that is sensed by the patient and observed clinically.[18]

Clicking and popping do not necessarily indicate joint pathology, but rather a momentary obstruction of disc movement. Patients with MPD often report clicking and popping and these are easily verified clinically. Grating sounds (crepitus), however, are indicative of degenerative changes in the articular surfaces or actual deterioration of the disc.[18]

## Physical Examination

The temporomandibular joints can be palpated easily by placing the fingertips lightly over the joint areas. Pain over the TMJs may indicate intrinsic joint pathology. The condyles should move smoothly in a forward and slightly downward position when the mouth is opened.[18]

Next, the tips of the little fingers should be placed in the external auditory canals and pulled forward gently. This allows the examiner to feel the distal surfaces of the condyles. The patient is asked to open, move the jaw from side to side, and move the jaw anteriorly. Pain may indicate intrinsic joint pathology. Myofascial pain dysfunction syndrome will not cause pain over the joints upon palpation or when the fingers are placed in the ears over the distal surfaces of the condyles.[18]

With the bell of a stethoscope placed over the temporomandibular joint areas, sounds such as clicking, popping, or crepitus can be heard. The grating sound of crepitus is usually a symptom of joint pathology and warrants further radiographic and clinical evaluation.[18]

### Palpation of Muscles

Palpation of the muscles of mastication and of other muscles of the head and neck is very important in the clinical diagnosis of temporomandibular joint disorders.

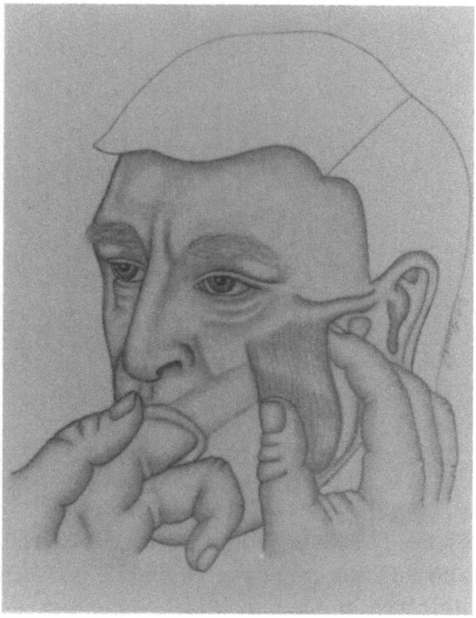

**Figure 11.4.** With the index finger intraorally, the finger is pressed laterally inside the cheek. With the fingers extraorally, pressure is placed medially down on the masseter muscle to its insertion at the angle.[19]

*Masseter Muscle*

With the index finger intraorally, the finger is pressed laterally inside the cheek. With the fingers extraorally, pressure is placed medially down on the muscle to its insertion at the angle (Fig. 11.4).[19]

*Internal Pterygoid Muscle*

The index finger is pressed laterally just distal to the hamular process and the muscle is traced down the medial side of the ramus to its insertion. Then the index finger is pressed laterally inside the angle of the jaw (Fig. 11.5).[19]

*External Pterygoid Muscle*

The index finger is pressed medially behind the tuberosity of the maxilla (Fig. 11.6).[19]

*Digastric Muscle*

Anterior belly of the digastric: At a point halfway between the angle of the mandible and the chin, pressure is applied extraorally in an upward and medial direction. Posterior belly of the digastric: Pressure is applied medially and upward, beginning just distal to the angle of the mandible (Fig. 11.7).[19]

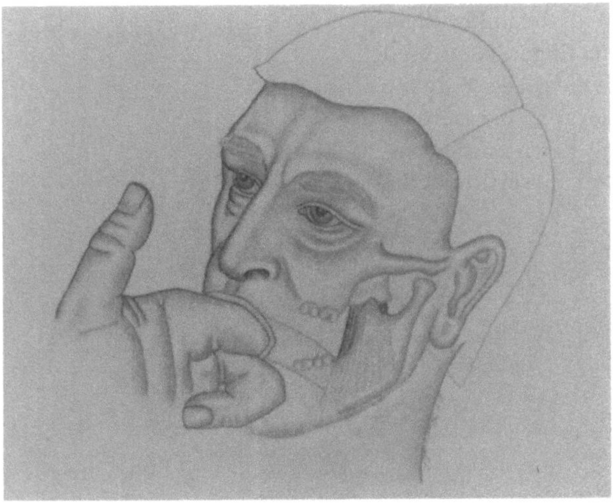

**Figure 11.5.** The index finger is pressed laterally just distal to the hamular process and the internal pterygoid muscle is traced down the medial side of the ramus to its insertion. Then the index finger is pressed laterally inside the angle of the jaw.[19]

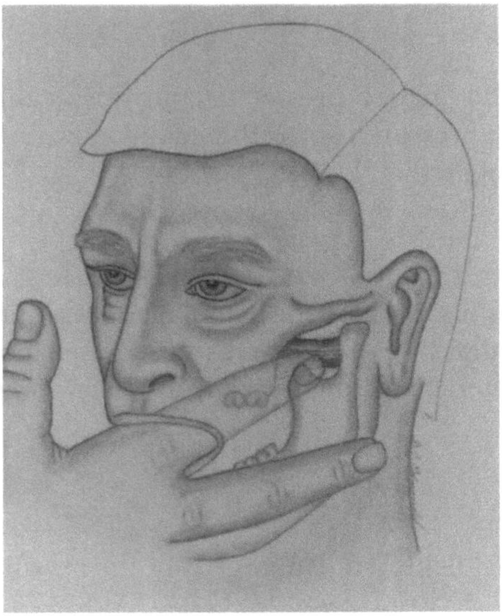

**Figure 11.6.** To palpate the external pterygoid muscle, the index finger is pressed medially behind the tuberosity of the maxilla.[19]

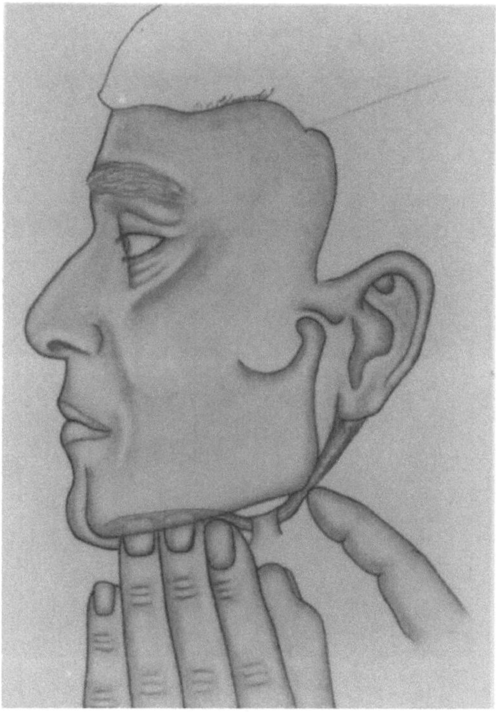

**Figure 11.7.** Anterior belly of the digastric: At a point halfway between the angle of the mandible and the chin, pressure is applied extraorally in an upward and medial direction. Posterior belly of the digastric: Pressure is applied medially and upward beginning just distal to the angle of the mandible.[19]

*Temporal Muscle*

There are three muscle heads in the temporal fossa that are easily palpated (Fig. 11.8).

*Sternocleidomastoid Muscle*

The patient is asked to roll the head to the side being tested.[19]

ORIGIN: The muscle can be palpated at the sternum.
INSERTION: The muscle can be palpated at the mastoid process.
BODY: The muscle can be palpated at the midpoint between the sternum and the mastoid process (Fig. 11.9).

*Occipitalis Muscle*

This muscle is easily palpated at the back of the head (Fig. 11.10).

## Neck and Shoulder Muscles

*Trapezius Muscle*

The trapezius muscle is a large triangular muscle with three portions: an upper portion can be palpated in the neck, a middle portion can be

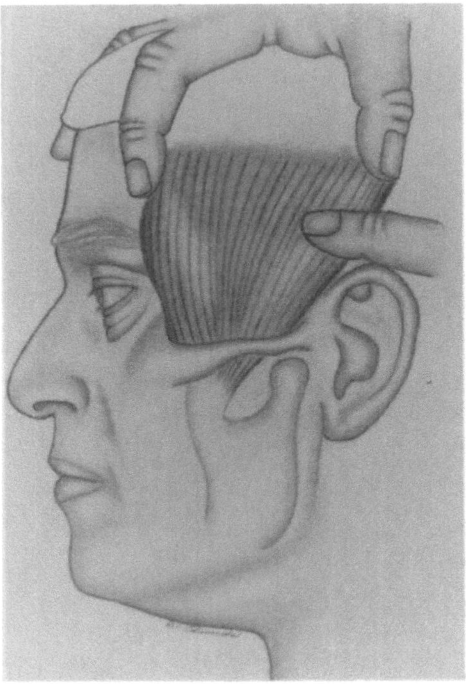

**Figure 11.8.** The three heads of the temporalis muscle in the temporal fossa are easily palpated.[19]

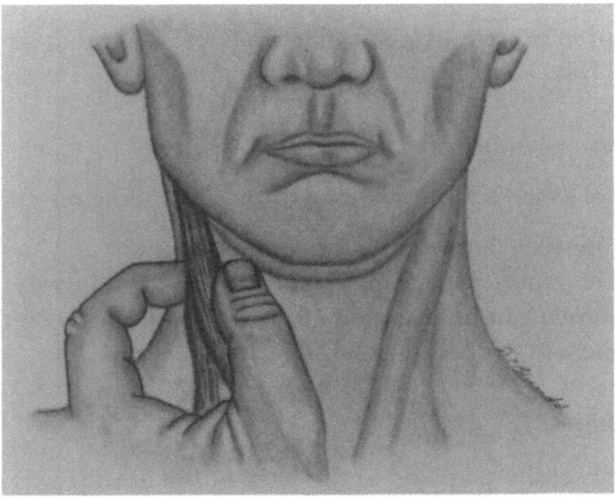

**Figure 11.9.** ORIGIN: The sternocleidomastoid muscle can be palpated at the sternum.
INSERTION: The muscle can be palpated at the mastoid process.
BODY: The muscle can be palpated at the midpoint between the sternum and the mastoid process.[19]

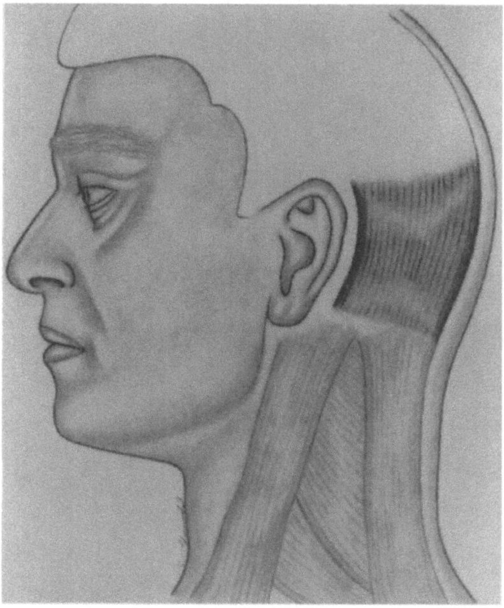

**Figure 11.10.** The occipitalis muscle is easily palpated at the back of the head.[19]

palpated in the shoulders, and a lower portion can be palpated in the middle of the back (Fig. 11.11).

*Splenius Capitus Muscle*

This muscle can be palpated between the insertion of the sternocleidomastoid muscle and the origin (in the neck) of the trapezius (Fig. 11.12).[19]

## Examination of Teeth

A careful examination of the teeth should be made that includes radiographs, periodontal probing, mobility testing, and occlusal analysis.[20]

Stress-induced muscle activity often results in grinding or clenching of the teeth in either conscious or sleep states. There is a forceful rubbing together (bruxism) or application of pressure (clenching) by opposing teeth. Such force is exerted by the contraction of the elevator muscles of the mandible. Excessive and prolonged contraction of the masticatory muscles can cause spasm and MPD.[20]

The interaction of psychological stress and occlusal (bite) imbalance can occur as follows: Ideally, there is a state of harmony and balance between the occlusion of the teeth, masticatory muscles, and the temporomandibular joints, as there might be in one's emotional life. Such an ideal condition allows the individual to clench and grind teeth evenly. However, when the state of equilibrium between the component parts of the masticatory system is lost or altered, these parts are then in a state of imbalance.

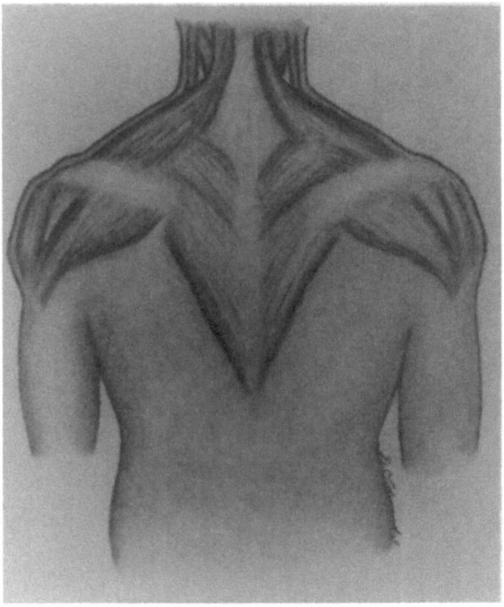

**Figure 11.11.** The trapezius muscle is a large triangular muscle with three portions: an upper portion can be palpated in the neck, a middle portion can be palpated in the shoulders, and a lower portion can be palpated in the middle of the back.[19]

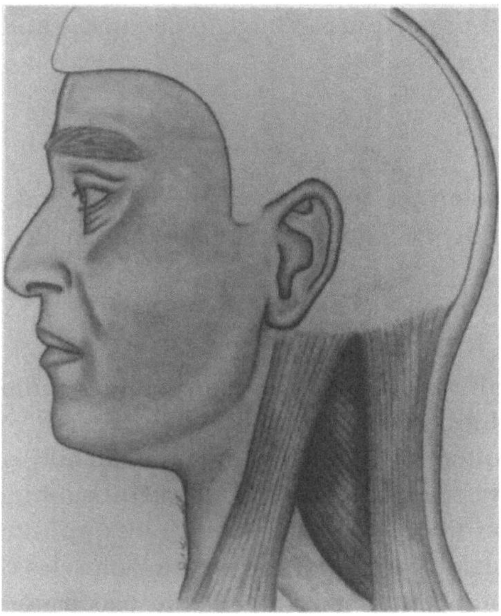

**Figure 11.12.** The splenius capitus muscle can be palpated between the insertion of the sternocleidomastoid muscle and the origin (in the neck) of the trapezius.[19]

In the case of tooth loss, the teeth adjacent to and opposing the resultant space will drift and rotate, causing abnormal pressures to be exerted on them. The application of such pressure to a tooth initiates a response in the proprioceptors of the periodontal membrane. Through proprioception, the resulting stimulus activates the muscles of mastication to move the mandible so that the teeth occlude in a less traumatic position. In this manner, proprioception can be viewed as a defense mechanism of the teeth.[20]

If the mandible moves into an abnormal position, the masticatory muscles are placed under stress and tension. Often the muscle goes into spasm. Prolonged and sustained hyperactivity of the masticatory muscles past the adaptive capacity of a well-balanced dentition can create the MPD syndrome.[20]

### Acute Malocclusion

Acute malocclusion (i.e., sudden change of the bite) is an abrupt change in the way the teeth come together. As a consequence, the observed occlusion at the time of examination may be quite different from the patient's actual occlusion.[21] Acute malocclusion is an important symptom of a temporomandibular disorder and should be carefully evaluated.

#### *Loss of Posterior Occlusion*

The posterior teeth when in occlusion determine the position of the condyle in the glenoid fossa. Loss of posterior teeth unilaterally or bilaterally will cause the condylar head to have a posterior-superior displacement as compared to its normal centrally placed condyle-to-fossa relationship. In addition, loss of posterior teeth can lead to collapse of the vertical dimension causing muscle spasm and pain.[22]

## Intrinsic Disorders of the Temporomandibular Joint

The temporomandibular joint is subject to all the same disorders that may affect any of the other joints of the human body. The list is long and beyond the scope of this book. There are, however, several discrete and frequently seen types of problems that would be of particular interest to the practitioner involved in a pain clinic (Table 11.1). It must be understood that although these entities will be discussed separately, intrinsic disorders of the TMJ (especially those pertaining to disc derangements) are usually associated with some extraarticular component of pain and dysfunction (e.g., muscular disorders). It is incumbent on the practitioner to look for and properly diagnose this condition prior to considering treatment of the intrinsic disorder. Treatment of one without the other will usually be disappointing.

**Table 11.1.** Internal Derangements of the Temporomandibular Joint

| |
|---|
| I. Abnormalities of the meniscus |
| a. Meniscal dislocation |
| 1. with reduction |
| 2. without reduction |
| b. Meniscal perforation |
| II. Tumors of the joint |
| a. Benign |
| b. Malignant |
| III. Arthritic conditions of the joint |
| a. Osteoarthrosis |
| b. Rheumatoid arthritis |
| IV. Fractures of the joint |
| a. Intracapsular |
| b. Extracapsular |

## Derangements of the Articular Disc

The pathophysiology of articular disc derangements is not yet completely understood, and continues to be an area of intense speculation and research. There are, however, at least two principal, recognized derangements that have been well documented clinically, radiographically, and histologically. These are disc displacement and disc perforation.

### *Disc Displacement*

This occurs when the disc, which normally has its thin central or intermediate zone situated between the condylar head and the posterior slope of the articular eminence, becomes displaced, usually slipping anteriorly and medially. The condyle will then articulate at rest on the posterior band, or, when the displacement is severe or long standing, on the posterior attachment (this is related to the extent of the anterior displacement).

While the etiology of this process is unclear, it is currently thought to be related to a combination of muscular imbalance (uncoordinated lateral pterygoid function on the disc or condyle), laxity of the elastic retrodiscal attachment, and adhesion in the joint space (which may hold the disc in a malposed position). Alternatively, a traumatic incident may precipitate an acute disc displacement or bony abnormality which may then lead to a chronic disc derangement.[23]

In an early, mild displacement the condyle may reseat itself into the central zone of the disc by jumping over the posterior band during opening (displacement with reduction). This usually manifests clinically as a click-

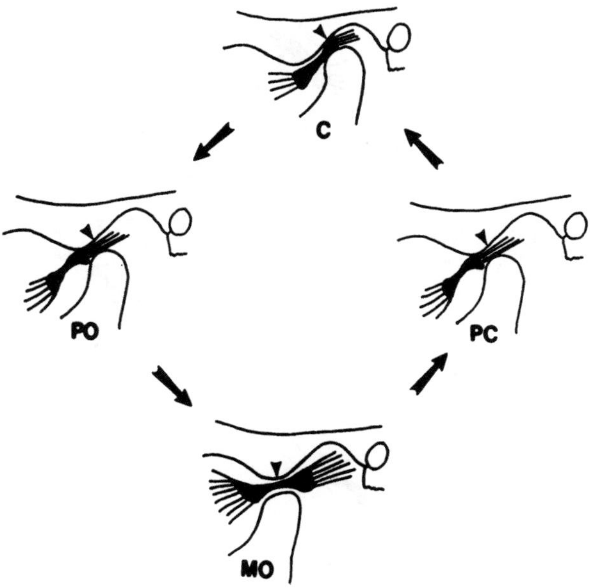


**Figure 11.13.** Anterior dislocation of disc with reduction on maximum opening (mo). Small arrows indicate points of maximum function, (c) closed portion, (po) partial opening, (pc) partial closing.

ing or popping sound that can be heard and felt during opening. Often there will be a similar sound heard on closing as the disc displaces anteriorly again. These sounds have been defined as a *reciprocal click*, and may be accompanied by pain (Fig. 11.13).[24]

Disc derangements usually show progressive changes in joint function. With the initial displacement there may only be an early, mild click with little pain and lack of opening. With time the click will come later in the cycle and the patient may need to manipulate the jaw from side to side to reduce the disc (let the disc slip back over the posterior band into the central zone) and allow for mandibular opening.

As the disorder progresses the disc can move further forward, forming a deformed mass anterior to the condyle. This may prevent any translating type motions of the condyle (displacement without reduction), although rotating movements may still occur. As the condyle attempts forward translation it is physically restricted by the displaced disc, or by secondary adhesion formation in the joint. This restriction leads to the condition of *closed lock* (Fig. 11.14).[25]

Clinically, these patients will have pain on opening and closing that may, or may not, be associated with a painful popping or clicking of the joint. There will also be joint tenderness to cutaneous or endaural palpation. In the patient with closed lock (displacement without reduction) there will usually be an inability to open beyond the point of condylar rotation, about 20 to 25 mm, since the mandible is prevented from

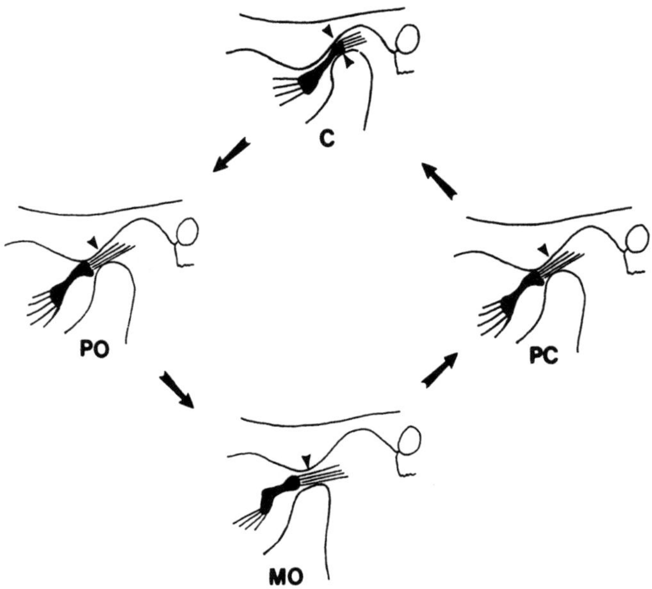


**Figure 11.14.** Anterior dislocation of disc without reduction. Disc remains ahead of condyle during all excursions leading to limitation of movement ("closed lock").

translating down the eminence by the displaced disc (although the mandible may open further if the disc becomes deformed enough). There may also be mandibular deviation on opening (toward the affected side) as the normal side translates, rotating about the nonmoving, affected condyle.

If the condyle articulates directly on the highly innervated retrodiscal tissue (as it would in a severe anterior meniscal displacement) pain often ensues. This pain will be exacerbated by movement of the condyle, but may also exist at rest from pain emanating from stimulated stretch receptors in the retrodiscal tissue. Another significant source of pain is the capsule. If the condyle is situated on, or rides over, the posterior band, it widens the joint space and stretches the capsule. [26,27] This stretching of the highly innervated capsule leads to a painful joint.[28]

The treatment of disc dislocation is related to the degree of displacement and the presence of pain. Once the diagnosis of internal derangement is made (by history, physical exam, or one of the diagnostic modalities mentioned later in this chapter), the patient is initially placed on a regimen of therapy designed to eliminate any associated muscular symptoms that could hamper the post-surgical rehabilitation. This regimen is discussed in detail in the section on extraarticular disorders.

If appropriate, the joint can then be explored surgically by a variety of approaches.[29] Most oral and maxillofacial surgeons use a small vertical incision in the crease of the ear to expose the joint. Once exposed, the extent of the dislocation may be ascertained, as well as the presence of any other intrinsic problems, e.g., disc perforation, condylar head abnormalities, joint adhesions, etc. If the disc is not badly deformed and is only moderately displaced, it can be pulled back into position and secured with sutures (meniscal plication). Alternatively, a portion of the posterior attachment may be resected, with the meniscus repositioned and secured posteriorly with sutures (meniscoplasty).

If the meniscus has been severely deformed and deemed not repairable, it is removed and may be replaced with an alloplastic implant (e.g., silastic sheet or a proplast-teflon laminate), autogenous transplant (e.g., fascia lata, dermis, etc.), or nothing.[30] This implant may be wrapped around the condylar head or affixed to the roof of the glenoid fossa and articular eminence.

*Disc Perforation*

Disc perforation may occur as the result of condylar pressure on a weakened area of a chronically dislocated disc, or erosion of the disc by a roughened articular surface (as might be seen in degenerative joint disease). It may occur in the retrodiscal tissue, the avascular central zone, or, less commonly, in the anterior or posterior bands.

Clinically, these patients may show any of the signs and symptoms seen with disc dislocation, but they will almost always have distinct crepitus. This grating sound may be heard by auscultation of the joint, and is also usually heard and felt by the patient.[31] These patients often present with significant pain and limitation of movement.

The treatment of painful meniscal perforation must be prompt if damage to the articular surfaces is to be avoided. Treatment by the oral and maxillofacial surgeon most commonly involves meniscectomy (removal of the disc) with, or without, plant or transplant replacement. The prognosis following menisectomy is guarded, as patients often return within a few years with repeat symptoms of pain and dysfunction. Much research is currently being done to find an ideal disc replacement that will have better long-term success.

## Benign and Malignant Tumors of the Temporomandibular Joint

Tumors, especially malignant tumors, of the TMJ are fortunately rare. When they do occur, however, they may cause symptoms similar to, or even identical to, other intrinsic disorders and should therefore be included in any discussion of the differential diagnosis of TMJ pain.[32] Because of the similarity in presentation it is incumbent on the astute practitioner to rule out these diagnoses prior to instituting treatment for any other intrinsic disorder. When one suspects a possible tumor of the TMJ, immediate referral to an oral and maxillofacial surgeon for biopsy and diagnosis is indicated.

While benign tumors are usually treatable with simple excision and reconstruction, malignancies, due to the proximity of the joint to nearby vital structures (middle cranial fossa, middle ear, carotid arteries, etc.), are complicated lesions to treat, requiring major surgery, radiation therapy, chemotherapy, or a combination of these modalities.

Following resection of a benign or malignant tumor of the TMJ, immediate or delayed reconstruction of the joint by the oral and maxillofacial surgeon may include bony arthroplasty, meniscal replacement, glenoid fossa replacement, or even total joint replacement. The physical therapist and the maxillofacial prosthodontist are indispensable in the postoperative management of these patients, in order to achieve maximal neuromuscular adaptation to the surgery.[33]

## Arthritic Conditions of the Temporomandibular Joint

The arthridities represent a significant percentage of painful conditions that afflict the TMJ. Of even greater importance is that they manifest themselves with many of the same signs and symptoms as both muscular disorders and disc derangements. Although less frequently seen than these other two entities, the arthridities must be considered in the differential diagnosis of TMJ pain.[34-39]

Osteoarthrosis (DJD) is a non-inflammatory degeneration of the TMJ. It represents approximately 10% of all temporomandibular joint related pain.[40-43] It is primarily a disease of middle to old age. This factor often helps in differentiating DJD from muscular disorders, a disease process with which it shares a multitude of signs and symptoms.[44] It has been estimated that 85% of cadavers over the age of 70 demonstrate clinical evidence of degenerative disease.[9] Despite the fact that the disease is undoubtedly inevitable with advancing age, very few patients are clinically symptomatic to any significant extent (probably less than 5%).[14] When symptoms do occur, they usually run an acute and limited course of one to three years, and result in little or no lasting disability. This is true despite the often impressive radiographic changes.[45,46]

The clinical symptoms of DJD are often similar to those of other internal derangements, which make the history and radiographic examination the primary diagnostic factors. There is gradual onset of dull pain, which is usually isolated to just one joint. This is a very important factor in the differential diagnosis. Joint noises are common, especially grating sounds (which may be both heard and felt by the examiner). Stiffness and loss of motion become increasingly severe, and sometimes worsen after periods of rest. Pain on direct or endaural (within the ear canal) palpation of the joint is also evident.

The treatment for degenerative joint disease of the TMJ is usually palliative, controlling the disease until it has run its course.[47-49] However,

**Table 11.2.** Comparison of Osteoarthritis and Rheumatoid Arthritis

| | Osteoarthritis | Rheumatoid Arthritis |
|---|---|---|
| Mechanism | Non-inflammatory | Inflammatory |
| Peak age range | >40 | Any age |
| Primary tissue affected | Articular fibrocartilage | Synovial membrane |
| Primary sites affected | Isolated joints, usually unilateral | Polyarthric, often bilateral |
| Joint type usually affected | Weight bearing | Nonweight bearing |
| Course of disease | 1 to 3 years, often "burns out" without disability | Intermittent with progressive destruction |

when nonsurgical therapy (which is performed by either a general dentist or an oral and maxillofacial surgeon) is inadequate to control the patient's pain or dysfunction, then an arthrotomy (open surgical procedure) may be indicated.

Unlike osteoarthrosis, which primarily affects the articular surfaces, rheumatoid arthritis is an inflammatory disorder that initially affects the synovial lining of the joint. It is characterized by intermittent periods of acute activity with progressive joint involvement and damage. Rheumatoid arthritis is a generalized, systemic, polyarthric disease that tends to affect the smaller, nonweight-bearing joints. The age of onset is usually in the third or fourth decade but varies widely. The incidence of TMJ involvement in patients diagnosed with rheumatoid arthritis is unclear. Some authors have reported as few as 3% of RA patients with TMJ symptoms, while other authors have reported as much as 75%.[50,51] On initial clinical presentation one may see stiffness, swelling over the joint, pain on movement, limitation of motion, and tenderness to direct or endaural palpation. As the disease progresses to its chronic stage, crepitus (grating) becomes the prominent symptom, while pain and restricted opening may diminish (or even disappear).[52–57]

The differentiation between rheumatoid arthritis and the more common osteoarthrosis of the TMJ is a relatively simple task based on history and physical examination (Table 11.2), except when complicated by coexistence of the two diseases.

The treatment of rheumatoid arthritis of the TMJ is usually coordinated with the general medical care (by the internist or rheumatologist) of the patient's systemic manifestations and consists of palliative therapy during active periods of the disease (e.g., analgesics and anti-inflammatory drugs, moist heat, rest, and physical therapy).[1] Should conservative measures fail to control the disease, arthrotomy may be indicated.[58–61]

Finally, because of the systemic nature of RA, it lends itself well to the concept of team management. The internist or rheumatologist, anesthesiologist (who may be consulted prior to surgery regarding the most appropriate anesthetic techniques for the patient with extremely limited opening), dentist, oral and maxillofacial surgeon, and physical therapist (for presurgical and postsurgical mouth opening physiotherapy) all have a role in treatment.

## Diagnostic Modalities for Diseases of the TMJ

It is generally agreed that the diagnosis of temporomandibular joint disease and specifically the differentiation between extrinsic joint disease (i.e., muscular disorders) and the various intrinsic disorders can often be made by the astute clinician using only the history and physical examination. While there is clearly no substitute for an adequate clinical evaluation, a number of diagnostic tools are available to the practitioner to aid in the verification of the clinical diagnosis or to shed light on the more obscure case.

The temporomandibular joint is a difficult anatomical structure to visualize radiographically. Its location at the base of the skull surrounds it with other dense bony structures that makes isolation of joint elements troublesome. In addition, one of the main sources of joint pathology, the articular disc, is radiolucent. This creates the need for more elaborate studies to render it visible on radiographic examination. Obviously, a well-trained radiologist can be invaluable in these endeavors. The object for the clinician is to choose the most appropriate film study for each individual patient. This is defined as the study that will best show the pathology suspected by the clinician, with the least radiation dose and at the least cost.

### Panoramic Radiograph (Panorex)

The panoramic film is one of the most commonly used screening radiographs in oral and maxillofacial surgery. It is essentially a curvilinear tomogram of the lower and middle face, taken in a single thin focal trough (depth of focus). That is, it provides a two-dimensional (flat) view of the entire mandible and maxilla, including the TMJ. This provides a relatively clear picture of these structures as a whole, but represents only a small percentage of their total thickness. In other words, one might see a normal condyle in the particular plane of the film, while on either side of the focal trough considerable pathology may exist. Also, although the condyle may be satisfactorily imaged on a panorex, the glenoid fossa and joint space are usually not visualized well enough to be of clinical use (Fig. 11.15).

While there are certainly inherent disabilities in the use of the panoramic radiograph, there are clearly several advantages to its use. It is a widely available tool, owned and routinely used in most oral and maxil-

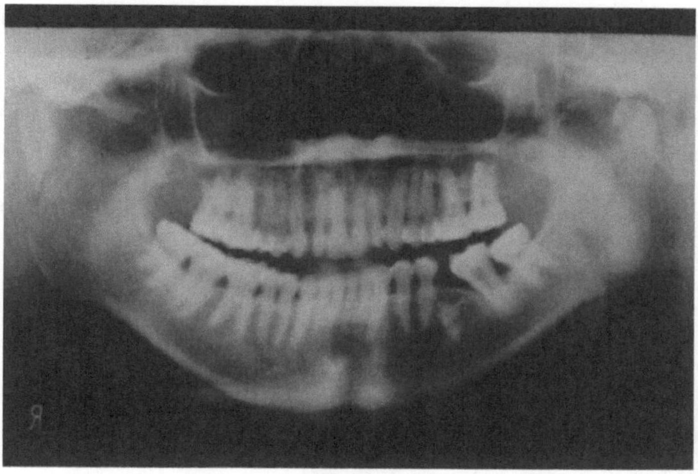

**Figure 11.15.** Panoramic radiograph. Note intracapsular condylar fracture on patient's left side, and subcondylar fracture on patient's right side. Resolution of joint anatomy makes this useful only as a screening film.

lofacial surgeons' offices and hospital outpatient clinics. This widespread use has made the panorex a relatively inexpensive machine to purchase and use. In addition, the radiation dose is quite moderate.

The panorex is an excellent screening radiograph to visualize gross pathology of the jaws, or to rule out gross articular pathology in the case of diagnosed extraarticular disease. Its limitations, however, make it less than ideal for use as a diagnostic tool for internal derangements.

## Conventional TMJ Radiography

To minimize the overlap of the joint with other nearby radiodense structures, one can choose the particular beam angle that will best elucidate the most desired joint components. Specifically, one can order a submental-vertex projection, lateral transcranial projection, or transmaxillary projection. These views, which are static, are usually taken in the closed, partially open, and fully open mouth positions. Although there is still considerable overlap, they may provide a particular view of the articular surfaces that is better than the panorex (Fig. 11.16). Additionally, although they are static films, by obtaining films in the three different stages of opening one can gain some insight into the motion dynamics of the condyle. The information gained by these films can be useful in arthritic conditions or where significant bony pathology of the joint exists.[62,63]

It has been questioned as to whether any information may be ascertained regarding meniscal derangements by assessing condylar position on this type of film (e.g., condylar retropositioning from an anteriorly

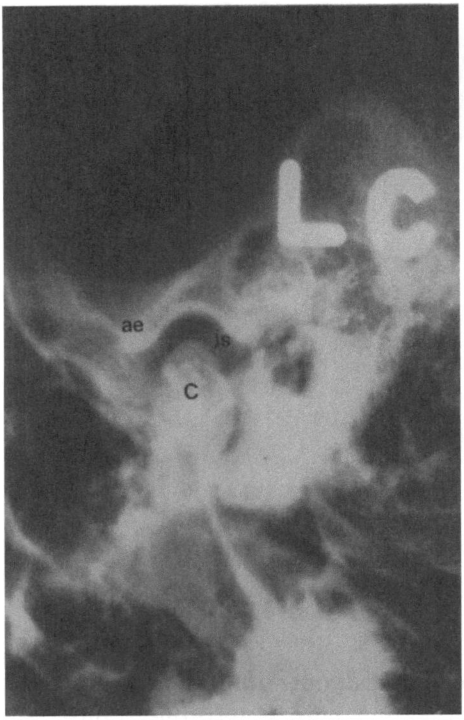


**Figure 11.16.** Transcranial radiograph of TMJ. Resolution of joint structures is improved over the panorex, more clearly demonstrating the condylar head (c), articular eminence (ae), and joint space (js). (Courtesy Dr. Guttu, Richmond, VA).

displaced meniscus). This concept has not met with universal acceptance, however, and it is generally felt that these are not ideal films for the diagnosis of meniscal derangement.

Because of the two-dimensional compression of the image, accurate information regarding the entire articular surfaces is still lacking.[64,65] These films do, however, have the advantage of being widely accessible, inexpensive, non-invasive and expose the patient to a minimal radiation dose.

*Tomography*

If taken correctly, tomograms virtually eliminate the problem of overlap of bony structures. By viewing multiple thin-section X rays, taken sequentially by depth into the joint, it is possible to adequately examine the entire articulating surfaces, as well as the nearby surrounding bony structures (e.g., the articular eminence).[66] This clarity is of great use in the diagnosis of articular surface disease (e.g., osteoarthrosis, late rheumatoid arthritis), and of bony ankylosis. This is especially true when the X-ray beam is paralleled to the long axis of the condyle (axially corrected tomogram) to eliminate the distortion caused by angulation of the condyle within the fossa.[67] This correction is done by measuring the condylar

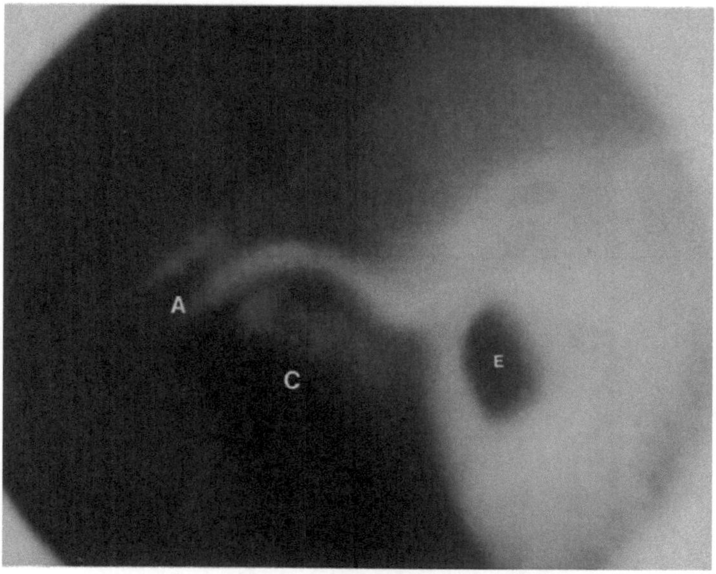


**Figure 11.17.** Axially corrected tomogram of TMJ. Excellent resolution delineates minute degenerative changes in the condylar surface (c). (A) Articular eminence, (e) ear canal. (Courtesy Dr. R. Guttu, Richmond, VA).

angulation to the frontal plane on a submental-vertex view, and then adjusting the tomographic plan accordingly (Fig. 11.17).

The disadvantages of tomography include the lack of universal availability, the relatively high radiation exposure and cost, and the lack of soft tissue and disc visualization.

*Arthrotomography*

To view the articular disc it is possible to inject a small amount (about 1 cc) of radiopaque dye into the upper and lower joint spaces. The dye will outline the disc, which may then be examined statically using conventional tomography, or dynamically using fluoroscopy. While dual space arthrography is preferred, an inferior joint space injection is often sufficient for diagnostic purposes (Fig. 11.18).

This technique has been found to be highly useful in detecting, both qualitatively and quantitatively, meniscal derangements as well as meniscal perforation (which is visualized as upper joint space opacification after the initial lower joint space injection).[68,69]

The clinical correlation between the arthrographic findings and the clinical findings at the time of surgery has been shown to be very high, and the arthrotomogram is generally considered the standard against which

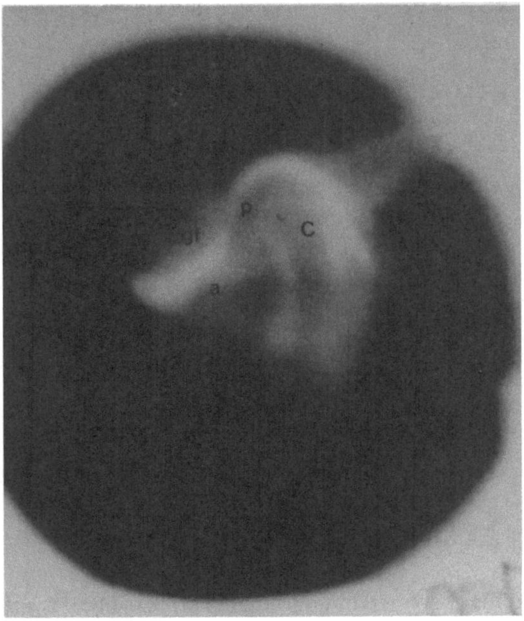

**Figure 11.18.** Arthrogram of TMJ. Injected dye will outline the anterior (a) and posterior (p) bands of the disc, and the glenoid fossa (gf). (c) Condyle. Using fluoroscopy, one can perform a dynamic arthrogram that can demonstrate reduction of the disc and any associated popping or clicking.

all other modalities designed to demonstrate soft tissue changes are compared.[70]

The procedure may be done under local anesthesia with fluoroscopy control for placement of the needle. Depending on the particular institution and equipment availability, it may be performed by either an oral and maxillofacial surgeon or radiologist.

By obtaining preinjection routine tomographic films (i.e., "scout films") it is possible to examine both the articular surfaces and the meniscus with the arthrotomogram. This is a distinct advantage over most other modalities that look at only one or the other. It also has the ability to provide either a static or true dynamic (real-time) study of the joint. The dynamic view (fluoroscopic study) can be diagnostically correlated to joint clicking or noises during function, offering excellent clinical evidence of any uncoordinated movements of the meniscus.[71]

Disadvantages of arthrotomography include the relatively high cost and radiation dose, lack of universal availability of equipment and personnel, and the fact that it is an invasive procedure (with the attendant, although minimal, risks of infection, pain, edema, hemarthrosis, and articular surface damage from the needle). Occasional systemic reactions to the dye have also been reported.

From a historical perspective, it is important to note that the ability to visualize the disc radiographically has greatly enhanced our abilities to diagnose joint pathology, as well as make possible the formulation of a logical, consistent protocol of treatment based on an accurate diagnosis (i.e., performing surgery for an intrinsic disorder as opposed to providing medical therapy for a muscular disorder).

*Computerized Tomography Scanning (CT)*

In recent years much research has been done on the use of CT scanning for diagnosis of internal derangements of the TMJ.[72–74] Although technically more difficult, scanning is best done in the sagittal view (rather than the usual axial view) to provide the examiner with a picture similar to the other radiographic modalities of this joint.[75] Utilizing advanced techniques (e.g., "Blink Mode"), it is possible to obtain diagnostic images of both the hard and soft structures of the joint. However, interpretation of these films may be difficult, especially regarding the soft tissue components.[76] Hard tissue diseases, however, are usually well delineated by CT and include osteoarthrosis, late rheumatoid arthritis, and ankylosis.

Advantages of CT scanning include the modest radiation dosage and relative availability (compared to standard tomographic studies). However, the use of CT scanning appears to be dwindling in the face of a newer modality, magnetic resonance imaging.

## Magnetic Resonance Imaging (MRI)

This comparatively new technology involves applying a strong electromagnetic field to the involved tissues, and then observing changes in the thermal interactions between the nuclei and their local environment. These changes can then be interpreted by computer and a three-dimensional image view similar to a CT scan, but much higher in soft tissue resolution, can be produced. Unfortunately bony resolution is poor (Fig. 11.19).

MRI scanning is extremely effective in delineating soft-tissue abnormalities of the joint (pathology of the meniscus, synovium, posterior attachment, etc.). Perforation of the disc, however, may not be as well visualized as with arthrography.[77] Recent research has demonstrated that the findings on MRI studies can be well correlated to findings at the time of surgery, although not all positive findings upon surgical exploration can be retrospectively diagnosed on MRI.[78]

Because of the lack of radiation exposure (and the concomitant biologic hazards), MRI has the distinct advantage of being usable to monitor progress throughout the course of treatment. Ideally, after a new therapy is instituted, an MRI could be used to assess its effect without fear of excessive radiation exposure. Although the MRI is rapidly becoming one of the

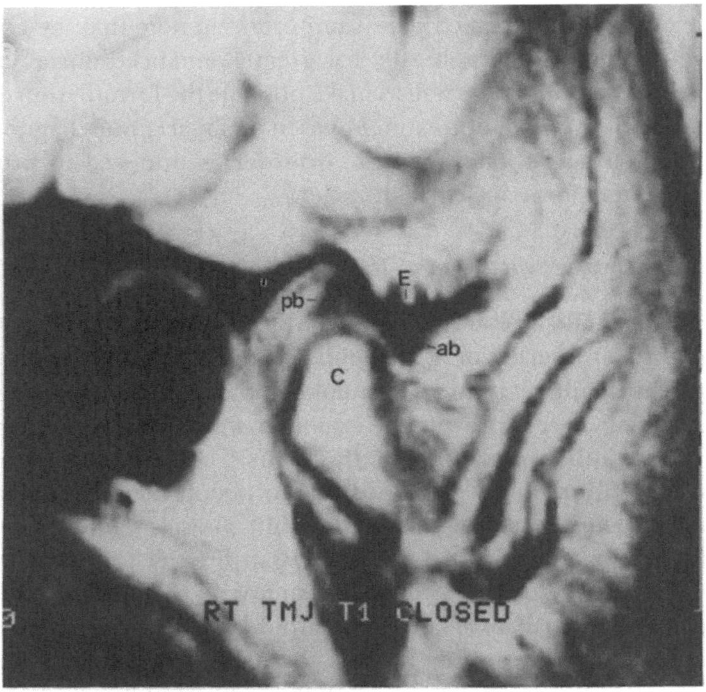


**Figure 11.19.** Magnetic resonance image of TMJ (MRI). Note butterfly appearance of disc with its anterior (ab) and posterior (pb) bands. The cortical bone of the condyle (C) and eminence (E) are seen as a low signal density (dark) while the medullar bone is seen as higher signal density (light).

most useful tools in the definitive diagnosis of temporomandibular joint disease, the current high cost (around $800 at the time of printing) precludes such routine use throughout the treatment period. As the cost decreases, the continuous assessment of the effects of various treatment modalities will probably become more common.

*Arthroscopy*

For several years one of the principal diagnostic and therapeutic tools used for larger joint disease (e.g., knee, shoulder) has been arthroscopy. Advances in fiberoptic technology allowed Oshnishi in 1975 to report the first use of arthroscopic examination for accurate diagnosis of internal derangements of the TMJ.[79] Utilizing a 1.7 mm to 2.3 mm (O.D.) arthroscope inserted into the superior joint space under general anesthesia, it is possible to examine the glenoid fossa, meniscus anatomy and location, joint adhesions, and any perforations (all of which are visible with this technique).[80,81]

Until recently, treatment options using the arthroscope within the TMJ have been limited mainly to diagnostic examination and sweeping the joint of adhesions (in the hope that an anteriorly displaced meniscus would slip back in place when released of any adhesive restrictions).[82] Clinical research has now begun into the use of arthroscopy for therapeutic meniscoplasty, menisectomy, and articular surface surgery within the temporomandibular joint.

It is obvious that as more such techniques are shown to be possible and effective, arthroscopic examination and surgery may become a great tool in both the diagnosis and treatment of TMJ disorders. It must be noted, however, that several serious complications have been reported associated with this technique. These have included middle cranial fossa perforation, middle and external ear canal perforation, articular surface damage, hemarthrosis, and severe bleeding requiring arthrotomy.[83,84] Appropriate consultation with an otolaryngologist or neurosurgeon may be necessary in these instances.

### Nuclear Medicine

Bone scans utilizing bone-seeking radiopharmaceutical uptake may be quantitated by skeletal scintigraphy (radiation mapping) to provide insight into the metabolic activity of the joint. Materials labeled with Technetium-99 are most commonly used for this purpose.

The main purpose of bone scanning in temporomandibular joint disease is to determine the level of metabolic activity of arthritic and neoplastic conditions. For example, a presumed osteoma that shows no uptake on the bone scan is usually left untreated. Conversely, the asymmetric patient with positive uptake on bone scan is referred to the oral surgeon and examined for an active neoplastic process. Because of the lack of specificity, bone scanning is only rarely used as a diagnostic modality in the TMJ.

## Physical Evaluation and Sequencing of Treatment

When suspecting an intrinsic disorder of the TMJ, it is imperative for the practitioner to first begin with a complete history and physical examination, including searching for an extrinsic cause for the patient's symptoms. It cannot be emphasized enough that the majority of patients with internal derangements also have an extrinsic (muscular) component to their pain. It is very important, therefore, for the examiner to look for this, since treatment of the muscular component should precede any surgical treatment of the intrinsic disorder. Only after all sources of extrinsic pain have been eliminated or minimized can surgical treatment hope to be successful. Physical evaluation of the patient with specific emphasis on the signs and symptoms of an intrinsic disorder is done at this time as well. When an intrinsic disorder is suspected, this process is best performed by an oral and maxillofacial surgeon, although a general dentist, orthodontist, or prosthodontist will usually be consulted to aid in the dental examination and the initial nonsurgical therapy.

Following the initial history, physical examination, and establishment of a working diagnosis, appropriate consultation with other services should be obtained. The muscular component may require psychiatric and physical therapy consultations, along with the previously mentioned dental consultations. When the source of the pain appears to be centrally located, neurologic and neurosurgical evaluations may be useful. Since many TMJ diseases manifest as ear pain, an otolaryngology consult is often beneficial as well. Only after the preceding has been accomplished should surgical treatment of an internal derangement be initiated.

The patient is usually then sent for the most appropriate radiographic examination that will confirm or rule out the working diagnosis (e.g., arthrography or MRI for disc displacement, tomography for arthritis, etc). Once the definitive diagnosis has been made, conservative medical and splint therapy is instituted to remove any muscular components. If deemed appropriate, surgical treatment may be performed at this point. Lastly, postsurgical physiotherapy is instituted as recommended by the physical therapist to maintain ideal neuromuscular adaptation to any surgical changes. Long-term (lifetime) follow-up is required to intercept at an early stage any return of anatomic pathology.

## Symptoms of Temporomandibular Disorders

Bell[22] classified temporomandibular joint disorders into five categories:

1. Acute muscle disorders.
2. Disc-interference disorders of the joint.
3. Inflammatory disorders of the joint.
4. Chronic mandibular hypomobilities.
5. Growth disorders of the joint.

For simplicity, Bell's classification can be broken down to two main categories: (1) acute muscle disorders of the temporomandibular joint (extraarticular or extrinsic disorders) and (2) disorders of the temporomandibular joint itself (structural joint disease, intraarticular or intrinsic disorders).

The majority of temporomandibular joint disorders are of the muscular type. Acute muscle disorders of the temporomandibular joint are also known as temporomandibular joint pain dysfunction syndrome (Schwartz, 1956) and myofascial pain dysfunction syndrome or MPD (Laskin, 1969).[22] Because the latter term is so widely used in the literature, acute muscle disorders will be referred to as myofascial pain dysfunction syndrome (MPD) in this chapter.

Symptoms of acute muscle disorders of the temporomandibular joint or MPD[16] are:

1. Pain of unilateral origin is the most common symptom, although pain can be bilateral.
2. Dull ache of the ear or preauricular region that frequently radiates to the temporal region, the angle of the mandible, or the lateral cervical or occipital regions.
3. Masticatory muscle tenderness.
4. Clicking or popping in the TMJs.
5. Limitation of mandibular movement.
6. Absence of clinical, radiographic, or biochemical evidence of organic changes in the TMJ.[16]
7. Tinnitus, hyperacusia, or pain of the ear.

The most frequent areas of tenderness in myofascial pain dysfunction syndrome (MPD) are found over the neck of the condyloid process, in the area distal and superior to the maxillary tuberosity, and in the anterior temporal crest.[16]

Patients with only the symptom of clicking or popping are not considered to have MPD. Not all persons with this symptom develop MPD syndrome. To establish the diagnosis there must also be accompanying symptoms of pain, muscle tenderness, or both.[16]

In myofascial pain dysfunction syndrome (MPD), 85% of the temporomandibular joint pain or discomfort can be traced to involvement of the musculature directly and indirectly used in the movements of the jaw.[85]

The muscles that may be involved in myofascial pain are the masseter, internal and external pterygoids, temporalis, occipitalis, diagastric, sternocleidomastoid, trapezius, and splenius capitus.

Pain in the muscle in and around the TMJ has been described as dull, but also as sharp, stabbing, and oppressive. The pain is unilateral or bilateral and occurs in one or several muscles.[86]

Pain can also occur in the shoulder and neck muscles in 62% of patients with MPD.[86]

Almost all reports agree that limitation of movement and/or deviation of the mandible are very common complaints. The deviation of the mandible is toward the affected side and a forced deviation to the nonaffected side is painful. Limitation of opening is also commonly seen in patients with MPD.[86]

Another symptom of masticatory dysfunction is acute malocclusion. The patient may complain of a sudden change in the occlusion and this symptom often accompanies other symptoms of masticatory dysfunction or pain.[22]

Acute malocclusion can result from either muscle spasm or a sudden change in the relationship of the disc-condyle complex with the articular eminence.[22]

Spasm of the lateral pterygoid muscle is the cause of most muscle-induced malocclusion. The condyle is drawn forward on the affected side, thus causing disocclusion of the posterior teeth and premature contact of the anterior teeth contralaterally.[22]

Myospasm of the masseter muscle (displaces the mandible laterally) or the medial pterygoid (displaces the mandible medially) may also induce malocclusion but not of a magnitude that can be easily detected clinically. The patient's subjective remarks pertaining to the malocclusion are sometimes the only indicator of the acute malocclusion.[22]

Acute malocclusion can also be caused by a sudden change in the relationship of the disc-condyle complex with the articular eminence. This malocclusion, therefore, is caused by an intrinsic joint problem rather than a muscular, or extrinsic disorder of the TMJ. Such a malocclusion can occur as a result of trauma, rapid deterioration of the osseous surfaces of the condyle, dislocation of the disc from the condyle, swelling of the retrodiscal tissue, or accumulation of excessive fluid within the joint from an inflammatory process, etc.[22]

It is important to realize that muscle spasm that is part of the myofascial pain dysfunction syndrome can predispose the patient to intrinsic joint disorders of the TMJ if not treated early or effectively.

When myospastic activity develops, it can become an independent, self-perpetuating, cycling myospasm that can go on indefinitely. Spastic activity of the elevator muscles can increase the passive intraarticular pressure, thus altering or interfering with normal biomechanics of the joint. As such, it predisposes to discal interference during mandibular movements. In addition, spastic activity in the lateral pterygoid muscle induces acute malocclusion that can begin a chain of masticatory problems that involve the temporomandibular joint itself and the musculature in and around the joint. A simple muscle disorder (MPD) can therefore activate a much more serious masticatory problem involving the temporomandibular joint proper. Consequently, it is important to manage MPD early and effectively to prevent intrinsic joint pathology.[22]

The preponderance of patients who seek help for temporomandibular joint disorders are women between the ages of 20 to 40 years of age. As reported in the literature the percent of women varies from 58% to 89%.[87] The reason for the preponderance of women suffering from TMJ disorders is not well understood.

## Management of Myofascial Pain Dysfunction Syndrome

Management of MPD syndrome is founded on certain basic principles that include the establishment of an accurate diagnosis and avoidance of irreversible forms of treatment.[88] It is also based on the clinician's understanding that psychological factors play an important role in the etiology of the disease and that the results of treatment must be considered in the light of placebo effects and the contributions of a good doctor-patient relationship.[88]

## Home Therapy

There are a number of simple yet effective ways of managing MPD that the patient can do at home to reduce muscle fatigue, spasm, and pain, increase mandibular mobility, and restore good masticatory function. These include proper diet, the limitation of jaw movement, avoidance of parafunctional habits, and use of heat and massage. The diet should be of a soft, nonchewy character. Food should be cut into small pieces so that excessive chewing is not necessary. Jaw motion should be limited and wide opening, such as yawning, should be avoided or consciously controlled by placing the hand under the chin.[88]

Heat and massage are beneficial to patients with MPD. Moist heat applications should be used for a half hour at least twice daily. These applications should be placed over the involved masticatory muscles for 10 minutes, followed by a 5-minute pause, and then reapplied for two more times in the same manner. Between heat applications and mild exercise, using hinge motion within the limit of pain may be used to maintain muscle function.[88]

## Bite-plane (Splint) Therapy

Parafunctional habits, such as clenching or bruxism, should be avoided. Many patients, however, are usually not aware of these habits, especially if they occur at night. Patients should be instructed to keep the teeth apart if they recognize such activity. Other parafunctional habits such as fingernail biting, lip biting, cheek biting, and the holding of pipes or cigars in the mouth for prolonged periods must also be avoided since these habits can include masticatory muscle fatigue.[88]

Bite-plane appliances are effective orthotic devices (Fig. 11.20) used for the treatment of acute and chronic TMJ/MPD disorders. Bite-planes are the most widely used method for reducing muscle activity in these disorders.[89]

Electromyographic research has shown that hyperactivity in the masticatory muscles diminishes within a short time following the insertion of a biteplane.[90] Patients generally report a decrease in pain and improvement in mobility after wearing an appliance for several days or weeks.

Currently, several types of occlusal splints are used in the treatment of TMJ/MPD disorders.

Only hard appliances should be utilized. The soft appliances, which are often fabricated from thermoplastic resin materials employed in a suck-down vacuum technique, may contribute to continued muscle spasms

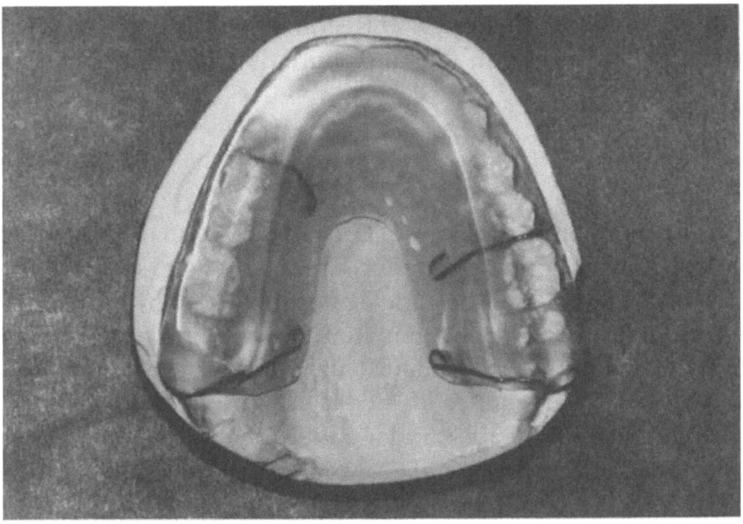

**Figure 11.20.** A bite-plane appliance is an effective orthotic device.

instead of eliminating or reducing the spasms. However, soft appliances can be used for short periods of time to relieve acute symptoms.[91]

The flat plane, full-arch occlusal bite-plane has a long history of effectiveness in the management of pain of TMJ/MPD disorders. The flat platform allows the mandible to position itself in response to the reduction of muscle hyperactivity and the healing of the joint(s) provided the splint is properly adjusted. The adjustments should be done as often as necessary to accommodate for vertical as well as horizontal changes in condylar position.[89]

Full-arch bite-planes are best utilized to prevent any supereruption of posterior teeth and are best fabricated for the maxilla. Bite-planes made for the mandibular arch can cause intrusion of the bicuspids and molars if used for extended periods of time.[89]

Mandibular orthopedic repositioning appliances (MORA) are essentially bite-raising appliances that have been modified functionally to attempt to "recapture the disc" when the disc is considered to be anteriorly displaced. Although the device may give spectacular relief of pain in some patients, prediction is highly questionable and the end result is frequently severe malocclusion. Intrusion of posterior teeth and extrusion of anterior teeth often occurs, especially in patients who clench and brux. A posterior open bite resulting from the use of a MORA appliance may only take 1 to 2 weeks to develop.[92]

It is not unusual to see a patient who continues to have severe pain and dysfunction after the use of a MORA. It is also not unusual to see severe malocclusion and pain develop after the use of a MORA when the initial diagnosis was painless clicking.[92]

## Short-term Medication

Clinicians will often face the dilemma of treating a patient with acute TMJ/MPD pain. Patients present with different degrees of painful symptoms with some acute pain patients suffering to such a degree that a thorough TMJ evaluation may not be possible at the initial visit.[89]

In addition, some patients may not only have acute pain, but may also display trismus. These patients are best managed by prescribing short-term drug therapy. Muscle relaxants and nonsteroidal anti-inflammatory agents with analgesic properties given for 10 days usually relieve the acute symptoms and decrease trismus.

Muscle relaxants interrupt muscle spasm that causes pain. The benzodiazepines are the drugs most often prescribed as muscle relaxants. The best known and most widely used drug in this category is diazepam (Valium), which is prescribed in the range of 2 mg twice a day to 5 mg four times a day. It should be taken in conjunction with an analgesic for the best effect.[89]

Cyclobenzaprine HCL (Flexeril) and chlorzoxazone with acetaminophen (Parafon forte) are effective muscle relaxants; cyclobenzaprine HCL is a compound that is related to the tricyclic antidepressants and, as such, has some of the same side effects that can be distressing to some patients. Some of these side effects are xerostomia, blurred vision, nausea, and constipation. Chlorzoxazone with acetaminophen seems to be well tolerated by most patients and is probably as effective as the benzodiazepines.[89]

The usual dosage of cyclobenzaprine HCL is 10 mg three times a day and of chlorzoxazone with acetaminophen (each tablet contains 250 mg of chlorzoxazone and 300 mg acetaminophen) is 2 tablets four times a day.[89]

The use of drugs with only muscle relaxant properties and no sedative or tranquilizing effects, such as carisoprodol (Soma) and methocarbamol (Robaxin), have generally not been as successful for the treatment of TMJ/MPD disorders.[89]

Mild analgesics are effective for treatment of acute pain when, as mentioned, they are prescribed along with muscle pain.[89]

Examples of analgesics that may be used effectively are: aspirin, 10 grains buffered or coated three times a day; acetaminophen, 650 mg three times a day; diflusinal (Dolobid), initial dose of 100 mg followed by 500 mg every 8 to 12 hours; and ibuprofen (Motrin), 400 mg every 4 to 6 hours. Diflusinal and ibuprofen are quite effective analgesics for treatment of TMJ/MPD disorders and for acute pain; either of the drugs coupled with a muscle relaxant such as chlorzoxazone with acetaminophen (Parafon forte) can manage pain in the majority of patients.

Most patients respond to analgesics and/or muscle relaxants within 10 days and then can be administered other therapeutic modalities on a longer term basis.[89]

## Relaxation Techniques

Because MPD is basically a problem related to increased muscle tension and spasm, any technique designed to induce muscle relaxation can be helpful. Biofeedback and conditioned relaxation are among the more effective and well-accepted modalities available.[88]

Electromyographic biofeedback involves supplying the patient with visual or auditory information about the moment-to-moment contractile status of the muscle being monitored. The patient then concentrates on relaxing the muscle, and, if effective, this condition is reflected by a corresponding reduction in the level of the graphic representation or the audible sound. The patient thus learns to produce muscle relaxation. Although the procedure concentrates on only one muscle at a time, learning to reduce its activity has a generalized relaxing effect.[88]

Condition relaxation is similar to biofeedback in its end result but differs in that the patient does not have the benefit of a feedback indicator. This is actually an advantage because the person does not become dependent upon a machine to indicate relaxation, but instead develops a definite awareness of how the state of relaxation actually feels. The patients are taught to contrast and relax the various muscle of the body, including the muscles of mastication, learning to appreciate the contrast between the two states.[88]

Conditioned relaxation can be taught by the clinician, or the patient can learn it by using instructional audiocassette tapes. In the latter instance, the patient should still have personal instruction initially to assure that the instructions are understood.[88]

## Physical Therapy

Physical therapy plays a vital role in the treatment of TMJ disorders. It has been well established that muscular involvement plays a major part in TMJ disorders. Physical therapists have in-depth training in the musculoskeletal system and in patient rehabilitation. Moreover, growing numbers of therapists have become specialized in therapy for TMJ disorders and work closely with other health professionals to improve the patient's condition. Because most TMJ sufferers respond to conservative treatment, therapy has provided excellent results and valuable input into this complex disorder.[93]

Patients are instructed in various exercises to restore muscle coordination, balance, and strength. Exercises are also used to restore proper shoulder, neck, and head posture, as well as proper tongue positioning.[93]

Physical therapists may use any or all of the following techniques in the treatment regimen.[93]

*Massage Therapy*

Gentle rubbing of the muscles helps them to relax, increases circulation, and decreases muscle spasm.[93]

*Moist Heat Therapy*

Heat increases circulation to the muscles, causes relaxation, and decreases pain.[93]

*Ice Therapy*

Lowers tissue sensitivity, decreases edema, relaxes muscles, and lessens pain. Cold penetrates two to three times deeper than heat.

*Vapocoolant Spray and Stretch*

A spray, such as fluoromethane or ethyl chloride, may be used over the painful area. The coolant relieves pain and muscle spasm, allowing for gentle stretching of the painful muscle.

*Ultrasound*

High frequency sound waves are used to create a deep heating effect. Muscles relax in response to the rise in tissue temperature. Ultrasound can also be used to increase the resorption of adhesions and calcification deposits.

*Acustimulation*

Acustimulation (Neuroprobe) is a low frequency, high galvanic electrical stimulus that is applied over various trigger points to increase the body's production of natural pain killers (endorphins) to decrease pain.[93]

*Transcutaneous Electrical Nerve Stimulation*

The use of transcutaneous electrical nerve stimulation (TENS) is based on the concept that stimulation of the cutaneous branches of the fifth nerve creates an inhibitory effect on the trigeminal spinal tract nucleus and thereby not only reduces awareness of pain but also helps indirectly to induce muscle relaxation. Patients are treated by placing the electrode directly over the area of most discomfort (care in avoiding main branches of the facial nerve will reduce the twitching effect). Therapy sessions last 30 minutes and should be repeated daily. Patients can be taught to use portable units at home and may then perform several treatments each day. Analgesics may be used to aid in further reducing periods of discomfort between sessions.[88]

*Acupuncture*

Although recognized for centuries in Chinese medicine as an effective analgesic technique, acupuncture is relatively new to Western medicine.

Acupuncture seems to be a useful early form of therapy for patients with TMJ/MPD disorders that are expected to be largely functional and reversible and with evidence of psychophysiological or neuromuscular disturbances but not of any marked occlusal interference or joint damage. Acupuncture could well be complementary to other TMJ/MPD treatments, either preceding or following them, to achieve full neuromuscular rehabilitation, to ease other treatments, or to eliminate other possible contributory factors.[94]

### Doctor-Patient Relationship

Symptoms associated with MPD syndrome can be affected by the doctor-patient relationship.[88,95] Patients experiencing pain are likely to have higher levels of stress. The reassurance of a doctor and the belief that he or she can provide help have an immediate, positive effect on the stress a patient is experiencing.[95]

*Tricyclic Antidepressants*

Chronic pain can cause clinically significant reactive depression, and primary depression can also lead to chronic pain behavior. Because of the relationship between chronic pain and depression, tricyclic antidepressants have been used as part of the therapeutic approach to this complex problem.[96]

*Psychologic Techniques*

Operant conditioning and cognitive therapy that are administered by psychologists are valuable techniques in the treatment of chronic pain.[97]

## A Multidisciplinary Approach to the Management of Chronic Orofacial Pain (TMJ/MPD)

As any practitioner who treats chronic pain knows, these cases are challenging and frustrating. The practitioner often has difficulty trying to determine which symptom is part of the syndrome and which is not.[98]

Patients with chronic orofacial pain are often sad, hostile, anxious, frustrated, and tenaciously cling to dental and medical professionals. They often have extreme difficulty with sleep and pain becomes an all-encompassing fixation. These patients often have an extremely negative attitude toward their lives and they make no realistic plans for the distant future.[99]

The patient with facial pain may be so demanding that it is worth reiterating several cardinal rules regarding treatment of pain. First, pain is a symptom and not a disease. The causes of pain should always be investigated vigorously but objectively. Second, although analgesics are important in management of pain problems, they are not complete in themselves. There are only a few clearly established situations, such as pain from terminal cancer, in which narcotic analgesics are the primary form of treatment. Abolishing pain can delay determination of the underlying cause. Third, destructive procedures should not be done until the anatomic and physiologic basis for the pain is understood with maximum confidence. Finally, and most important, we must be careful in acknowledging professional limitation in achieving a diagnosis and in our providing continuing therapy that is appropriate.[100]

More often than not, numerous specialists have to be called in to consult on symptoms that appear to be relevant to the pain problem but do not fall into the area of expertise of the practitioner. Unless all aspects of the patient's pain are treated simultaneously, the dental practitioner's treatment eventually will become just another unsuccessful effort in the patient's search for relief.[98] To treat patients, the practitioner not only has to be an expert in dental therapies for these disorders but also must act as a conduit to, and interpreter for, numerous specialists whose opinions and advice are necessary for successful treatment.[98] An extensive background in differential diagnosis in otolaryngology, neurophysiology, rheumatology, trauma, anesthesiology, orthopedics, kinesiology, psychology, and psychiatry is necessary for the diagnosis and treatment of these pain problems.[98] Therefore, patients with chronic oral facial pain cannot be treated successfully by a succession of individual practitioners from their own isolated, limited point of view. The reason for this is that these patients have a multiplicity of causative factors present, all contributing to the total problem. Therefore, to achieve any success, a multidisciplinary approach is necessary so that the problem can be viewed and recommendations made from many different but closely related specialties.[99]

For the patient to benefit from the insights of appropriate specialists in many different areas, a team approach has been developed at many medical centers across the country. The multidisciplinary approach is proving to be the most effective way of managing chronic pain of all types. It is of great value in the treatment of TMJ/MPD disorders. By controlling all of the various psychological and physical manifestations of stress and chronic pain, management is becoming a reality.

## References

1. Kroening, R.J. (1984). Pain. In: *Dental Anesthesia and Analgesia. Third Edition.* Allen, G.D. Baltimore: Williams and Wilkins Co.

2. Fricton, J.R., & Kroening, R.J. (1982). Practical differential diagnosis of orofacial pain. *Oral Surgery, Oral Medicine, Oral Pathology* 54:628–634.
3. Donaldson, D., & Kroening, R. (1979). Recognition and treatment of patients with chronic orofacial pain. *Journal of the American Dental Association* 99:961–966.
4. Foreman, P.A. (1985). Temporomandibular joint and myofascial pain dysfunction—some current concepts, part 1: Diagnosis. *New Zealand Dental Journal* 81:47–51.
5. Costen, J.B. (1934). A syndrome of ear and sinus symptoms dependent on disturbed function of the temporomandibular joint. *Annals of Otolaryngology, Rhinolaryngology, Laryngology* 43:1–15.
6. Kotick, J.M. (1985). 25 years of TMJ. New York: *Journal of Dentistry* 55(3):111–115.
7. Sicher, H. (1960). *Oral Anatomy.* St. Louis: C.V. Mosby Co.
8. Muskin, D.J., Fourrier, J.L., Shelley, L.R., & Waid, L.R. (1986). A common sense approach for treatment of myofascial pain—dysfunction syndrome. *Journal of the Alabama Dental Association* 70(1):34–39.
9. Gibilisco, J. (1983). Management of temporomandibular joint disorders associated with systemic disease. *Dental Clinics of North America* 27(3):457–478.
10. Solberg, W. (1986). Temporomandibular disorders: functional and radiological considerations. *British Dental Journal* 160:195–200.
11. Osborn, J. (1985). The disc of the human temporomandibular joint: Design, function and failure. *Journal of Oral Rehabilitation* 12:279–293.
12. Rees, L. (1954). The structure and function of the mandibular joint. *British Dental Journal* 96:125–133.
13. McNamara, J. (1973). The independent functions of the two heads of the lateral pterygoid muscle. *American Journal of Anatomy* 138:197–206.
14. Toller, P. (1973). Osteoarthritis of the mandibular condyle. *British Dental Journal* 134:223–231.
15. Malkin, D. (1987). The role of TMJ dysfunction in the etiology of middle ear disease. *International Journal of Orthodontics* 25:20–21.
16. Laskin, D.M., & Sarnat, B.G. (Eds.) (1980). *The Temporomandibular Joint—A Biological Basis for Clinical Practice.* Third Edition. Springfield, Ill.: Charles C. Thomas.
17. Day, L. (1982). History taking. In: *Diseases of the Temporomandibular Apparatus—A Multidisciplinary Approach.* Morgan, D.H., House, L.R. Hall, W.P. and Vamvas, S.J. (Eds.). St. Louis: C.V. Mosby Co.
18. Bell, W.E. (1986). *Temporomandibular Disorders: Classification, Diagnosis, Management.* Second Edition. Chicago: Year Book Medical Publishers, Inc.
19. DeSteno, C.V. (1977). The pathophysiology of TMJ dysfunction and related pain. In: *Clinical Management of Head, Neck and TMJ Pain and Dysfunction—A Multidisciplinary Approach to Diagnosis and Treatment.* Gelb, H. Philadelphia: W.B. Saunders Co.
20. Cannistraci, A.J. (1977). Biofeedback—The treatment of stress induced muscle activity. In: *Clinical Management of Head, Neck and TMJ Pain and Dysfunction—A Multidisciplinary Approach to Diagnosis and Treatment.* Gelb, H. Philadelphia: W.B. Saunders Co.
21. Crandall, J.A. (1986). Evaluation of mandibular movement and range of motion in the diagnosis of craniomandibular disorders. *The Journal of Craniomandibular Practice* 4(3):235–245.

22. Bell, W.E. (1982). *Clinical Management of Temporomandibular Disorders*. Chicago: Year Book Medical Publishers, Inc.
23. Brooke, R., & Stenn, P. (1978). Post-injury myofascial pain dysfunction syndrome: Its etiology and prognosis. *Oral Surgery* 45:846–850.
24. Farrar, W., & McCarty, W. (1979). The TMJ dilemma. *Journal of the Alabama Dental Association* 63:19–26.
25. Scapino, R. (1983). Histopathology associated with malposition of the human temporomandibular joint disc. *Oral Surgery* 55(4):382–397.
26. Isberg-Holm, A., & Westesson, P. (1982). Movement of disc and condyle in temporomandibular joints with and without clicking. *Acta Odontologica Scandinavica* 40:165–177.
27. Isberg-Holm, A., & Ivarsson, R. (1980). The movement pattern of the mandibular condyles in individuals with and without clicking. *Dentomaxillofacial Radiology* 9:59–69.
28. Solberg, W. (1986). Temporomandibular disorders: Management of internal derangement. *British Dental Journal* 160(11):379–386.
29. Irby, W. (1980). *Current Advances in Oral Surgery*. Vol. IV. St. Louis: C.V. Mosby Co.
30. Bronstein, S. (1987). Retained alloplastic temporomandibular joint disk implants: A retrospective study. *Oral Surgery* 64(2):135–145.
31. Graham, G., Ferraro, N., & Simms, D. (1984). Perforations of the temporomandibular joint meniscus: Arthrographic, surgical, and clinical findings. *Journal of Craniomandibular Practice* 4(3):255–262.
32. Shafer, W., Hine, & M. Levy, B. (1983). *A Textbook of Oral Pathology*. Philadelphia: W.B. Saunders.
33. Nelson, A., & Cohen, S. (1987). The post-surgical TMJ patient: A protocol for treatment. *TMJ Update* 5(4):60–64.
34. Hall, E. (1982). Organic abnormalities of the TMJ. *Ear, Nose and Throat Journal* 61:632–637.
35. Schwartz, H. (1981). Sarcoid temporomandibular arthritis. *Oral Surgery* 52(6): 588–590.
36. Chue, P. (1975). Gonococcal arthritis of the temporomandibular joint. *Journal of Oral Surgery* 39:572–577.
37. Copenhaver, R., Dennis, M., et al. (1985). Fracture of the glenoid fossa and dislocation of the mandibular condyle into the middle cranial fossa. *Journal of Oral and Maxillofacial Surgery* 43:974–977.
38. Gross, B., Williams, R., et al. (1987). Gout and pseudogout of the temporomandibular joint. *Oral Surgery* 63:551–554.
39. Sanders, B., & Halliday, R. (1979). Psoriasis and rheumatoid arthritis: Their relationship in TMJ ankylosis. *Journal of Oral Surgery* 34:4–7.
40. Brooke, R. (1973). Secondary osteoarthrosis of the temporomandibular joint. *Canadian Dental Journal* 43(7):323–328.
41. Mejerso, C. (1987). Therapeutic and prognostic considerations in TMJ osteoarthrosis: A literature review and long term study in 11 subjects. *Journal of Craniomandibular Practice* 5(1):70–78.
42. Mongini, F. (1983). Influence of function on temporomandibular joint remodelling and degenerative disease. *Dental Clinics of North America* 27(3): 479–494.
43. Ogus, H (1980). Degenerative disease of the temporomandibular joint in young persons. *British Journal of Oral Surgery* 17:17–26.

44. Kopp, S. (1977). Clinical findings in temporomandibular joint arthrosis. *Scandinavian Journal of Dental Research* 85:434–443.
45. Trenwith, J., & Beale, G. (1977). Rheumatoid arthritis of the temporomandibular joint. *New Zealand Dental Journal* 73:195–199.
46. Hansson, L., Petersson, A., & Vallon-Christersson, D. (1984). Clinical and radiologic six-year follow-up study of patients with crepitation of the temporomandibular joint. *Swedish Dental Journal* 8:277–287.
47. Agus, B., Weisberg, J., & Friedman, M. (1983). Therapeutic injection of the temporomandibular joint. *Oral Surgery* 55(6):554–556.
48. Poswillo, D. (1983). Conservative management of degenerative temporomandibular joint disease in the elderly. *International Dental Journal* 33(4):325–331.
49. Poswillo, D. (1970). Experimental investigation of the effects of intra-articular hydrocortisone and high condylectomy on the mandibular condyle. *Oral Surgery* 30:161–173.
50. Ogus, H. (1975). Rheumatoid arthritis of the temporomandibular joint. *British Journal of Oral Surgery* 12:275–284.
51. Anderson, J., & Blair, G. (1975). Screening in a dental clinic for adult rheumatoid arthritis involving the temporomandibular joint using a discriminate function. *Journal of Oral Rehabilitation* 2:187–197.
52. Zide, M., Carlton, D., & Kent, J. (1986). Rheumatoid disease and related arthropathies. *Oral Surgery* 61(2):119–125.
53. Morgan, D. (1975). Surgical correction of temporomandibular joint arthritis. *Journal of Oral Surgery* 33:766–773.
54. Ganik, R., & Williams, F. (1986). Diagnosis and management of juvenile rheumatoid arthritis with TMJ involvement. *Journal of Craniomandibular Practice* 4(3):253–262.
55. Seymour, R., Crouse, V., & Irby, W. (1975). Temporomandibular ankylosis secondary to rheumatoid arthritis. *Oral Surgery* 33:766–773.
56. Resnick, D. (1974). Temporomandibular joint involvement in ankylosing spondylitis. Comparison with rheumatoid arthritis and psoriasis. *Radiology* 112:587–591.
57. Harvey, A., Johns, R., et al. (1976). *Principles and Practice of Medicine.* Edition 19. New York: Appleton-Century-Crofts.
58. Kent, J., Carlton, D., & Zide, M. (1986). Rheumatoid disease and related arthropathy (Part II). *Oral Surgery* 61(5):423–439.
59. Heir, G., Berrett, A., & Worth, D. (1983). Diagnosis and management of TMJ involvement in ankylosing spondylitis. *Journal of Craniomandibular Practice* 1(2):76–81.
60. Solberg, W. (1986). Temporomandibular disorders: Management of problems associated with inflammation, chronic hypomobility, and deformity. *British Dental Journal* 160(11):421–428.
61. Olsson, A. (1969). Temporomandibular joint function and functional disturbances. *Dental Clinics of North America* 43:643–658.
62. Jones, G., & Harn, S. (1979). Diagnostic value of transcranial radiographs of the temporomandibular joint. *Journal of Dental Research* 58:153 (abstract).
63. Mongini, F. (1981). The importance of radiography in the diagnosis of TMJ dysfunction. *Journal of Prosthetic Dentistry* 45(2):186–197.
64. Toller, P., & Glynn, L. (1976). *Degenerative Disease of the Mandibular Joint, Scientific Foundations of Dentistry.* Chicago: Year Book Medical Publishers.

65. Omnell, K., & Petersson, A. (1976). Radiography of the Temporomandibular Joint Utilizing Oblique Lateral Transcranial Projections. *Odontologisk Revy* 27:77–92.
66. Dunn, M., Rabinov, K., et al. (1981). Polycycloidal corrected tomography of the temporomandibular joint. *Oral Surgery* 51(4):375–384.
67. Bussard, D., Kerr, G., et al. (1980). Technique and use of 'corrected axis' tomograms of the mandibular condyles. *Oral Surgery* 49:394–397.
68. Katzberg, R., Keith, D., et al. (1980). Correlation of condylar mobility and arthrotomography in patients with internal derangements of the temporomandibular joint. *Oral Surgery* 54(6):622–627.
69. Helms, C., Katzberg, R., et al. (1982). Arthrotomographic diagnosis of meniscus perforations in the temporomandibular joints. *British Journal of Radiology* 53:283–285.
70. Bronstein, S., Tomasetti, B., & Ryan, D. (1981). Internal derangements of the temporomandibular joint: Correlation of arthroscopy with surgical findings. *Journal of Oral Surgery* 39:572–584.
71. Murphy, W. (1981). Temporomandibular joint arthrography. *Radiology Clinics of North America* 19:365–378.
72. Roberts, D., Pettigrew, J., et al. (1984). Three dimensional imaging and display of the temporomandibular joint. *Oral Surgery* 58:461–474.
73. Helms, C., Morrish, R., et al. (1982). Computed tomography of the temporomandibular joint: Preliminary observations. *Radiology* 145:719–722.
74. Helms, C., Katzberg, R., et al. (1983). Computed tomography of the temporomandibular joint meniscus. *Journal of Oral Maxillofacial Surgery* 41:512–517.
75. Manzione, J., Seltzer, S., et al. (1983). Direct sagittal computed tomography of the temporomandibular joint. *American Journal of Radiology* 140:165–167.
76. Tilds, B., & Miller, P. (1987). Radiographic pathology of the temporomandibular joints, and head pain. *Headache* 27:427–430.
77. Donlon, W., & Moon, K. (1987). Comparison of magnetic resonance imaging arthrotomograhy, and clinical and surgical findings in temporomandibular joint internal derangements. *Oral Surgery* 64(1):2–5.
78. Wilk, R., Harms, S., & Wolford, L. (1986). Magnetic resonance imaging of the temporomandibular joint using a surface coil. *Journal of Oral and Maxillofacial Surgery* 44:935–943.
79. Oshnishi, M. (1975). Arthroscopy of the temporomandibular joint. *Journal of the Stomatognathic Society of Japan* 42:207–213.
80. Murakami, K., Matsuki, M., et al. (1986). Diagnostic arthroscopy of the TMJ: Differential diagnosis in patients with limited jaw opening. *Journal of Craniomandibular Practice* 4(2):118–126.
81. Liedberg, J., & Westesson, P. (1986). Diagnostic accuracy of upper compartment arthroscopy of the temporomandibular joint: Correlation with postmortem morphology. *Oral Surgery* 62:618–624.
82. Sanders, B. (1986). Arthroscopic surgery of the temporomandibular joint: Treatment of internal derangement with persistent closed lock. *Oral Surgery* 62(4):361–372.
83. Westesson, P., Eriksson, L., & Liedberg, J. (1987). The risk of damage to facial nerve, superficial temporal vessels, disk, and articular surfaces during arthroscopic examination of the temporomandibular joint. *Oral Surgery* 62(2):124–127.

84. Gross, A., & Bosanquet, A. (1986). Temporomandibular joint arthroscopy. *Journal of Oral and Maxillofacial Surgery* 44(8):614–617.
85. Vamvas, S.J. (1982). Differential diagnosis of TMJ disease. In: *Diseases of the Temporomandibular Apparatus—A Multidisciplinary Approach*. Second Edition. Morgan, D.H., House, L.R., Hall, W.P. and Vamvas, S.J. (Eds.). St. Louis: C.V. Mosby Co.
86. DeBoever, J.A. (1979). Functional disturbances of the temporomandibular joint. In: *Temporomandibular Joint Function and Dysfunction*. Zarb, G.A. and Carlsson, G.E. (Eds.). St. Louis: C.V. Mosby Co.
87. Hijzen, T.H., & Slangen, J.L. (1985). Myofascial pain-dysfunction: Subjective signs and symptoms. *Journal of Prosthetic Dentistry* 54(5):705–710.
88. Laskin, D.M., & Block, S.B. (1986). Diagnosis and treatment of myofascial pain-dysfunction (MPD) syndrome. *Journal Prosthetic Dentistry* 56(1):75–83.
89. Fattore, L., & Strauss, R. (1986). A review of the practical concepts and treatment of temporomandibular joint disorders in the dental office. *Illinois Dental Journal* 55(6):514–519.
90. Dahlstrom, L., Carlsson, G.E., & Carlsson, S.G. (1982). Comparison of effects of electromyographic biofeedback and occlusal splint therapy on mandibular dysfunction. *Scandinavian Journal of Dental Research* 90:151–156.
91. More dental udpate—TMJ questions and answers. (1984). *Indian Health Service* 23(3):54–58.
92. Ash, M.M. (1986). Current concepts in the aetiology, diagnosis and treatment of TMJ and muscle dysfunction. *Journal of Oral Rehabilitation* 13:1–20.
93. Wolf, C. (1987). Early detection and treatment of TMJ disorders. *Dental Assistant* 56(2):19–23.
94. Raustia, A.M., & Pohjola, R.T. (1986). Acupuncture compared with stomatognathic treatment for TMJ dysfunction. Part III: Effect of treatment on mobility. *Journal of Prosthetic Dentistry* 56(5):616–623.
95. Okeson, J.P. (1981). Etiology and treatment of occlusal pathosis and associated facial pain. *Journal of Prosthetic Dentistry* 45(2):199–202.
96. Hersh, E.V. (1987). Tricyclic antidepressant drugs: Pharmacologic implications in the treatment of chronic orofacial pain. *Compendium of Continuing Education in Dentistry* VIII(9):688–693.
97. Singer, E. (1987). Pain control in dentistry: Management of chronic orofacial pain. *Compendium of Continuing Education in Dentistry* VIII(2):114–120.
98. Harte, L.S. (1984). The TMJ center: Filling a gap in chronic pain treatment. *Journal of the Massachusetts Dental Society* 33(4):205–218.
99. Quinn, J.H. (1980). Chronic orofacial pain. *Journal of the Louisiana Dental Association* 38(4):8–10.
100. Lazar, M.L., Greenlee, R.G., & Naarden, A.L. (1980). Facial pain of neurologic origin mimicking oral pathologic conditions: Some current concepts and treatment. *Journal of the American Dental Association* 100:884–888.

# 12

# Bringing It All Together: Developing the Clinical Team

*Kathleen Blindt Segraves*

The literature concerning chronic pain is replete with the term "multidisciplinary team" to describe the collaboration of professionals from various fields. There is, however, little mention of the ways in which the disciplines become a team and where work becomes teamwork.

The purpose of this chapter is not to provide a "cookbook" for setting up a multidisciplinary team or pain clinic. Rather, its purpose is to stimulate a way of thinking about the formation of such a team, and to address some of the issues that may have been taken for granted, or never considered, when designing a collaborative effort. Given that there is no one model of teamwork that is appropriate for all situations, this chapter will provide ways of understanding various team models.

## The Planning Process

With limited resources, planning has become a crucial, albeit often neglected, aspect in the health care field. Service providers, who often stress the importance of stating the problem, the treatment, and the evaluation in observable or concrete terms, often do not apply the same strategies in designing new programs or services. Abstract goals of health teams serve little management function. Operationally defining tangible objectives to fit the defined goals of the program permits effective planning and decisions making.

### Team Planning

Team planning begins in the identification of problems, goals, and objectives. Problems are often articulated in terms of the prevailing value system (e.g., societal what "should" or "ought" to be). Discrepancies between "what should be" and "what actually is" often lead to the identification of goals. Such goals are typically broad statements that are made more cogent by the generation of specific objectives. Tasks, or service activities, are then designed to satisfy the objectives.

The process thus far serves to establish a specific and measurable focus for the activities of the "service idea." This initial phase of planning usually involves a core group of professionals who have the capacity to recruit and allocate resources. The people involved in the initial phase are concerned with the what, why, and to whom questions of program development.

In the second phase of planning, the core individuals, who have identified a problem, begin to consider strategies to achieve the initial goals and objectives. Selection of program/service approaches designed for the greatest impact on the problem, given the available resources and political climate of the existing organization, requires dynamic and creative thinking. Exploring the wide range of options, rather than immediately gravitating toward the "tried and true" service strategies, will often yield programs that are most appropriate for a particular organization and target population.

Stating program objectives in concrete and measurable terms facilitates both the identification of required tasks and the measurement of outcomes. The tasks or activities, when performed in a specific manner, should result in the achievement of the operationalized objectives. The service strategies when stated in precise terms, help to determine the policy of the program (e.g., necessary actions, target population, quality assurance, personnel, etc.). The planning implementation process addresses the practical questions of where, when, how, and by whom.

The final phase of the process concerns evaluating the impact of selected activities on the identified problems. The strengths and weaknesses of each component are identified and these findings form the basis of program decision and revisions. The ongoing concerns of the evaluation process include: (1) the appropriateness of the tasks for the stated objectives; (2) the cost effectiveness; and (3) overall efficacy of the services.

## How Teams Begin

As the process of planning, development, and evaluation continues it becomes obvious that most problems are very complex and intervention can occur at many levels. Chronic pain frequently has an enormous impact on the psychological, social, financial, and behavioral aspects of the individual. Multidetermined, chronic-pain conditions require the knowledge base and skills of a variety of disciplines. A team approach is thus a reasonable way to address the complex problem of chronic pain. This approach allows tasks to be divided so that members do what they are best suited for, given their individual area of expertise.

Recruitment of team members is a critical function for effective team development. Effectiveness of a team is potentiated when its membership possess the necessary skills to meet the goals of the organization.[1] The mere assignment of a group of people to work as a team does not guarantee effective collaboration since teaming is a dynamic concept where people come together to plan, coordinate, and implement activities for a specific purpose.

## Teamwork

According to Brill (1976), "A team is a group of people each of whom possesses particular expertise; each of whom is responsible for making individual decisions; who together hold a common purpose; who meet together to communicate, collaborate, and consolidate knowledge, from which plans are made, actions determined and future decisions influenced" (p. 22).[2] Members of the team come together to establish working procedures and processes with the purpose of either formulating a new service or improving the current system.

### *Problems of Teamwork*

The nature of teamwork is not without certain difficulties including individual differences, time constraints, and conflicts. The individual members bring to the team both their personal and their role identities. As Brill (1976) observes: "The individual uses his unique personal characteristics to affect his work, and these attitudes and behaviors can be an asset or a liability, both to him and to the group" (p. 31).[2] The individual characteristics of team members will exercise tremendous influence on the team's nature and effectiveness.

In addition, teamwork is not only demanding on the individual members, it can be time consuming and ponderous. For example, a pain clinic that includes representation of all disciplines in the assessment and treatment planning may require members to keep weekly blocks of time open for team meetings. When one or more members cannot attend a scheduled meeting, additional time may need to be allocated for the purpose of meeting as "a team." Late test results or other evaluation information also may require an additional meeting before treatment decisions can be made. Participatory democracy tends to be a cumbersome and slow-moving process. Emerging situations may require a shortcutting of the process and substitution of more authoritarian action. Problems in conflict resolution and communication within the team can limit the effectiveness of the work. In fact, teamwork can lead to increased fragmentation of services. Differences in status of members and service requirements, as well as friction between the various disciplines, can lead to team work difficulties.[2] Selecting a specific organizational team design can minimize some of these liabilities.

### Rationale for Teamwork

Several factors justify a teamwork approach to chronic pain. First, a greater number of patients can receive the concerted efforts of many specialists within a short period of time. This is important, given the fact that the demand for the special services needed in treating the problem of chronic pain often exceeds the supply of specialists. A team practice provides a medium where a greater number of patients can receive consultation by specialists then might be afforded through a private practice. Second, a multidisciplinary practice increases the effective use of pooled specialized knowledge through a more comprehensive and integrated range of activities. A team provides a forum for the assessment and evaluation of treatment plans in light of the differing frames of references. A multidisciplinary clinical practice promotes the treatment and integration of all aspects of patient functioning. This results in a comprehensive analysis of the person-situation complex. The biological, psychological, environmental, financial, and behavioral components that contribute to and maintain the chronic pain condition can be better analyzed and addressed through a team approach.

## Organizational Design

Most people in the field of health care do not automatically attend to organizational design when planning a team. Professionals are frequently unaware of the many design options and the strengths and weaknesses of each. The complex issues of designing multidisciplinary services for a broad range of problems can be simplified using the metaphor of team sports.

Most people have been exposed to the strategies of sports from a very early age. Every sport presents a game with rules for interacting. The rules dictate patterns of communication and compliance gaining behaviors. All teams present with their own "culture." The culture, or prevailing style, of a sports team is very comparable to the types of health care delivery systems or clinics. The "culture of a complex health care organization influences the perception and exercise of social power and identifies the patterns of communication which are used by members of the organization to sustain a functional system in light of the competing ideological systems."[3] Although membership interactions are dynamic, the prevailing way in which things get done are often ritualized, thus becoming the culture of the organization.

Organizational structure, important in designing pain clinics, will be described using a sports analogy. This analogy will serve to: (1) make the basic design concepts concrete; (2) demonstrate its applicability to many team endeavors; (3) keep the focus on design without the distraction of discipline bias; and (4) offer a method of understanding team models to demonstrate design options. Relating the organizational design of a specific team sport to the multidisciplinary pain clinic might help planners select the right team sport strategy to address the specific goals of a pain clinic.

A specific sport requires the recruitment of people to fill the roles and functions of the team. Although all teams may have the same basic roles, it would be erroneous to say that all baseball, football, or basketball teams are the same. The differences among the teams are due to many factors including: (1) the organizational structure; (2) the team strategy; and (3) the personality, skills, and knowledge of both the coach and individual players. This is quite analogous to the many chronic pain clinics. Although the literature is replete with descriptions of pain clinics that offer comparable discipline representation (e.g., anesthesiology, neurosurgery, occupational therapy, physical therapy, psychiatry, psychology, social work, etc.), the type of service offered and methods used vary considerably.

## Pick Your Sport

Three sports that can be used to describe the organizational structure of most of the pain clinics reported in the literature are football, baseball, and basketball. The organizational design of each sport will be described to demonstrate how the tasks central to all teams (e.g., staffing, planning, operating) differ according to the strategy of the sport. The sports model can be applied to any organization, regardless of its size. Using the sports model developed by Keidel,[4] each team metaphor will demonstrate organizational design.

### *Baseball Teams*

Baseball is a game of individual effort. Players function independently with minimal interaction. Scoring plays relates to individual effort rather than to hierarchically designed strategies. The team manager is concerned with "batting order." He makes sure that the players are in the game at the appropriate time and in the right order. The basic unit is the individual. The design of the game creates spatial separation among the players throughout the geographic area (field). Performance is the sum total of every team member. Situations may call for some actions that resemble teamwork (e.g., walks, steals, sacrifices, etc.). Although such strategies may help to contribute to the score, the team members are autonomous and the game (score) is dependent on individual effort and initiative. Coordination is essentially controlled by the rules of the game. In baseball design priority is to get the players right.[4]

A multidisciplinary pain team consisting of a collection of specialists available for consultation and referrals can be viewed using the baseball model. The clinic director schedules the appropriate referral "line up" and recruits experts from many diverse fields. Finding the best players or stars enhances the success rate of both the individual and the team. The director would select and assign team members, as needed, for the given situation. The baseball model requires only a minimal amount of interrelating, allowing for a wide range of personalities to work as an effective team. People who might not wish to form close collaborative relationships might consider the baseball model of teamwork. The rules and strategies of baseball are more conducive to tolerating personality extremes such as extroverts and introverts than either football or basketball (p. 24).[4]

The baseball model might be an appropriate design choice when the core members of the clinic are recognized specialized professionals and are highly visible in the community. This design permits both member autonomy and a summative recognition through team affiliation. Successful treatment within each specialty would add rather than detract from the success of the team. The game plan of baseball allow a dispersed field arrangement. In applying this plan to a pain clinic, a central geographic location is not as important as the recruitment of specialized consultants. An organizational design that is predominately representative of the baseball team model can be found in the literature.[5-7] Patients are often seen in the health care provider's own office or clinic. The patients' activities are usually connected through a path of sequential tasks. For example, a patient might first be sent to an internist, then to the neurologist, then to a social worker, etc. Specialists will analyze the situation and provide treatment according to their area of expertise. The individual professional contributes to the pain clinic independently with little interaction between disciplines.

The responsibilities of the coordinator might include the recruitment of members and services and scheduling the order of consultations throughout the delivery of service. The consultants or team members can relate autonomously to one another as well as to the coordinator. The coordinator may control the line up; however, the individual team members are the producers. Expansion of a team using this model would generally be through recruitment of more specialists or an affiliation with other centers, where new services could be offered. Delegation of authority is central to this model. Independent and often unrelated units or members are brought together by a coordinator who directs the order of patient contact. Once the players are in place they make the decisions without consulting continuously with the manager or other team members.

One example of a baseball-organized pain team would be a service that includes a rehabilitation center, medical departments of a hospital, auxiliary services such as psychology, social work, nursing, a day hospital, and outpatient service. The affiliation may be more on paper than in location. The primary method of communication is through referral notes and the clinic or medical chart.

Keidel (1985) observes that: "players on a baseball-organization rarely interact with each other, are likely to be geographically dispersed, and render discrete, quantifiable contributions to the whole. They relish being on their own and being evaluated for their individual performance" (p. 36).[4] These might be individuals who do not have the time to meet frequently. Success with one specialist is not contingent on success with other consultants. Hence a "team" service is provided without developing a central clinic facility as treatment would take place within the existing individual settings.

*Football Teams*

In contrast to baseball, football demands systematic teamwork. The design of the comprehensive game plan is primarily done in hierarchical direction from the coach to the players. The head coach coordinates the game plan and every player is involved in executing this plan. Although the quarterback may have some ability to "call the plays" in a last-minute adjustment on the line, these calls are usually within the general framework prescribed by the coach.

This is a sport that requires more team member interaction. The basic unit is a large group consisting of the offense, defense, and special teams. There are also smaller groups within the defense and offense that must function as individual units (e.g., the linemen and backs on offense, the linemen, linebackers, and backs on defense).[4] There is a tight sequencing of tasks and these tasks are usually complex and interdependent.

The literature suggests that certain clinics have a predominant organizational design analogous to a football team.[8-11] This approach is sometimes known as the medical model. The clinic director (e.g., physician, psychologist, nurse specialist, etc.) is often high in the hierarchical structure of the hospital or clinic and the team is organized around this central figure. This person usually determines the total operation of the team and the strategy of the program. He or she maintains control of the team through lines of communication, reporting requirements, organizational support, and professional authority. Individual and team evaluations are made by this person.[2] The director usually determines the strategy of the program and is ultimately responsible for patient care.

The football model combines the skills of many disciplines or fields and creates a coordinated, hierarchical service. Tasks are sequential and may be viewed as efficient when they are organized by a single coordinator who has knowledge of the whole program. Communication often includes team meetings where individual reports are shared and discussed. The final decision, however, is most often made by the director.

Referring to this organization design, Spengler (1983) pointed out that "after obtaining a thorough assessment of the patient with chronic back pain and reviewing all previous records, the physician is in a position to discuss management with other members of the team. In the majority of cases all members of the team will usually agree to an approach even if one or two members of the team harbor some skepticism. A unified front is essential during presentation of further treatment options to patients who have chronic pain" (p. 76).[8]

A football team approach would be appropriate when the organization is large and consists of many independent services. The hierarchical structure requires that decisions be made by a single person or a small core group. This is efficient for large programs, where issues of ultimate responsibility are important. Roles are clearly delineated and tasks and activities specified. The success of this team approach depends on the ability of each member to accomplish the assigned task.

In summary, the football team strategy has a central administrative plan and the director assigns discrete tasks to individual team members. The strength of such an approach rests on the assumption that the individual components of the team can accomplish the assigned tasks. Because decisions are made by one or two high-ranking members, this represents an efficient system. Although this hierarchical method of decision making is sometimes experienced as very controlling or authoritarian, it can enhance system efficiency and control.

*Basketball Teams*

Basketball is a sport requiring continuous team member awareness, cooperation, adjustment, and spontaneous reaction. "Professional basketball at its best is the quintessential display of patterned, yet spontaneous, teamwork."[4]

The coach functions as an enabler rather than as a director, as in football, or as an organizer/coordinator, as in baseball. In this role, the coach "carries out the tasks of promoting and sustaining or strengthening people's motivations . . . responding to signals of distress, providing legitimate support, identifying transactional patterns; legitimizing concerns; validating strengths; conveying hope; reducing ambivalence and resistance" (pp. 100–110).[12]

The strategy of basketball, from a coach's perspective, is to enable the team to coordinate itself. "The universal property of basketball-organizations is their integrative nature. They not only bridge different disciplines or competencies, they also bring together the worlds of planning and doing" (p. 56).[4] Flexibility and quick adjusting of one's actions in relation to other team members are important elements to this strategy. Unlike football, which has a week to prepare for the game, basketball players compete against several opponents each week. There is no time to prepare for the opposing team; instead the team must adjust to each new situation as it presents itself.

Pain clinics using a basketball team approach usually have a manageable number of professionals who coordinate treatment plans by combining resources in creative ways.[13–19] For example, such a team might be a centrally located inpatient pain rehabilitation center. Meetings concerning patient care might occur informally as well as in daily team sessions. Under this model, a social worker and rehabilitation therapist might exchange impressions, ideas, and strategies for new treatment approaches. A physician and behavioral therapist might collaborate to create a portion of the plan. Members of the team work together as equals in designing, adjusting, and readjusting the treatment approach and each member of the treatment team is aware of the treatment goals and how a particular patient is responding in all aspects of the treatment program. For example, when the team decides that abnormal pain behaviors will be ignored and coping behaviors reinforced, all members of the team (e.g., physician, psychologist, social worker, nursing staff, etc.) follow this reinforcement schedule. Operating on the basis of common decisions, the collaboration is more informal, resulting in less structured lines of communication. The leadership of such a team is often on a revolving basis.[2,4] The director coordinates the process according to the plan of the program.

In summary, basketball is an example of flexible, dynamic interacting. A basketball team approach often has a horizontal dynamic environment rather than a strict hierarchical structure with a single line of communication. The horizontal communication lines encourage open discussions among various disciplines and a more egalitarian approach to teamwork. Tasks are more cooperative and members have more flexibility in accomplishing the tasks according to the discretion of team members. The strength of this model is synergy, innovation, and dynamic flexibility.[4] Its primary drawback is size limitations. A process that relies on total collaboration and democracy is efficient and effective when the number of participants is small enough to facilitate interaction and large enough to accomplish the needed tasks. Given the blending and overlap of roles and function, this method may result in organization ambiguity.

## Differential Diagnosis of the Team

What team sport would you or other members of your team use when describing your present or future service team? The differences among the sports is in the way that they achieve teamwork. Several areas must be analyzed to determine the teamwork organizational structure, including: (1) the team member relatedness and roles; (2) the type of tasks needed to provide the services of the program; (3) the lines of communication, power, and responsibility; (4) the size of the organization; (5) the value system of the team; (6) the leadership style; and (7) the type of "teaming."

Baseball best describes a pain service where individual experts pool their specific services to create a special program. The power resides at an individual level and the members may be located in various geographic areas within a medical center. Success of task accomplishment depends on self-initiative and self-motivation. The status of such a model is one of horizontal separation, where every expert is autonomous and contributes a specific expertise and/or skill as determined by the program director. The style of leadership most descriptive of this model is laissez-faire.[3,4] This model is often seen in the coordination of referrals to specific consultants in a large medical center.

Football best depicts a pain service that combines the skills of diverse fields in a coordinated manner under the direction of a primary administrator. The director determines the path of tasks as well as the timing or sequence in which they will occur. This model relies on a central administration, usually operating on a hierarchical system. Team loyalty motivates task completion. Coordination of activities aimed at accomplishing the goal occurs in a systematic, sequential fashion. The leadership is authoritarian. This is often called the medical model in health care facilities. Status of team members can be seen as vertical with hierarchical separation.

Basketball best describes a pain service in which the team consists of a manageable number of members who meet regularly to coordinate treatment plans. Roles often overlap and tasks are usually reciprocal. Treatment plans are coordinated through mutual cooperation and adjustment. The prevailing attitude of the team is egalitarian or mutualistic. A basketball organized pain team would be centrally located, as proximity of team members is essential to the sharing of information and the adjustment of treatment plans. The teamwork is reinforced by a cooperative spirit. The lines of communication occur in three directions: (1) team leader to members; (2) member to member; and (3) members to team leader. The status of the team is egalitarian.

## Team Hybrids

Teams can be conceptualized on a collaboration continuum. At one end, every member is essentially autonomous, working within a specifically defined area, in a parallel manner. The method of communication across these two parallel positions is formal, limited, and defined. Boundaries are often guarded. At the other end of the continuum is the integrative practice, characterized by a united effort, with greater flexibility of boundaries and freedom to exchange roles and responsibilities according to need.[2,4] Many variations can be found along this continuum, resulting in a hybrid form of sports team.

Analysis of a specific organizational structure, as determined by the sports analogy, may reveal a combination sport. Some aspects of the multidisciplinary team may be analogous to baseball, while others may more resemble football. The politics of the institution where the pain center is housed may dictate a specific model. For example, a medical center or hospital may have a policy stating that all clinics must have a medical director who is ultimately responsible for patient care. The director, however, might delegate authority for decision making to members of the team. Such a delegation might result in an overt structure of a football team with an operational covert basketball treatment team. Another example might be where a baseball-team-organized department is used for one portion of the service, such as diagnosis or evaluation, and then patients are transferred to a basketball-organized-treatment team.

Knowing the organizational structure of a pain service helps the director to effectively motivate and direct the team toward the goals of the organization. For example, when all the team members are baseball players, it might be more successful in delivering a service that uses a baseball strategy rather than attempting to deliver one that employs a football strategy.

## Team Development

Most work teams go through a development process. As with human development, maturity is not something outwardly bestowed on an individual. Instead, maturity is a process of trial and error, evaluation, assimilation, and adaptation. Every team develops at its own rate and transitions to new stages depend on prior levels of development. Skipped tasks may lead to problems later.

The beginning of a team may reveal ambiguities and uncertainties that affect how people relate to one another. Team members may begin to experiment with ways of approaching problems. The success or failure of this step in team development is often related to the strengths and expertise of team members as well as the pressure and politics of the external system.

Understanding group process and development helps to understand how multidisciplinary teams are formed. In most situations, teams begin with a pre-affiliation period. Here, interested individuals begin to identify a problem, service need, target population, and/or an area of practice interest. The task of this phase is to formulate a purpose for collaboration. The next phase is orientation where the purpose of collaboration is defined. The group begins to define the purpose, boundaries, and related systems.

Newly formed teams need to address role concerns. Where interdependence among members is vital for a successful working team, roles must be defined and areas of overlap addressed. The first action might be to have team members discuss what they consider to be the focal role of an individual and the individual's obligation to the team. This might seem unnecessary, as some roles are self evident. Such an assumption, however, can create problems in the early development of a team. For example, what if a patient calls the physician stating that he or she has been put on a fixed schedule of pain medication and "needs" more than allowed. Although the physician is the person to field medical questions, any recommendation may be counterproductive to the ongoing treatment plan. In this case, the patient might best be served if directed to the substance abuse management team who set the detoxification schedule.

Becoming a member of a very interactive team does result in some loss of autonomy. It results in the need to communicate with members openly and honestly. Newly formed teams, where members have not worked together prior to "teaming," may find it more difficult to trust the judgments of others during the early phase of team development. With time, the experience of working together creates a more trusting and workable environment. All teams need to work out ways of handling disagreements, anger, and competitiveness. The submergence of self into the team and the necessity for sharing and collaboration may not come easily to some individuals.

The mature team develops its own culture, resulting in a common language and pattern of effective communication. Roles are defined and responsibilities are understood. Territories or boundaries associated with roles often overlap for the purpose of flexibility. Such overlap should be nonthreatening and accepted by the team members. Brill (1976) describes a mature team as a special kind of group whose energies are devoted to problem solving and whose members have attained maximum interaction. The group has a clearly defined purpose, with stated goals and objectives and with an organizational design capable of proceeding toward these goals effectively.[2]

The mature team has achieved its gestalt when the necessary functional elements are in place and integrated, acting and reacting with dynamic responsiveness. Such a team functions as a unit. The team supersedes the summation of its elements. The efficient mature team has developed its own system, energy, and relatedness which allows it to adapt and change according to the demands placed on it. This unity is not at the cost of individual thought. The relatedness is a form of freedom and conflicts are treated as points of evaluation and growth (pp. 46–47).[2]

Team development often represents changing from one team sport to another as the team matures. When blending specializations to produce a consorted effort, consultation, referral, and collaboration are often utilized. The preaffiliation stage of a clinical team often involves the loose association of "consultants." Patients are often referred to other specialists with whom they begin to become acquainted. The overlap in treatment may lead to an interest in forming a clinical service for the treatment of chronic pain. A baseball team organization may be most effective for this early affiliation. Each specialist would continue to practice independently; however, some administrative planning regarding the sequence of referrals to provide a more comprehensive service might be warranted. As the team matures and the members begin to trust and respect one another, a new organizational design might be considered. This point of team maturity might necessitate a football or basketball strategy. The choice would depend on the newly formed goals and objectives.

In summary, designing and revising the organizational structure of a multidisciplinary clinic service is determined by the following considerations: (1) the immediate and long-range goals of the organization; (2) the tasks that need to be accomplished; (3) the location of each component of the service; (4) the level of team development; (5) and the composition of membership. The numerous choices of "game plans" and strategies make ongoing team evaluation important when planning or maintaining a multidisciplinary pain clinic.

## Staffing

Values or attitudes play a large part in determining what disciplines will be included in the service of patients with chronic pain. How the clinic defines and understands the problem of chronic pain determines its assessment and treatment approach. The approaches provided by pain clinics that are represented in the literature fall into three primary categories, including: (1) clinics that offer a medical or surgical treatment for chronic pain;[20–22] (2) psychosocial emphasis where no surgery is offered—the focus is instead on the psychological and behavioral aspects of pain;[9,13,14,17–19,23–27] and (3) an integrated program where medical, psychological, and behavioral treatments are emphasized.[6,7,8,10–12,15,16,28–32]

The literature concerning pain clinics reveals a wide range of disciplines represented in pain teams. Of the 24 teams reviewed for membership,[5,6,8–11,13,15–17,20–24,28,29,31,33–38] the reported specialties and frequency of inclusions were: medical consultants, not regular members of the team (44%); psychologist (68%); social worker or social service department (56%); clinical nurse specialist (36%); nursing staff (64%); physician or what was cited as a "medical doctor" (56%); psychiatrist (50%); anesthesiologist (36%); orthopedic surgeon (20%); neurosurgeon (40%); physical therapist or physiotherapist (60%); recreational therapist (32%); rehabilitation therapist (40%); vocational or occupational therapist (44%); biofeedback therapist (24%); behavioral medical specialist (28%): oral surgeon (4%); family medicine physician (4%); music therapist (4%);

pharmacist (16%); radiologist (8%); neurologist (16%); chaplain (8%); dietitian (8%); residents and fellows (13%).

The predominant structure found in the literature is a team consisting of a medical representative from one of a variety of medical specialties (e.g., anesthesiologist, psychiatrist, family medicine, etc.), and a psychologist, social worker, physical therapist, rehabilitation specialist, and a nurse specialist with additional staff. With this type of structure, roles often overlap and the team tends to have frequent staffings with all participants involved in the treatment process.[13–17,19] More specialized pain centers, such as in the treatment of the terminally ill, tend to have a more medical emphasis.[20–22]

## Values and Assumptions Affecting Assessment and Treatment

Treatment of chronic pain evokes many issues that may present ethical dilemmas for health care providers. The interrelationship among values, ethics, moral judgment, and assumptions are important concepts to consider and recognize when developing and providing services to patients with chronic pain. A clinician who views the problem as a learned condition and does not attend to new information may miss a new development. A patient who experiences chronic pain may also develop cardiac problems, diabetes, arthritis, or other physical conditions that might require a revision in the treatment plan.

Health care providers may articulate that their ethical framework is stable for all conditions. In examining clinical decisions, however, often one finds more complexity to their ethical behavior. For example, a clinician may decide to include in the pain management program only those patients who are not currently taking addictive pain medication. This decision may stem from the belief that continuous use of addictive pain medication is inappropriate for the treatment of a chronic condition, and that patients who depend on pain medication may be less motivated to try behavioral methods of pain management, etc. A dilemma might present itself when a terminally ill cancer patient, who has been prescribed morphine for pain, seeks treatment to learn behaviors that may improve the quality of his or her life. The team might justify its change in policy by suggesting that this situation presents competing considerations. The broad ethical decision then becomes amended to include the case of a terminally ill patient receiving a narcotic agent for pain control. This narrow ethical view reflects the results of novel situations where "exceptions" have been added through weighing relative values.

Teams that avoid the discomfort and anxiety of working through ethical dilemmas by creating broad moral decisions operate under an over-simplistic view of the world. The working-through process facilitates team consensus regarding actions. The moral actions taken are determined by the balance of relative weights assigned to all the competing facts and values relevant to the specific case. Therefore, each new dilemma helps to develop practice principles.[39] Analyzing why something is or is not done is an attempt to find this balance.

Values concerning functional pain, work, medication, and exercise shape the treatment program. In the treatment process, each team member's set of personal values blend with societal values which, in turn, interact with the patient's own set of values regarding treatment. Problems arise when there are discrepancies in values, or when any option available necessitates a compromise in values.

## Functional Pain and its Treatment

Functional vs. organic pain is an issue for clinicians as well as patients. Individual beliefs are often found at the extreme ends of the organic vs. psychogenic issue. Patients are often labeled according to the beliefs held by the therapist or clinic. Some clinics will give a functional diagnosis to patients when discrepancies exist between the subjective experience and the objective pain measures. Such a diagnosis often represents a value judgment that might lead to the labels of malingerer or hysteric.

Others argue that the exclusive use of pain measures gives primary importance to physiological data while ignoring operant conditioning or patients' learning histories.[40] How one defines the problem directly affects what treatment that will be offered. For example, the prevailing value system under the operant approach[9,34,36] is "that patients' pain behaviors are maintained by social consequences (e.g., attention from a solicitous spouse or family, avoidance of unwanted work or home responsibilities) rather than underlying tissue damage" (pp. 67–68).[35] Fordyce adds that pain is not caused by operant conditioning. Rather, pain behaviors occurring subsequent to the presentation of a presumed noxious stimulus are maintained and modified by the principles of learning theory. When patients emit overt pain behaviors, people in the environment typically respond with actions aimed at relieving the pain. If "Those around the patient engage in minister behaviors in response to pain signals, they may observe some favorable effect on his pain behavior by their actions" (p. 180).[10] Under this assumption, both the person with pain and the person responding to the pain behaviors are experiencing something positive within the interaction, including such factors as temporary relief, distraction, kindness received by the person emitting pain behaviors, and the special feeling associated with care giving. This reciprocal pattern demonstrates the operant learning model where behavior is believed to be controlled by its consequences. In this example, both sets of behaviors are being reinforced by the consequence of both the sender's and responder's experience.[9]

Some centers are designed to provide only noninvasive treatment. Such clinics might be staffed primarily by nonmedical professionals. The assumption held is that the medical community is not trained to address the patient with chronic pain. "The population with chronic back pain appears to be one of the most highly refractory to medical care by either conservative management or surgical intervention . . . failure of conventional medical treatment (might be explained) by suggesting that chronic back pain does not conform to the stimulus-response model of medicine" (pp. 1294–1295).[24] Traditionally, medicine looks for a physical condition and a physical cure. "Few physicians are trained to view pain as "legitimate" without clear evidence of tissue damage . . . in short, patients without "objective" signs do not receive prompt or appropriate treatment" (p. 996).[41]

Gottlieb et al. support their cognitive and psychological treatment emphasis by citing the literature that relates procedures used to treat high-risk individuals who experience chronic pain suggesting that "these (medical) procedures are ineffective and may be iatrogenic" (p. 996).[41] Some programs emphasize the individual psychological component, with the assumption that chronic pain is associated with "personality problems and payoffs in the home and job situation for adopting a sick role" (p. 767).[42]

## Work

Some centers have very strong biases on the value of work. Program success is often measured by the patient's return to work and remaining employed upon follow up.[8,34,42] "In this society the occupational role has a paramount place, and its loss is seen as perhaps the greatest of all role losses, transcending at times the loss of the sexual role" (p. 288).[38] This value judgment is further articulated: "By returning to work, he could earn more money and enhance the quality of his family life more than if he accepts the invalid role" (p. 998).[41]

## Medication

Medication is another area where values influence how patients will be served. Some programs do not exclude patients from treatment if they are not willing to reduce their pain medication. This perspective is based on the assumptions that this approach is ineffective. As Hallet and Pilowsky state, "It is fairly clear from clinical experience that any treatment contract which insists that pharmacotherapy is not used is quite unrealistic and, indeed, inappropriate as a basis for initiating a therapeutic alliance" (p. 373).[29] Other behavioral programs reviewed have the reduction of medication as one of the primary goals for all patients.[6,7,9–11,14,15,19,23,30,32,34,35] How this belief system is implemented varies among clinics. Some centers believe that it is appropriate to use placebo pills or pain cocktails, whereas others have a strong bias against such methods. This dichotomy appears related to the operating value of the clinic. In clinics where external control is fostered, the team members regulate the medication for the patients through time-contingent schedules. In clinics where the emphasis is placed on self-control, the patient is responsible for the reduction in medication.

### Exercise

Another goal often found in clinics using a behavioral perspective is increasing a patient's level of activity.[5,9,15,34,36] The literature describes many attitudes regarding the types of exercise determined as important. Programs range from very structured to the promotion of recreational activities. Some centers believe that "good" exercise is active exercise, whereas other centers view many forms of activities (walking, moving vs. sitting, stretching etc.,) as representing "appropriate" exercise goals.[5,34–36]

## Summary

In conclusion, awareness of one's biases, beliefs, and values is important. It affects the recruitment of team members as well as the types of services offered in the clinic. If the basic assumption held by the team is that chronic benign pain is maintained by inactivity, learned pain behaviors, medication patterns, etc., then the team will be quite different form one where the basic assumption is that such pain is maintained exclusively by physiological causes.

All decisions concerning assessment and treatment communicate something to a patient. For example, the decision to send a patient for all the medical tests technology has to offer might communicate to the patient that the problem is indeed physical. Centers that do not repeat or perform high technology assessments may run the risk of litigation if a physical problem is overlooked.

A few team meetings held with the agenda of making preconscious assumptions conscious and shared will aid in building a collaborative team. A team, like an individual, has a value system. This enduring set of beliefs is reflected in what members consider to be preferable and appropriate team behavior. Open discussions regarding prevailing assumptions promote group cohesion. Communications will be less confusing to patients when all team members have the same goals and treatment priorities. Basic assumptions and values will affect all policies set forth in the organization, treatment delivery, and evaluation of the treatment team.

The literature concerning the treatment of chronic pain supports the utilization of multidisciplinary teams. This chapter has attempted to address the issues of forming a team and stimulate a way of thinking about teams. The team sports analogy was used to demonstrate organizational structures and strategy options. Many factors enter into the type of collaboration that develops including: (1) the target population, (2) the target problems; and (3) the available resources (e.g., team members, facilities, adjunctive services, affiliations, reimbursement, funding, etc.). It is important to be aware of the options and to question and evaluate the appropriateness of what is being chosen when developing a pain service. Begin to think about the team sport that best describes your current team and become aware of how value judgments affect practice. Question what is and what is not being offered within your setting. Lastly, make evaluation an ongoing part of the planning and implementation process. Administrators, team members, and consumers who continue to evaluate the services offered will aid in developing appropriate services.

## References

1. Burk, W.W. (1982). *Organization Development Principles and Practices.* Boston: Little Brown.
2. Brill, N.I. (1976). *Teamwork: Working Together in the Human Services.* Philadelphia: J.B. Lippincott.
3. Perley, M.J. (1987). *Organizational culture and Social Power: Analysis of a Health Care Organization.* Paper presented to the Speech Communication Association. November. Boston.
4. Keidel, R. (1985). *Game Plans: Sports Strategies for Business.* New York: E.P. Dutton.
5. Hudson, J.S., & Pratt, T.H. (1979). Pain clinics: Their value to the general practitioner. *Southern Medical Journal* 72(7):845–847.
6. Berns, J. (1978). Team approach to chronic pain. *Health and Social Work* 3(2):182–192.
7. Gorsky, B.H. (1979). Chronic pain: A management plan based on experiences in a pain clinic. *Postgraduate Medicine* 66(4):147–154.
8. Spengler, D.M. (1983). Chronic low back pain: The team approach. *Clinical Orthopedics and Related Research* October (179):71–76.
9. Fordyce, W.E., Fowler, R.S., Lehmann, J.F., & DeLateur, B. (1968). Some implications of learning in problems of chronic pain. *Journal of Chronic Disease* 21:179–190.
10. Donovan, W.H., Dwyer, A.P., White, B.W.S., Batalin, N.J., Skerritt, P.W., & Bedbrook, G.M. (1981). A multidisciplinary approach to chronic low back pain in western Australia. *Spine* 6(6):591–597.
11. Ghia, J.N., & Gregg, J.M. (1982). The University of North Carolina Pain Center—I. Organization and function. *Anesthesia Progress* 29(2):41–46.
12. Germain, C.B., & Gitterman, A. (1980). *The Life Model of Social Work Practice.* New York: Columbia University Press.
13. Coyle, N. (1987). A model of continuity of care for cancer patients with chronic pain. *Medical Clinics of North America* 71(2):259–270.

14. Hudgens, A.J. (1977). The social workers' role in a behavioral management approach to chronic pain. *Social Work in Health Care* 3(2):149–157.
15. Cairns, D., Thomas, L., Mooney, V., & Pace, J.B. (1976). A comprehensive treatment approach to chronic low back pain. *Pain* 2:301–308.
16. Aronoff, G.M., Wilson, R.R., & Sample, S.S. (1978). Treating chronic pain the team approach. *Journal of Nursing Care* 13:12–13.
17. Seres, J.L., & Newman, R.I. (1976). Results of treatment of chronic low back pain at the Portland Pain Center. *Journal of Neurosurgery* 45 (July):32–36.
18. Newman, R.I., Seres, J.L., Yospe, L.P., & Garlington, B. (1978). Multidisciplinary treatment of chronic pain: Long term follow-up of low-back pain patients. *Pain* 4:283–292.
19. Seres, J.L., Painter, J.R., & Newman, R.I. (1981). Multidisciplinary treatment of chronic pain at the Northwest Pain Center. In *New Approaches to Treatment of Chronic Pain: A Review of Multidisciplinary Pain Clinics and Pain Centers.* NIDA Research Monograph 36. Lorenz K.Y. Ng (Ed.). Rockville, MD: National Institute on Drug Abuse, pp. 41–65.
20. McEwen, B., DeWilde, F., Dwyer, B., Woodforde, J.M., Bleasel, K., & Connelly, T.J. (1965). The pain clinic for the management of intractable pain. *Medical Journal of Australia* 1:676–682.
21. Evans, R.J. (1970). Intractable pain associated with malignancy. *Applied Therapy* 12:21–23.
22. Swerdlow, M. (1967). Four years' pain clinic experience. *Anesthesia* 22:568–574.
23. Gottlieb, H., Strite, L.C., Koller, R., Madorsky, A., Hockersmith, V., Kleeman, M., & Wagner, J. (1977). Comprehensive rehabilitation of patients having chronic low back pain. *Archives of Physical Medical Rehabilitation* 58:101–108.
24. Tollison, C.D., Kriegel, M.L., & Downie, G.R. (1985). Chronic low back pain: Results of treatment at a pain therapy center. *Southern Medical Journal* 78(11): 1291–1295.
25. Maruta, T., Swanson, D.W., & Swenson, W.M. (1979). Chronic pain: Which patients may a pain management program help? *Pain* 7:321–329.
26. Swanson, D.W., Maruta, T., & Swenson, W.M. (1979). Results of behavior modification in the treatment of chronic pain. *Psychosomatic Medicine* 41:55–61.
27. Roberts, A.H., & Reinhardt, L. (1980). The behavioral management of chronic pain: Long term follow-up with comparison groups. *Pain* 8:151–162.
28. Simpson, D.A., Richbeith, R.H.C., Rees, V.E., Burnell, A.W., & Cramond, W.A. (1965). Experience in a pain clinic. *Medical Journal of Australia* 1:671–676.
29. Hallet, E.C., & Pilowsky, I. (1982). The response to treatment in a multidisciplinary pain clinic. *Pain* 12:365–374.
30. Carron, H., & Rowlingson, J.C. (1981). Coordinated outpatient management of chronic pain at the University of Virginia Pain Clinic. In: *New Approaches to Treatment of Chronic Pain: A Review of Multidisciplinary Pain Clinics and Pain Centers.* NIDA Research Monograph 36. Lorenz, K.K. Ng (Ed.). Rockville, MD: National Institute on Drug Abuse, pp. 84–91.
31. Rosomoff, H.L., Green C., Silbret, M., & Steele, R. (1981). Pain and low back rehabilitation program at the University of Miami School of Medicine. In: *New Approaches to Treatment of Chronic Pain: A Review of Multidisciplinary Pain Clinics and Pain Centers.* NIDA Research Monograph 36. Lorenz, K.K. (Ed.). Rockville, MD: National Institute on Drug Abuse, pp. 92–111.

32. Anderson, T.P., Cole, T.M., Gullickson, G., Hudgens, A., & Roberts, A. (1977). Behavior modification of chronic pain: A treatment program by multidisciplinary team. *Clinical Orthopedics* Nov–Dec (129):96–100.
33. Crue, B.L., & Pinsky, J.J. (1981). Chronic pain syndrome—four aspects of the problem: New Hope Pain Center and Pain Research Foundation. In: *New Approaches to Treatment of Chronic Pain: A Review of Multidisciplinary Pain Clinics and Pain Centers.* NIDA Research Monograph 36. Rockville, MD: National Institute on Drug Abuse, pp. 137–168.
34. Floer, A., Naxon, E., Jones, R.E., & Mooney, V. (1981). An occupational therapy program for chronic back pain. *American Journal of Occupational Therapy* 35(4):243–248.
35. Houpt, J.L., Keefe, F.J., & Snipes, M.T. (1984). The clinical specialty unit: The use of the psychiatry inpatient unit to treat chronic pain syndromes. *General Hospital Psychiatry* 6(1):65–70.
36. Kientz, J.H., Fitzsimmons, D.S., & Schneider, P.J. (1983). Reducing medication use in chronic pain management program. *American Journal of Hospital Pharmacy* 40(12):2156–2158.
37. Lutz, R.W., Silbret, M., & Ohshan, N. (1983). Treatment outcome and compliance with therapeutic regiment. *Pain* 17(3):301–308.
38. Roy, R. (1984). Psychosocial assessment of chronic headache. *Health Social Work* 4(9):284–293.
39. Hundert, E.M. (1987). A model for ethical problem solving in medicine, with practical applications. *American Journal of Psychiatry* 144(7):839–846.
40. Cinciripini, P.M., & Floreen, A. (1983). An assessment of chronic pain behavior in a structured interview. *Journal of Psychosomatic Research* 27(2):117–123.
41. Gottlieb, H.J., Alperson, B.L., Kollner, R., & Hockersmith, V. (1979). An innovative program for the restoration of patients with chronic back pain. *Physical Therapy* 59(8):996–999.
42. Chapman, C.R. (1977). Psychological aspects of pain patients treatment. *Archives of Surgery* 112:767–772.

# Author Index

# Subject Index

MIX
Papier aus verantwortungsvollen Quellen
Paper from responsible sources
FSC® C105338
FSC
www.fsc.org

If you have any concerns about our products,
you can contact us on
**ProductSafety@springernature.com**

In case Publisher is established outside the EU,
the EU authorized representative is:
**Springer Nature Customer Service Center GmbH**
**Europaplatz 3, 69115 Heidelberg, Germany**

Printed by Libri Plureos GmbH
in Hamburg, Germany